INTRODUCTION TO
HEALTHCARE DELIVERY

MARY BETH BROWN

D1283396

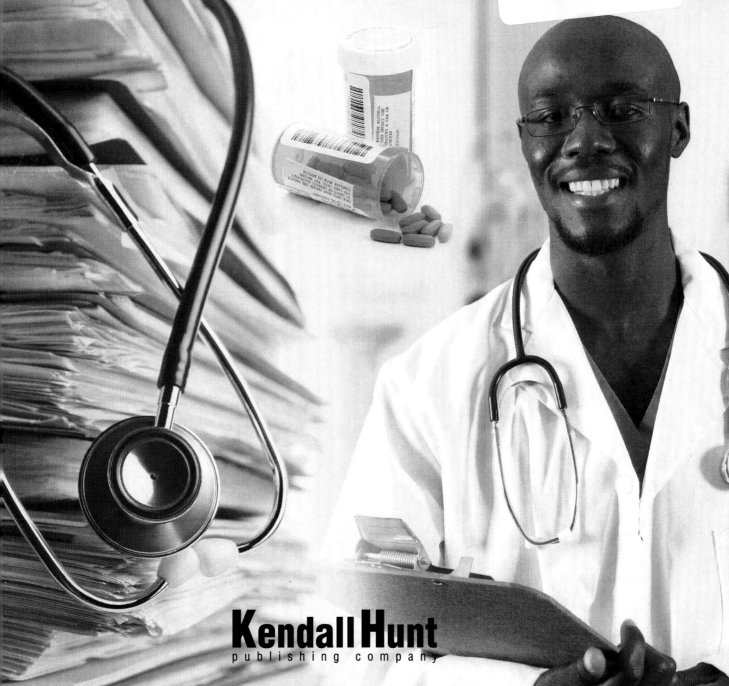

Kendall Hunt
publishing company

Cover images © 2012 Shutterstock, Inc.

Kendall Hunt
publishing company

www.kendallhunt.com
Send all inquiries to:
4050 Westmark Drive
Dubuque, IA 52004-1840

Copyright © 2012 by Kendall Hunt Publishing Company

ISBN 978-1-4652-0014-3

Printed in the United States of America
10   9   8   7   6   5   4   3

BRIEF CONTENTS

CONTENTS

ACKNOWLEDGEMENTS

I must say I never intended on being involved in a project to compile a book. But as they say "necessity is the mother of invention" and the need for a book for our Introduction to Healthcare Delivery class led to the development of this book. And please notice that I did say compile and not write. I need to start by thanking all of the authors whose work is now part of this book. This book would not have been possible without the work included from each of you.

Next I want to thank my colleagues at Sinclair Community College: Jennifer L. Spegal, MT, M.Ed., CMA (AAMA), Assistant Dean, Life and Health Sciences, Chairperson, Allied Health Instruction and my boss, for her support and assistance with this; Jeri Layer, A.T.S., CCBE, CD, my teaching partner for many years, together we ironed out so many of the details for the new course; Joseph Gregory Dudash, M.D., Associate Professor in the Department of Allied Health Instruction and Sheranita Hemphill, RDH, MS, MPH, Professor, Dental Health Sciences, who were truly instrumental in the building of the new course, and Christine A. Steineman, AAS, AA, our administrative assistant, who is, as I always say, the keeper of all knowledge great and small and saved me more time than I can ever count!

To Glenn Hammersmith, Lynne Rogers, and Mary Melloy at Kendall Hunt Publishing for guiding me through this maze you call publishing. I truly would not have known where to start, yet alone get this to completion, and for always being there to answer the constant stream of questions I had throughout the process. You all ARE THE BEST!

And last, and definitely not least, my wonderful husband Randy, who always sticks by me when I seem to get myself involved in these large 'projects'. I could never do it without his support!

This book is for the students of the Life and Health Sciences Division at Sinclair Community College. Here is to creating a foundation on which to build your future in your chosen allied health profession.

CHAPTER **1**

Personality and Personality Traits

The Individual Subsystem: *Personality*

Learning Objectives

- Examine the two sides of personality preferences—temperament and character.
- Identify the different personality types.
- Examine the role of personality type in choosing an appropriate career in healthcare.

Key Terms

Activity level	Goodness of fit	Personality type
Adaptability	Intensity of reaction	Quality of mood
Approach and withdrawal	Introvert	Response threshold
Attention span	Judger	Shadow
Character	Perceiver	Situational difference
Cooperators	Persona	Temperament
Distractibility	Personality	Typewatching
Extrovert	Personality theory	Utilitarians

INTRODUCTION

Differences in physical features can easily be seen in people. One person is taller than another; one has blue eyes, another brown; one has blond hair, one black. Just as people are different in their outward physical features, so they are different in many aspects of their individual system which includes such features as temperament, birth order, and personality. Temperament, birth order, and personality type are composites of an individual's distinctive personal qualities and make each of us unique.

An aspect of diversity is prevalent in the variety of individuals we encounter. In the family and the work place, we find ourselves continually challenged and confronted by differences. Recognizing differences, accepting individuality, and learning how to optimize everyone's unique talents is a challenge that can be most rewarding in family interactions and in the environments outside the home. In working with other people, it becomes clear that our individual pursuits will be more productive only if we can understand these differences, and also actually value and capitalize on them. Our satisfaction is increasingly dependent on our skills and abilities in building relationships with a wide variety of people. Those with whom we share a similar perspective are often easy to get along with and those with differing perspectives are often more challenging. Yet in these interactions and relationships with people who are different from us are a wealth of traits and perspectives that provide a richer experience for ourselves and others, if only we can learn how to appreciate this diversity and work together.

Physiologically, our nervous systems are different; one person is more sensitive or excitable than another (Asher, 1987). One person seems to have a higher activity level, while others have longer attention spans and can be more persistence. Temperaments and personalities of individuals are different, and cause different types of behaviors in people.

People's response patterns differ not only because they are unique human beings with individual personalities, but also because each is in a different stage of development, making their needs and perceptions of the environment very different. For example, a two-year-old, ten-year-old, sixteen-year-old, and thirty-year-old will all exhibit different needs, and different behaviors, because of different personality types and differing developmental needs. People think differently: they perceive, gather information, conceptualize, process it, understand, comprehend, and make decisions differently because of personality differences and differing developmental stages. Manners of acting and showing emotions, governed as they are by wants and beliefs, differ greatly—even in a small group such as a family system. Many of these differences are believed to be due to personality type.

An exploration of some aspects of personality follows. Three major components are believed to come together to influence the composite of what we call personality; one aspect of the internal environment. These three components are temperament, birth order, and personality type.

TEMPERAMENT

Human beings are believed to bring into the world an array of behavioral dispositions that interact with the environment with mutual modification (Carey, 1990). These behavioral dispositions known as one's temperament are believed to be the precursor of personality. The well known studies in temperament are those by Thomas and Chess (1977). These researchers observed nine characteristics in newborns as early as two months of age. These nine characteristics appeared to be present in all babies with differing degrees of intensity on a continuum from low to high. These nine characteristics describe ways individuals respond to their environment, and provide a framework for understanding reaction patterns. The nine response types include activity level, rhythmicity, approach and with-

drawal, adaptability; response threshold, intensity of reaction, quality of mood, distractibility, and attention span. The ways in which people respond within the continuum of response patterns are neither good nor bad; they are just differences in people's responses. When extremes of these response patterns are present in a family system, it is especially challenging to balance differing needs in order to create a cohesive family system. A brief summary of each behavioral characteristic follows.

Activity level refers to the frequency of spontaneous motor activity. Depending on a person's activity level on a continuum from low to high, one individual may seem to be in constant motion, while the opposite behavior on the activity level continuum will see a person moving very slowly or not at all. Variations of this are almost sure to be present in families, and the extremes are challenging in any environment, especially when the person in perpetual motion is paired with a slow mover in a family environment.

Rhythmicity manifests itself in a preference that life be in sequence, on a distinct time schedule, such as: breakfast at seven, dinner at six, bedtime at ten, with little or no deviation in daily routine. For the person who likes rhythmicity, all activities follow a similar schedule on a daily basis. The opposite of the scheduled individual is a person with no scheduled daily routines, but rather one with a haphazard sequence of events throughout the day.

Approach and withdrawal behaviors are those that represent an individual's approach to another individual to initiate social interactions, or the opposite, withdrawal from social encounters. This is a distance-regulating mechanism affecting relationship development, intimacy, and cohesion inside as well as outside the family.

The **adaptability** continuum is a range that stretches from having the ability to adapt and give up old reference points to the need for having the requirement of the same things in the environment all the time. Adaptability refers to adjusting to changes in space, time, objects and people. Opposites on this continuum are people enjoying changes and new things in their environment to people demanding the same rather inflexible routine.

Response threshold refers to the responsiveness of individuals through the use of their senses. A person may be slow to respond (having a high tolerance for noise) or be very sensitive and quick to respond (seeming to overreact) showing a low tolerance for sensory inputs and stimulation from the environment.

Intensity of reaction refers to impulse control under stress and how individuals react under stressful circumstances. We usually react in one of three ways: we adapt by managing the stimuli, withdraw by shutting down, or explode.

Quality of mood refers to a continuum of responses that range from happiness to sadness. This is often a difficult quality to deal with in a family system because of the perception that everyone should be happy and in a good mood. In families, parents tend to blame themselves if their children are unhappy and try to fix the situation.

Distractibility is the ability to concentrate even with distractions in the external environment. The opposite is a person who is easily distracted by any noise or activity. This has implications for design and spacing in classrooms and work sites. Some individuals work best in contained, rather closed areas, while others enjoy open environments in which to work. This individual response also has implications for planning home and room designs, spacing, and boundaries.

Attention span is the ability to be persistent or stay with a task; the opposite end of the continuum might reveal a person who quickly goes from one project to another. As might be expected, distractibility and attention span are closely related. In fact, these nine response types are interrelated; one response type influences the response of another.

After reviewing the variety of temperamental response patterns, it is tempting to compress the data into a summary that could be easily remembered. One could conclude that a person's social competence and adjustment are primarily influenced by the difficult/easy or sociability/flexibility aspects of temperament, especially approach, adaptability and mood. Task performance in school or the work setting appears to be predominantly affected by the task orientation aspects of temperament that include persistence/attention span, distractibility, and activity.

Appealing as this summary might be, it would not reflect the complexity of the actual interactions. Other characteristics such as persistence are important in social adjustment (Thomas, Chess, and Birch, 1968). Sociability (approach and adaptability) is a significant factor in school performance (Martin, 1988) and temperamental difficulty has been related to colic and excessive weight gain, both in infancy

and middle childhood (Carey, 1985). The principal reason that we cannot demonstrate simple linear relationships between risk factors and clinical conditions is that much of the individual's outcome depends on the contribution of other factors in the physical make up of the individual and the environment, particularly in the social cultural environment. An important aspect of this interaction is a component called the "goodness of fit", a term suggested by Thomas and Chess.

Impact Depending on Goodness of Fit

Temperamental behavior is important for the optimal development of the individual. Temperament is an important component because the child's care givers and others in the environment may find these characteristics challenging and sometimes difficult to deal with because of their own expectations of what the child should be.

Goodness of fit is a concept describing an interaction that results when the properties of the environment and its expectations and demands are in accord with the organism's own capabilities, motivations and styles of behavior. When there is harmony between the organism and the environment, optimal development in a progressive direction is possible. Conversely, "poorness of fit" involves dissonances between the environmental opportunities and demands and the capacities and characteristics of the organism producing distorted development and maladaptive functioning. Goodness of fit occurs between personalities inside the family and also within the social cultural environment in terms of values and demands. When a poor fit generates excessive stress in the system, conflict in relationships occurs. This stress may lead via the individual's physiological predispositions and psychological defense mechanisms to various clinical problems (Carey, 1990).

A number of specific factors can influence the goodness of fit and the impact of temperamental risk factors. These include: (1) strength and duration of the behavioral characteristic of the child (organism), (2) other individual attributes, (3) the outcome of the relationship between the individual and the environment, and (4) the environment in which the individual is embedded. Note these are a direct application of the four elements of a system discussed earlier: the organism, its attributes, the relationship of the system elements, and the environment. An ecological perspective is clearly evident in the goodness of fit concept.

The stronger and more pervasive the behavior of the risk factor in the environmental setting, the greater the chances of conflict. Little is known now about the changeability of temperament characteristics but, those that are less modifiable will present a greater challenge to care givers. However, we do know the most difficult infants become "easier" as they get older, but we have little understanding of how and why this happens (Carey, 1990).

The individual attributes of the child play a role in influencing a fit between the child (organism) and the environment. For example, inattentiveness is not as big a problem in toddlers as it is in school age children. Intelligence also plays a role, since an inattentive bright child may be able to keep up with school work while the less well-endowed child may not. It also appears that the inattentive child who is adaptable may be better able to attend when it really matters (Carey, McDevitt, & Baker, 1979).

The relationship outcome of the individual with the surrounding environment is the third important consideration in how temperament impacts the individual's development. For example, diverse educational requirements and teacher preferences for performance make different characteristics more congenial or more disruptive in the classroom situation. So too, the perception of the child's characteristic by the family, and especially the care givers, impacts the type of interaction whether congenial or irritable. Interactions between adult and child will influence individual development.

The environment, the fourth element of the system that determines the organism's goodness of fit, has many variables to be considered. The family's social economic status, the culture, the birth order of the child, maternal and family support systems and stresses within the family affect the impact of temperamental risk factors. From an anthropological perspective throughout the various cultures of the world, certain kinds of infants and children are regarded as troublesome or difficult, but the cultural ecological niche into which the child is born determines how the specific characteristics will be nurtured or discouraged.

Each individual is born with a diverse repertoire of temperamental traits that are manifest through behavioral interactions with the environment. The goodness of fit between individuals and their environment plays a major role in how individuals will develop, perceive themselves and perceive their world.

Birth Order

A second variable considered influential in explaining differences in individual systems is birth order. While a child is born with a predisposition for temperament and over time develops a personality style, the order in which a person is born into the family system is unchangeable. Birth order, or the individual's sequence of birth into the family, is believed to make a difference in how an individual develops behavioral and relationship interaction patterns with others. In other words, who we are is influenced by where we fit into the family, who is there ahead of us, and who comes after us.

From this family base siblings get their earliest perspectives of themselves in relation to parents and each other, and eventually to people outside the family. Placement in the family environmental system influences how an individual learns to interact with people. Family placement influences perceptions and provides opportunities for learning skills, such as how to get along with others in relationship to responsibility, decision-making, negotiation, mediation, and intimacy.

The big problem with assessing birth order is the almost impossible task of getting a clear focus on what is being studied. The family system environment is complex, made up of innumerable interdependent threads, some are apparent and some are not. This complexity makes it difficult to assess. Even if you could extract that one birth order thread it would only be one factor in a very complex system of family traits.

What we do know is that the family experience is a different environment for each child. Temperament, birth order, and personality type interact with that environment to create a unique individual. With this background we can consider what is influential in the child's development by virtue of birth order.

There are usually three "typical" birth order positions that are most influential in personality development: first born, middle born, and last born. These characteristics ascribed to birth order assume there is no more than five to six years between siblings. When there is a span of five to six years, a child is assumed to take on first born characteristics. Keep in mind these are not the patterns of all first born, but general patterns observed in many first born children. There are always exceptions to the patterns described.

The first borns are the achievers in life. They tend to be goal oriented, more adult oriented, helpful, self-controlled, conscientious and do not like surprises. To them, life is earnest. Parental demands and high standards established for first borns may result in their realizing higher education and professional accomplishments than their siblings (Furman & Lanthier, 2002). First borns cannot be ignored. If you are not one, you will have to deal with one in your life. They can also be extremely competitive, tense, and driven. In some cases this can mean friction. This is where the environment influences the individual system. First borns tend to spend more time with adults so it is natural that they grow up faster. They have learned their share of responsibility and they often hear, "I expect more of you because you are older" or "you have to be grown up, you're the oldest." In reality, they are not quite as driven as first borns who also turn out to be only children. "Only children" are extremely reliable and conscientious and have many of the same perfectionistic tendencies as first borns, but more so (Leman, 1984).

Children born later have the advantage of parents who have had some practice. These second born children are either middle children or last borns. Unlike first and last borns, middle children's characteristics are often difficult to describe or generalize. The term middle can mean several things. The middle child may be second or third, but a middle child could also be fourth, fifth, and so on. Middle and second borns have much in common, so we will talk of them together.

When observing the characteristics of middle children, each child looks around and sizes up their older sibling, and tries to develop a very individual style. If second borns sense they can compete with their older sibling, they may do so. However, if the older brother or sister is stronger, smarter, or excels in other characteristics, the second born typically chooses another direction.

No matter when second born children enter the family, their lifestyle is greatly influenced by their perceptions of the environment. This is an example of environment-organism interdependence. Middle children feel pressure from above and below, but often do not find a place that is their special spot or ecological niche. Middle born children all seem to playoff either the first born or the older sibling. For example, if the first born is a compliant person, the second born might be a challenger. The general conclusion of studies completed on birth order is that second borns will probably be at least partly the opposite of first borns. Since later borns are greatly influenced by siblings directly above them, there is no

way to predict how their personality might develop. Middle born children often associate more with their peer group than other children. Because they could not have Mom and Dad all to themselves, they learn to negotiate and compromise, and often become mediators or seasoned diplomats in childhood. They are compromisers, good negotiators, very sociable and make loyal friends. The skills of socialization developed with siblings and their peer group and skills of mediation learned in the family and with peers are quite useful skills in life.

As can be seen, it is difficult to come up with a clear picture of middle children. They have empathy for people, usually turn out to be tenacious adults, and are more accepting in relationships. They are not as driven as first borns, but then, they are not as compulsive, either. Perhaps the best description of middle children is balanced.

Finally, the last born, the youngest, who is often called the baby of the family. The position may be known as last, but these youngest members of the family system, get a sixth sense that tells them they are not going to be least! Youngest children in the family are typically the outgoing charmers, who are fun-loving, personable, spontaneous, caring, tolerant and affectionate. The last born is usually more carefree and vivacious, and seems to be a "people person" who is usually popular.

The typical last borns have a burning desire to make an important contribution to the world. From the time they are big enough to figure things out, last borns are acutely aware that they are the youngest, smallest, and least equipped to cope with life. They often hear "you're not big enough" or "you're not old enough." Studies show that last borns of the family gravitate toward vocations that are people-oriented, while first borns and only children tend to like jobs involving the handling of data, materials, or other "things."

What does come through as valid in affecting siblings are "power interactions" between older and younger children in a family—aggressiveness, competition, power struggles and attempts to dominate, but also power to help one another and to intervene for each other with adults when necessary. When we look at siblings in actual families, and not just at large statistical comparisons, it becomes clear that the emotional, intricate, ambivalent interplays among them—their "power interactions"—have a much greater and more lasting impact on their personalities and attitudes than does the simple fact of birth order (Klagsburn, 1992).

More important, what comes through as valid in birth order studies is the strong connectedness of later children to earlier ones. Later borns do not know a world that does not include siblings, and those siblings become the standard against which they measure themselves—idolizing them, imitating them, and trying to break loose from them. And just as the power interactions with younger siblings help shape the images and self-concept olders have of themselves, those interactions help form the self-views and concepts youngers will carry within them, views of themselves very different from those the olders hold (Klagsbum, 1992).

Although these general descriptions of birth order are interesting, position is not as important as the recognition that a particular birth order means you had a certain environment in which to develop. As an adult you can recognize your important characteristics, take practical steps to emphasize and utilize your strong points, and accept and strengthen those you wish to develop.

Family form and structure is greatly influenced by children and birth order. The first child in the family system not only breaks in new parents to parenting, but also in restructuring the family system to include an additional person. In this process of resolving such issues as how to parent, maintain family cohesion, remain connected, deal with power issues, redefine roles, reallocate resources, and maintain some degree of system homeostasis, the family system is stressed, adapts, and changes to accommodate the new individual. The family system that emerges is different from the couple relationship, because in the shifting and adapting individuals influence their environment and the environment influences them.

Typical family birth-order positions and behavioral characteristics have been described in terms of the family system environment's influence on personality development. Birth order clearly shows the O–E relationship. The organism (individual) is influenced by the environment of the family, just as the family environment is influenced by the individuals in the family.

Personality Attributes

Studies of temperament inform us about reaction patterns in individual systems. These patterns although modifiable, tend to remain with us for a lifetime. Birth order, in some way, is believed to influence how a person develops behavior and relationship patterns. Both contribute to personality development which is con-

sidered to be a composite of traits that develops after birth and continues to be modified throughout life. For some time, there was a belief that people were fundamentally alike. This appears to be a twentieth century notion. Probably the idea is related to the growth of democracy in the Western world. If people are equal, the belief seemed to follow that we must be alike (Kiersey & Bates, 1984). This changed as psychologists and educators questioned and observed individual differences.

In infancy, it is believed that personality traits develop on the basis of primary drives and emotions like hunger, thirst, fear and pleasure. These reactions are based on the physiology of the central nervous system, characteristics of individual temperament, and responses from environments in which individuals are embedded. Later in life, personality continues to be molded through experiences and interactions in the social-behavioral environment and the environment of the family system.

A number of theories of development have evolved by those who studied human behavior. A theory is a coherent set of ideas that are organized about an issue which describes and explains a phenomena. Additionally, there are theories that attempt to define unique categories or types of behavior that characterize individuals. These include trait theory, which attempts to define individuals by unique traits such as happy, sad, achievers or losers. There are theories based on developmental tasks, growth patterns, psychoanalysis, behaviors, cognitive development, social learning, and contextualism (the environments).

Perhaps the best known of the personality theories is the psychoanalytic approach of Freud. He believed we are all driven from within. This driving refers to the continuous struggle between the id, ego, and superego (our conscience) as the motivator of personality development. The observations from which he developed this idea were made with his clients who were considered mentally ill. Although he had a limited clinical sample as the basis of his theory, it has been influential in the literature of human development.

Erik Erikson (1950, 1968) recognized Freud's contributions but believed there were other dimensions of human development. He believed we developed in psychosocial stages. Erikson emphasized developmental change throughout the human life cycle, whereas Freud argued that our basic personality is shaped in the first five years of life. In Erikson's theory, eight stages of development unfold as we progress through the life cycle. Each stage consists of a unique developmental task that confronts individuals with a challenge of crisis that must be faced. Although Erikson called these a crisis, he considered them less a crisis than a turning point. He believed these to be a point of increased vulnerability with opportunities of enhanced growth and potential. The more successful individuals are in resolving their challenges, the healthier their development.

Behavioral theories developed by such social scientists as Rotter (1971), Bandura and Walters (1977) also value the importance of learning in personality development by explaining how individuals react to a stimulus, generalize from one experience to another, and focus on events of the present as opposed to the past.

A search for developmental patterns in children's cognitive and verbal skills and for the mechanisms that bring about these patterns with their subsequent influence on development is the basis for Piagetian theory. Piaget asked how does knowledge develop in children and was especially interested in the process that led children to produce the answers they gave (Thomas, 1992).

A search for patterns of environmental influence and for biological templates of human nature led to the development of ecological theory. Thus, many aspects of personality development have been explored and developed to construct a way to understand personality.

With this background in temperament, birth order, and personality theories, we move on to explore personality. What is personality? **Personality** is the distinct composite of personal qualities. Also described as one's individuality, they are the attributes or distinctive characteristics of the person. The range of individual personality traits are part of what makes each individual unique. This underscores the importance of recognizing individual differences in order to understand ourselves, as well as understand other people. It also speaks to the importance of learning how people develop relationships, learning how to appreciate differences, and learning how to work with other people.

Tests and theories that categorize people are controversial, so there are those who will be skeptical. This is not meant to draw a narrow picture of people, but to broaden it. Discussing attributes is used here to create a systemic framework for thinking about people (how they perceive, process information, develop values, make decisions, utilize resources, order their lives, and relate to others), to expand our perspective, and to promote understanding of ourselves and others.

In reality, it is very common for us to categorize people or use expressions to describe certain types of people. Terms such as "quiet", "loud", "winner", "underachievers" ... are used frequently. These expressions are usually used when we become aware that someone displays an identifying characteristic (Kroeger & Thuesen, 1988). This is a part of what we earlier described as "trait theory." All of these terms convey mental images that provide a kind of shortcut for communication. This is particularly true with people we know well. In fact, families develop their own private language that characterizes people and things.

As common and convenient as this may be, people tend to have mixed feelings about categorizing and labeling. This framework of categories describing personality type, is based on the work of an early psychologist, Carl Jung, a student of Freud. He suggested that human behavior is predictable and, therefore, classifiable (Jung, 1923, 1971). Jung's suggested categories of personality types are based on behavior as a result of individual preferences in ways to interact with the environment. These behavioral preferences for how we "function" emerge early in life, forming the foundation of our personalities. Subsequent perceptions and issues of life are translated and interpreted through each of our basic personality preferences.

Katharine Briggs read much of Jung's work and became interested in the personality differences she noticed. In observing people in the work force, she noticed that some individuals were assigned to tasks unsuited to their abilities and, therefore, they were not productive. Later, her daughter, Isabel Myers, became involved in the study of people. Myers believed that what we do is what we have "in mind". She observed different "types" of people and tried to understand their patterns of thinking or what they "had in mind." Their initial observations, combined with readings of Jung's work, led them to design an instrument (Myers-Briggs Type Indicator, 1962) that would explain differences according to Jung's personality preferences. They believed their indicator could be used to identify individual preferences, leading to an understanding of these preferences. This set the stage for people to get a word portrait of themselves and others. They believed this could promote a constructive blending of individual differences among people in the work force. In addition, individual preferences could be better matched to jobs, and people could be assigned to tasks to which they were well suited. For example, due to personality preferences, some people are better able to do repetitive tasks, while others enjoy working on a variety of tasks in their jobs.

Authors, Kroeger and Thuesen (1988), observed personality differences and call it "Typewatching."

Typewatching is one way of observing people's behaviors and their reactions to the environment. Looking at behaviors in relationship to personality types enables us to think a little more objectively about actions that we might otherwise take personally. Thus, we learn as much about ourselves and our interactions in environments as we learn of others. In observing behaviors with this perspective, the tendency for a person to be frequently silent or say very little can now be viewed as a "type characteristic" rather than a character defect or a personal affront. The goal here is a better understanding of people with the potential for finding ways to create harmony among those with whom we interact.

These theories include a combination of temperament, personality characteristics, and birth order. They are interrelated and build on one another to increase understanding of each individual as a unique system.

Personality Preferences

To further understand people and the systems in which we interact, it is important to understand that much of our attraction to others is the result of our personality preferences. There are two sides to personality; one is temperament and the other character. **Temperament** is our inborn form of human nature; **character** is the emergent form, which develops through interactions of temperament with the environment.

Each of us is born with a predisposition for certain personality preferences. Isabel Myers (Kiersey, 1998), worked with these preferences and developed portraits of personality. The four types are most likely derived from the interweaving of the two most basic human actions, how we communicate with each other, and how we use tools to accomplish our goals. Human beings have two advantages—words and tools. What sets one person apart from another is the way we use words and tools. The great majority of us are predominately concrete in our word usage, the rest abstract. About half of us are utilitarian in our choice and use of tools, the other half cooperative.

Cooperators try to get what they want and where they want to go by getting along with others. They are law abiding and accommodating with those around them. **Utilitarians** tend to go after what they want in the most effective way possible. They do live within the law, but go outside of the group to pursue their ambitions.

There are four pairs of preference of how people interact with their environment. In studying Jung's theory, Meyers used the traditional words from Jung's description of types, but in thinking and organizing them she used her own words. Box 1.1 shows the preferences patterns. The words in parenthesis are the words Myers used in developing the categories.

These preferences are developed by interactions with the environment and reflect both genetic predispositions and whatever else is part of the earliest experiences of life. As life unfolds, our environment, especially interactions within the family system, greatly influences the direction these preferences will take.

A word of explanation about preferences. Think of being right- or left-handed. If you are right-handed that does not mean that you never use your left hand. It merely means that you have a preference for using your right hand. Even in the use of a preferred hand, there are degrees of preference. A very strong preference means that a person uses one hand almost exclusively. Another person may not have such a strong preference, and will use both right and left hands almost equally. In behavioral personality preferences, some are very strong while others are very close to being equal. You may have a very strong preference for one characteristic, and only a slight preference for another. However, it is believed that within each pair, we do have a preference for one category over another, even if it is ever so slight in some people and very prominent in others.

According to **personality theory,** each of us is born with a predisposition for a certain personality preference. In every personality type, there is a basic form in which the prevailing personality type begins to develop, and its modes of adaptation are still being tentatively explored. The feedback mechanism of the system plays a role here; the more we use personality

Box 1.1 A person is either:

(Expressive)	Extroverted	or	Introverted	(Reserved)
(Observant)	Sensing	or	Intuitive	(Introspective)
(Tough Minded)	Thinking	or	Feeling	(Friendly)
(Scheduling)	Judging	or	Perceiving	(Probing)

preferences and receive feedback from our environment, the more confident we become and rely on our preferences, which in turn strengthens them. Similar to the analogy of hand preference, we still use our non-dominant preferences; however, they never take the place of our dominant preferences. So, introverts never become extroverts, and vice versa. However, the longer people live, the more they will learn to effectively use their non-preferred type, often called a **shadow,** but it is believed that people do not convert their preference. Development of both the **persona,** or preferred process, and the shadow, the auxiliary process, helps create a balance for people who are able to consider and use varying points of view (Kroeger & Thuesen, 1988). This enables them to see a greater variety of options to create solutions. Development and experience seem to lend breadth to the individual personality. Our preferences remain the foundation of our personality type, and the non-preferences give additional breadth and variety. For example, an extrovert will continue to have preferences for extroverted behavior, but can develop some qualities and understanding of the quieter introversive style.

What Are Types?

A **personality type** is developed by using one's personality preferences. These personality types develop from individual experiences in the near environment, primarily the family system. The essence of type development is the development of perception, information processing and judgment, and of the appropriate ways to use them.

Personality types differ in the kind of perception and the kind of judgment they develop. These predispositions for preferences can be encouraged through environmental factors that increase opportunities for people to develop their own unique qualities. Type research has shown that personality types differ in their interests, values, and needs. People learn in different ways, have different ambitions, and respond to different rewards. These basic differences have to do with the way people prefer to think about things and learn, and more specifically, with the way they perceive the environment, process information, and make decisions and judgments. Perceiving determines what people see and is the process of becoming aware of things, ideas, people, issues, and happenings. People with adequate perception see the relevant aspects of a situation. Adequate perception, information processing, and judgment make it possible for you to see what is relevant and to face and solve problems in a credible

manner. Together, perception and judgment, which make up a large portion of people's total mental activity, govern much of the way we learn and act. Therefore, basic differences in perception or judging often result in corresponding differences in behavior.

The material presented here gives an overview of personality types (Jung, 1923; 1970; Keirsey, 1998; Kiersey and Bates, 1984; Kroeger and Thuesen, 1988; Myers, 1980). As these personality types are summarized, look for similarities showing relationships between people's interactions within their environments, their perceptions (how they see things), information gathering (inputs of information that they believe important), information processing (their learning style) and outputs (decisions, judgments). Also begin thinking about your personality type, think about which of the characteristics from the lists of personality traits best fits you. The personality type with the most items that are similar to the way you interact with the environment will indicate your type. Each of us is strong in one mode, but everyone can learn all four styles.

The way people prefer to receive inputs from the environment and process information indicates a style called Extroversion (E) or Introversion (I). Introversion and extroversion are two complementary dispositions or orientations to life. **Extroverts** get their energy from outside themselves (friends and associates), while **introverts** get their energy from within themselves. This process determines how an individual gathers information and makes decisions. The introvert's main interests are in the inner world of concepts and ideas, while the extrovert is more involved with the outer world of people and things. The extrovert likes to focus on the outside environment. Introversion can be distinguished from extroversion by observing whether the individual gathers and processes information quietly and internally through a thinking process (introvert), or externally by talking (extrovert). No one is limited to the inner or outer world. Well-developed introverts ably deal with the world around them, but they do their best work reflecting. Similarly, well-developed extroverts can deal effectively with ideas, but they do their best work externally, usually in action. For both, the natural preference of the way they prefer to process information remains, but they utilize and adapt the preference as needed.

For example, readers who would like to see the practical application of this theory are looking at it from the extrovert standpoint. Others who are more interested in the insights the theory may provide for understanding themselves and human nature are seeing it from the introvert point of view, and waiting to process additional information as it is presented (see Box 1.2).

In American society, introverts are outnumbered about three to one (Bates and Kiersey, 1978). As a result, they must develop coping skills early in life. There is pressure on them to "shape up," and to act like the rest of the world. Thus, the introvert is pressured to respond and conform to the outer world (Kroeger & Thuesen, 1988; Myers, 1980).

After reading the preference characteristics for introversion and extroversion, perhaps you could agree with some, but not all the statements. The characteristics with which you agreed most reflect your preference for interacting with the environment and processing information.

The second description of the individual system of personality is the ways people perceive and prefer to gather information from their environment. The

Box 1.2   Characteristics of these complementary orientations of how people interact with their environments include:

Extrovert (E)	**Introvert** (I)
Talks first, thinks later. "Will I ever learn to keep my mouth shut?"	Thinks and rehearses before speaking. "I will think about that."
Knows many people and counts many as close friends.	Enjoys a small number of good friends.
Likes variety and action. Does not mind reading or having a conversation with the TV on. May become oblivious to noise and distractions.	Likes quiet for concentration. Enjoys peace and quiet. Tends to develop a high power of concentration that can shut out TV, conversation.
Dominates conversation.	Perceived as good listener. Often feels taken advantage of.
Approachable and easily engaged by friends and strangers.	Appears quiet, reserved, and reflective.
Likes going to parties and prefers to talk with many people.	Likes to share special occasions with just a few close friends.
Prefers generating ideas with a group. Bounces ideas off others.	Thinks of ideas, reflects on them and wishes he/she could get them out more forcefully.
Finds listening more difficult than talking. Likes to be in the limelight.	Likes to state ideas without interruptions.
Talks way through things. "I lost my books, has anyone seen them?"	Thinks through where misplaced items might be and looks for them on own.
Needs affirmation from friends. Enjoys feedback about accomplishments.	"Recharges" alone, especially after socializing with friends. When young, often told to "go out and play." Parents worried that you like to be by yourself too much.
Likes to talk at great lengths at any time.	Often gets suspicious if people are too complimentary or says something that has already been said.

preference of the way we gather information (perceive things) is called either Sensor (S) or Intuitive (N). Notice that the letter (N) is used to identify "intuitive" in the list below because "I" has already been used to designate introvert in the previous list of preferences.

Sensing and intuitive function influence our learning style. Sensing is the reality function. Our senses tell us things exist. Sensors are influential doers and are action oriented. Their learning style is hands on. Intuiting is a possibility function. Through hunches and guesses, they see possibilities inherent in objects. Their learning style is creating and experimenting (Robinson, 1995). Until recently intuitive qualities were often ignored, but now are considered to represent an asset of creativity and seeing the big picture (see Box 1.3).

Box 1.3

Sensor (S)	Intuitive (N)
Prefers specific answers to specific questions. Details are important.	Tends to think of many things at once; accused by others of being absent-minded.
Likes to concentrate on what he/she is doing. Does not wonder about what is next. Would rather do something than think about it.	Finds the future and its possibilities intriguing; more excited about where going than where you are.
Finds satisfying jobs that yield tangible results. Hates cleaning but would rather clean the office than think about where your career is headed.	Believes details are boring and redundant.
Believes if it is not broken, you do not have to fix it. Cannot understand why people have to try to improve everything.	Enjoys figuring out how things work just for the fun of it.
Likes to hear things sequentially instead of randomly; you would rather work with concrete facts and figures than ideas and theories.	Seeks connections and interrelatedness behind most things and ideas rather than accepting them at face value.
Does not usually engage in fantasy. Wonders about people who spend too much time "daydreaming" and imagining.	Spends time in reflective thinking, imagining, and looking for connections and interrelationships. "What does this mean?"
Reads magazines from front to back; does not understand why some people prefer to begin reading anywhere in a book or magazine.	Reads magazines anywhere there is an interesting topic.
Takes things literally and is very literal in the use of words. Gets frustrated when people (1) do not give clear instructions; (2) when someone says they will give you details later; or (3) if clear instructions are treated as vague guidelines.	Gives general answers, does not understand why so many people cannot follow directions given. Gets irritated when people push for specific details.
Sees details easier than the overall picture. Is happy to focus on the job, not how it fits into the overall picture.	Sees the overall picture with relationships and parts that make up the whole.
Believes "seeing is believing." Does not believe until sees evidence.	Would rather think about the possibilities, what could be.

Box 1.4

Thinker (T)

Does not show emotions readily, and is often uncomfortable dealing with people's feelings.

Stays calm, cool, and collected, even objective when everyone else is upset.

Settles a dispute based on what is fair and truthful rather than what will make people happy.

Enjoys proving a point for the sake of clarity; argues both sides in a discussion simply to expand intellectual horizons.

Appears more firm-minded than gentle-hearted. If you disagree with people, you would rather tell them than say nothing and let them think they are right. Prides self in objectivity. Often called cold and uncaring (you know this could not be further from the truth).

Makes difficult decisions and cannot understand why so many people get upset about things.

Thinks it is more important to be right than liked. Believes it is unnecessary to like people in order to work with them and do a good job.

Impressed with things that are logical and scientific. Remembers numbers and figures more readily than faces and names.

Feeler (F)

Tends to be very aware of other people and their feelings.

Considers a "good decision" one that takes others' feelings into account.

Over-extends self to others in considering a difference in opinion.

Prefers harmony over clarity; embarrassed by conflict in groups or family gatherings and tries to avoid it.

Does not hesitate to take back something said that offended someone; because of this they may be accused of being indecisive. Often takes things personally.

Wonders if people care what you want, although it is difficult to say this.

Over-extends themselves in meeting other people's needs.

People and feelings are more important in decision-making

This brief description of the way people perceive and gather information broadens the picture of personality types. As with the trait of extrovert and introvert, people usually have some traits of both preferences. Everyone has some sensing characteristics and some intuitive ones. The same person can also perceive things differently from one time to the next. This is called **situational difference.** For example, at bill paying time, even the most intuitive individual must rely on sensory processes to deal with objective facts and figures and attend to detail.

The third of the four preferences shows how people prefer to carry out the process of decision-making. People have preferences for making decisions as Thinkers (T) or as Feelers (F). Thinking is the logical function. Our thoughts interpret information, analyze and make sense out of facts or con-

cepts. Thinkers' learning is analytical and they try to make sense out of information and resources. Feeling is a value function. We make a value judgment about objects such as how we like or feel about them. The feeler's learning style is interactive and collaborative (Robinson, 1995). They are affiliative and promote participation (see Box 1.4).

One more preference set, judger or perceiver, completes the picture in the identification of types. This preference is the one believed to be the most common source of interpersonal tension and the one most easily observed (Kroeger et al., 1988). This is a preference for the functions of information gathering and decision-making most frequently used to interact with the outer world, verbally and behaviorally. People who prefer to orient their lives as structured, organized, scheduled, planned, and con-

BOX 1.5

Judger (J)	**Perceiver (P)**
Waits for others, who never seem to come on time.	Is distracted easily and gets "lost" between activities.
Puts everything in its place.	Loves to explore the unknown, even just a new way to class.
"Knows" that if people would do what they are supposed to when they are supposed to, things would be much better. Things are decided.	Does not plan tasks, but waits to see what the demands are. Often perceived as disorganized; (you know better). Things are pending.
Knows what the day will be upon waking; schedules things and follows the schedule. Difficult for you if things do not go as planned.	Depends on last minute spurts of energy to meet deadlines; makes the deadline, but drives everyone crazy in the process.
Does not like surprises, and makes this well known. Structured.	Believes creativity, spontaneity, and responsiveness are more important than order and neatness. Flows with the situation.
Keeps lists and uses them. Adds tasks to list just to cross them off.	Turns most work into play. A job probably is not worth doing if it is not fun.
Thrives on order; has a system to keep everything in its place, in drawers, or on a shelf.	Does not have a system for things. Changes conversation frequently. Topics include anything that enters his/her mind.
States opinion emphatically; often accused of being angry when merely stating opinion—often forcefully.	Does not liked to be pinned down about most things; would rather keep options open.
Likes to complete things and get them out of the way, even if they have to be redone to get things right. Closure.	Tends to make things less than definite, but not always—it all depends. Openness.

trolled with the ability to make decisions quickly are classified as **Judger** (J). People who prefer to allow their environment to be spontaneous, adaptive and responsive to a variety of situations, and who change decisions easily so others have difficulty knowing their position on issues are known as **Perceiver** (P). Although people must be both judgers and perceive when making a decision, both are usually not used at the same time. People shift back and forth between perceiver and judger preferences, sometimes quite abruptly, as when an adult with a high tolerance for children's noise suddenly decides that enough is enough (Myers, 1980).

There are many times when the use of either preference for how people prefer to orient their lives

might be appropriate. However, one preference is selected to use as often as possible when dealing with the outer world. For example, some readers are still following this outline of personality types with an open mind; they are for the moment using the preference of perceiver. Other readers decided that they agree or disagree with the information. They are using judgment. This preference distinguishes those who order their lives (judgers) from people who have a more flexible orientation (perceivers) (see Box 1.5).

Of the sixteen specific types that result from the various combinations of the preferences, (see Figure 1.1) each is the product of a dominant process, extroverted or introverted which is modified by the

		Sensing: Thinking	Sensing: Feeling	Intuitive: Feelings	Intuitive: Thinking		
Introverts	Judgers	**ISTJ** Serious, Quiet, Thorough, Practical Matter-of-fact, Logical, Orderly, Realistic	**ISFJ** Quiet, Friendly, Responsible, Conscientious Stable, Thorough, Accurate, Loyal	**INFJ** Perseverance, Originality, Quiet Forceful, Conscientious, Shows concern	**INTJ** Skeptical, Critical Determined, Independent	Judgers	Intuitive
Introverts	Judgers	Takes responsibility Works toward goals regardless of protest	Patient with detail and routine Concerned with how others feel	Desire to do what is needed Respected for firm principles Put best efforts into work Followed and respected for clear convictions to best serve common good	Has great drive for own ideas Power to organize job and carry it through Must learn to yield less important points to win most important	Judgers	Intuitive
Introverts	Perceivers	**ISTP** Cool onlooker, Quiet Observant, Reserved	**ISFP** Retiring, Does not force opinions, Quietly friendly Loyal followers	**INFP** Friendly Learns on own	**INTP** Quiet, Reserved Impersonal, Logical	Perceivers	Intuitive
Introverts	Perceivers	Analyzes life with detached curiosity and unexpected flashes of original humor Interested in how things work Exerts self no more than necessary—any waste of energy is inefficient	Modest about abilities Relaxed about getting things done Enjoys the present moment and does not want to spoil by undue haste or exertion	Absorbed in what he/she is doing Tends to take on too much Full of enthusiasm and loyalties but does not mention until knows you well Little concern for possessions or physical surroundings	Likes ideas—not small talk Enjoys theoretical or scientific subjects Has sharply defined interests Little liking for parties	Perceivers	Intuitive
Extroverts	Perceivers	**ESTP** Matter-of-fact, Conservative, May be blunt, Adaptable, Tolerant	**ESFP** Outgoing, Accepting, Practical Easy going, Friendly, Uses common sense	**ENFP** Warmly enthusiastic, Imaginative, High-spirited, Helping Ingenious, Capable	**ENTP** Quick, Ingenious, Good at things Stimulating company, Alert, Outspoken	Perceivers	Extroverts
Extroverts	Perceivers	Dislikes long explanations Works best with real things that can be taken apart	Enjoys everything and makes things more fun for others Knows what's going on and joins in eagerly Remembers facts easier than theory	Able to do almost anything that interests them Often relies on ability to improvise Quick with a solution	Apt to turn to new interests frequently May argue for fun or either side of a question Resourceful in solving new problems but may neglect routine	Perceivers	Extroverts
Extroverts	Judgers	**ESTJ** Practical, Realistic Matter-of-fact	**ESFJ** Warm-hearted, Talkative, Popular Born cooperator, Conscientious, Needs harmony	**ENFJ** Responsive, Responsible, Sympathetic Sociable, Popular	**ENTJ** Hearty, Frank, Well-informed Decisive, Leader, Public Speaker	Judgers	Extroverts
Extroverts	Judgers	Natural head for business or mechanics Likes to organize and run activities Good administrator—especially if considers other feelings	Always doing something nice for others Works best with encouragement and praise Little interest in abstract thinking or technical subjects	Feel real concern for what others think or want Tries to handle things with regard for feelings Can lead a group or present with ease	Good at anything that requires reasoning and intelligent talk May be more positive and confident than their experience in an area warrants	Judgers	Extroverts

Figure 1.1 Characteristics of Type (Adapted from Myers, I. 1980. *Gifts Differing*).

nature of the auxiliary process. This modification is especially influential in the introvert types, because it is the auxiliary processes that are primarily responsible for the individual's outer behavior. For example, introversion is not a trait, but a basic disposition or orientation. In each of the eight kinds of introverts, this orientation takes on a different personality style of interacting with others as a result of the other preferences involved.

SUMMARY OF THE FOUR PREFERENCES

Personality type is the result of an individual's own combination of preferences, which can be stated for convenience in four letters. For example, ISTJ means an introvert orientation with a preference for sensing and thinking and a predominately judging preference toward the outer world. ENFP means an extrovert orientation preferring intuition and feeling and an attitude toward the outer world as predominately a perceiver. Figure 1.1 shows the combination of the favorite and auxiliary processes for each of the sixteen types.

APPLICATION

The description of the four preferences of ways people interact with the environment were explored. The following is a review of an application of personality types showing the interaction of behaviors with one aspect of life that is observably influenced by it, the choice of an occupation or profession.

As might be expected, thinking types tend to work well in jobs using inanimate objects, and feeling types tend to prefer dealing with people. Sensing types with the judging preference function well in structured jobs with sharply defined procedures, but intuitive with a perceptive preference do not like such jobs, since the procedures restrict them from taking initiatives to pursue the possibilities they perceive.

The preference that seems to have the most influence on occupational choice, the SN preference, determines what will interest people (Myers, 1980). Those with sensing personality types are drawn to jobs that let them deal with a constant stream of facts, while intuitive like situations in which they can look at the possibilities. The intuitive wants to find fulfillment in the job itself, preferably by doing something creative. MacKinnon (1961), found that

especially creative groups, whether architects, writers, research scientists, or mathematicians, are almost entirely composed of intuitive.

The next most important preference, TF, determines the type of judgment process an individual prefers. Individuals who prefer the thinking preference are more skillful in handling issues that deal with inanimate objects, machinery, principles, or theories, none of which have any inconsistent or unpredictable feelings, and all of which can be handled with logical thinking. Individuals who prefer the "feeling" preference are better skilled in matters involving people, what they value, and how they can be persuaded or helped.

When individuals think about an occupational choice, it is useful to consider how the job and their preferred kind of perceptions and judgments match. When investigating a job, it is helpful for prospective workers to find out about what they will be doing, and how much time will be spent on each aspect of the job. Jobs that give individuals the opportunity to use preferred processes turn out to be more interesting and enjoyable for the worker.

People trying to make an occupational choice may find it helpful to look at the kinds of work that most appeal to people with the same favored perceptive and judging processes. Each of the four possible combinations of perception and judgment tend to produce distinct interests, values, needs, and skills. For example:

ST people focus on facts and handle these with impersonal analysis. They tend to be matter-of-fact, practical, and to use their abilities in technical skills dealing with facts, objects, and money. In a sample of students, the EF preference had a high percent of accountants and, in the fields of finance and commerce and bank employees, ST's made up over half of the individuals. ST's also do well in production, construction, applied science, and law (Myers, 1980).

SF's focus their attention on facts, but they handle them with personal warmth. They tend to be sympathetic and friendly, and they enjoy occupations that provide practical help and service to people. In the sales and customer relations sample, over three-quarters had SF preferences, and among nursing and education students, SF preferences represented just under fifty percent. SF's do well in medical specialties involving primary care, health-related professions, community service, education (especially elementary), and physical education. While students of law, counseling, and science, had a very small percent of SF's (Myers, 1980).

NF's prefer possibilities to facts, and they handle these with personal warmth. Their enthusiasm and insight bring them success in understanding and communicating with people. In a sample of students, over three-quarters of those in counseling and over one-half of the creative writers had NF preferences. Among theology students, the percent of NF's was over one-half, and health-related professionals, and journalism students were represented by just under one-half percent. NF's also do well in teaching, research, literature, and art; but among finance and commerce students, sales and customer relations people and accountants, NF's make up only ten percent or less (Myers, 1980; Koreger and Thursen, 1988).

NT people focus their attention on possibilities, but with a more impersonal style of analysis. They tend to be logical, and often use their abilities in theoretical and technical development. Among research scientists sampled, a large percent were NTs, and there is a large representation of NT people among science and law students. NT's also do well as inventors, managers, forecasters, and security analysts (Myers, 1980).

People should not be discouraged from pursuing a job or profession because they are not the usual personality found in that area. However, when an occupation is chosen in a field outside your preferred type, you should investigate the job thoroughly. If individuals make the effort required to be understood by their co-workers, they become valuable contributors of abilities that are rare among their co-workers. For example, among police there are probably few intuitive, but when a training course in human relations was instituted to aid the officers in handling domestic calls, those with intuitive preferences developed a higher level of skills than did the sensing types.

When people find a field of interest in which they are able to use their skills developed through personality-type preference, there usually turns out to be a variety of positions needing these skills. In addition, each job needs skills from the complimentary preference. Extroverts tend to find jobs more interesting and they work more effectively when things are happening all around them. They enjoy actively working with objects and people. Introverts tend to be more effective when their work involves ideas and the thinking activity can take place quietly in their head.

Among the sensing thinking (ST) people, for example, the introverts (IST) enjoy organizing facts and principles related to a situation, an important part of the work involved in economics and law. The extroverts (EST) like to organize the situation itself, which is useful in business and industry (Myers, 1980). Most people are happier when their work lies mainly in the world they know best, their dominant orientation preference.

The judger perceiver (P) preference can influence satisfaction. Judging people display their extroversion with people or situations, mainly with their best judging process, thinking or feeling. Perceiving people do their extroverting primarily with their best perceptive processes, sensing or intuition. As can be seen, J and P types approach situations differently. Judging types, those who prefer sensing (the S-J types); like to have their work organized and systematic, and need to know what is to come, often to the point of knowing what they will be doing a week away. Perceptive types, especially those who prefer intuition (NP types), want their work to be a response to the needs of the moment. Jobs differ greatly in these respects.

Jobs also differ in their decision-making demands. Judging types, especially those who prefer thinking, tend to see decision-making as an enjoyable feature of their job. Perceptive types, especially those who prefer feeling, often find routine decisions a burden, and difficult to make. They would rather see their way to a solution than deliver a choice between alternatives. Thus administrators tend to be judger (J) types and counselors perceiver (P) types.

Descriptions of personality types reveal opposite characteristics of given preferences. The various types tend to differ in their reactions to situations. Because these behaviors are general, they cannot describe every individual in every situation. One way to understand people as part of a system is by considering type theory.

The prescription for individually solving a problem is to exercise all four processes in succession: sensing to establish facts, intuition to suggest all possible solutions, thinking to determine all probable consequences of each course of action, and feeling to weigh the desirability of each outcome. This holistic perspective contributes to the comprehensiveness of decision-making. It is often difficult for one person to have all these views, but skills to coordinate such an inclusive thinking process can be developed.

In a work setting, ideally, co-workers constitute a team with a common goal. A variety of personality types can be advantageous because people bring their individual strengths. Especially on a team, differences can be assets. A job that may be boring and confusing to one personality type and (thus poorly done), may be interesting and exciting to another type. When people are well-suited to their jobs, they are much more effective in what they accomplish. For example, introverts with intuition think of new possibilities simply as ideas, they are the "idea" people on a team. Extroverts with intuition translate ideas into action, but they are not interested in carrying the action beyond the point where everything is worked out. Sensing types take over with great satisfaction and produce tangible results.

For a team to be effective, a variety of personality types are advantageous to perform the required tasks productively and with satisfaction for those involved. Opposite types will disagree on what should be done and how, but differing perceptions help people see various aspects of a situation. Team effectiveness will survive if members recognize that differing perceptions and kinds of judgments are essential to a sound solution.

A respect for differences not only contributes to effective teamwork, but also helps individuals recognize and cultivate their own best and least developed processes in interacting with others who have complementary preferences.

Similarly, family systems are composed of individuals with a variety of personality types. An effective family system is one in which differences and individual behavior preferences are respected. Diversity in the family system may be challenging when building relationships and developing family cohesion. Appreciating and respecting differences and the individual talents each has provide a richer experience for all. In the family system is where we initially are exposed to diversity in personality types. Relationship patterns and skills to interact positively with those who are different can be valued, encouraged and enjoyed.

SUMMARY

Personality, one aspect of the individual environment, was discussed. Each individual within the family has a unique personality based on temperament, birth order, sibling gender mix, and personality type. Temperament, with its nine response components of behavior, is believed to be the precursor of personality. Birth order and sibling gender mix are considered to be influential in describing how individual subsystem behaviors develop and influences personality development. Personality is considered a composite of traits that develops after birth and continues to be modified throughout ones life. The family environmental system (E) is influential in individual personality development (O). A number of personality preference types were described. Personality preferences describe different ways of perceiving and interacting with the environment. Appreciating differences and developing relationships with people with a variety of personality types increases not only our awareness of self, but also our understanding and ability to work well with others.

CHAPTER 2

History of Healthcare in the United States

Current Health Care System and Trends

Learning Objectives

- Discuss the history of healthcare.
- Discuss the impact of social influences on the development of healthcare.
- Describe the major forces in the health care industry today.
- Discuss the impact of history on the development of healthcare facilities.
- Identify the various types of health care facilities and describe the services provided.
- List the five challenges facing health care today and explain how the health care professional can contribute to their resolution.

Key Terms

Acupuncture	Holistic medicine	Osteopathy
Adult foster home	Homeopathy	Outpatient services
Alternative medicine	Hospice	Palliative
Ambulatory services	Inpatient	Pandemic
Assisted living residence	Integrative medicine	Psychiatric hospital
Baby boomers	Intermediate nursing care facility	Psychosomatic
Chiropractic		Skilled nursing facility
Complementary medicine	Massage therapy	Targeted drug therapy
Continuing care community	Medicaid	The Joint Commission
Expanding consciousness	Naturopathic medicine	Vital statistics
Gene therapy	Nursing homes	Wellness

THE CASE OF THE CONFUSED DAUGHTER

Until recently, Dora Freemont, age 87, lived alone in a small apartment. Last week she suffered a slight stroke. After several days in the hospital, she is ready to be discharged. Her daughter, Sally, is very concerned that her widowed mother is no longer capable of living alone and handling all her housekeeping and personal needs. She shares her concern with Angela Cisneros, one of the nurses who cared for her mother during her hospital stay. Sally is very worried and fears she will have to quit work in order to help take care of her mother. Angela knows that there are a variety of long-term care facilities and a number of options available for Mrs. Freemont. She refers Sally to the hospital social worker, who explains these options and discusses with her which might be most appropriate for her mother.

This chapter provides learners with important information they can use to assist their future patients. It also helps learners understand the many settings in which they can seek employment.

THE HEALTH CARE INDUSTRY TODAY

The health care industry is the largest service employer in the United States. Federal economists expect that in 2009, Americans will spend $2.5 trillion on health care (Arnst, 2009). Further, it is projected that by 2018, health care spending could nearly double to $4.4 trillion. Many factors are shaping the delivery of health care today. It is important for health care professionals to understand the characteristics of and forces behind this enormous industry. These will surely influence their working conditions, as well as determine what it takes for them to be successful on the job.

Technological Advancements

The long history of health care was marked by gradual change until the beginning of the 20th century. Table 2.1 contains a summary of significant events in the history of medicine. Starting about 100 years ago, the rate of discovery and change increased rapidly so that in the last 20 years, medical technology and diagnostic and treatment methods advanced more than in the previous 100 years. At the beginning of the 1900s, the major killers were infectious diseases. Physicians had a limited number of treatment techniques available. Because of the discovery of penicillin and antibiotics, along with the widespread use of immunizations, many of these diseases are almost unheard of today.

Table 2.1 History of Health Care

Time Frame	Event	Impact
Ancient Times (???–A.D. 400)	Study of fossilized bones and Egyptian mummies indicates many modern health conditions, such as arthritis, infectious bone diseases, appendicitis, arteriosclerosis, urine and intestinal diseases.	Health care problems and diseases have been with us from the beginning of human life.
	Belief system based on supernatural rather than natural laws. Causes of disease were expected to be supernatural (caused by spirits, ghosts, or gods).	Home remedies were used and rituals performed to drive away the evil spirits. Examples of rituals are creating loud noises, beating the ill person, or bloodletting. Preventive medicine consisted of wearing amulets and mutilating or painting the body to ward off evil spirits.
	Life span was only 20–35 years.	Chronic illnesses were rare.
	Hippocrates of Cos (460–379 B.C.) was the most famous Greek physician of ancient times. He stressed observation and conservative treatment. Believed that health was the balance of four humors.	Called the "Father of Medicine." He used dietetics as a means of balancing the humors. Only if diet failed would he resort to drugs or surgery.

Table 2.1 History of Health Care—cont'd

Time Frame	Event	Impact
Medieval Times (A.D. 400–1350)	Two plagues (in A.D. 543 & 568) killed majority of people and led to breakdown in civilization.	Monks preserved written medical texts and monasteries served as centers of learning to maintain knowledge
	Christianity became increasing center of power. Believed that disease was punishment for sins, possession by devil, or result of witchcraft.	Christians emphasized saving the soul, not the body. Treatment methods were prayer, penitence, and the assistance of saints. Any cure was considered a miracle.
	At the Council of Tours in 1163, the church proclaimed that they "do not shed blood."	Because most physicians were clergymen, they were no longer able to perform surgery.
	The title of Doctor became known and major medical legislation was written in 1140 and 1224 that specified a 9-year curriculum with state examinations and licenses.	Medicine became an official profession, although there were not enough physicians for the population. As a result, lower-class citizens still relied on barbers and lay healers.
	Black Plague of 1348 killed large percentage of European population.	Concept of quarantine as preventive measure was recognized.
	Network of hospitals built.	Marked a new and more humane approach toward the ill. Hospitals were primarily a refuge for the sick, old, disabled, or homeless.
Renaissance (1350–1650)	Revival of learning and science. Tremendous growth in inquiry of how the body was structured and how it worked. Numerous autopsies were performed.	First attempts to connect autopsy results with clinical observations made during life. Accurate anatomical drawings were now available for study.
	Despite the new advances, it was still a time of tremendous filth in the cities and their peoples, the spread of disease, and extreme superstitions.	Criticisms of the old ways were frequently met with hatred, such as toward Pierre Brissot, who spoke against bloodletting and died in exile.
	Study of botany (plants) greatly expanded as travel between countries increased.	Plants were the main source of drugs; 500 new plant species were categorized and first modern pharmacopoeia written.
	Girolamo Fracastoro wrote a book in 1546 in which he presented the first theory of contagious diseases.	Theory was not taken seriously and would not be proven for several centuries. High incidence of infections continued as hand washing and hygiene were not considered important (e.g., physician would perform autopsy and then go do surgery without washing his hands).
	Printing press invented.	Allowed for widespread distribution of new information and books.
	Invention of gun powder resulted in numerous gunshot wounds during frequent wars.	Need for surgical treatment of wounds elevated barber-surgeons to a higher status.
17th Century	Increasing interest in experimentation and observation.	Studies in anatomy continued, but the study of physiology (how the body functions) was also now investigated.
	William Harvey, an Englishman, stated that blood circulates throughout the body within a continuous network of vessels. Only the mechanical aspects of the system were addressed.	Vehemently opposed at first, this discovery led to the realization that medications could be injected into the circulatory system, and blood could be transfused. After many failed attempts, it fell out of favor for several centuries.
	In 1666, Anton van Leeuwenhoek invented the microscope.	Study of microscopic anatomy and visualization of organisms now possible. Germs were only viewed under the microscope; the connection with disease came several centuries later.

Continued.

Table 2.1 History of Health Care—cont'd

Time Frame	Event	Impact
	Quinine imported from Peru as a cure for malaria.	Separated malaria from other types of fevers. Confirmed the idea that specific diseases have specific cures.
	The study of the brain and psychology was of interest. (Prior to this time, a common belief was that the soul resided in the pineal gland and the rest of the body was purely mechanical in nature.)	Nervous system and stimulation of muscles discovered. The long-believed theory that mucus from a head cold was produced by the brain was disproved.
18th Century	Researchers and theorists still struggled with an explanation of how the body functioned.	Three theories were proposed. First, that the body functioned like a hydraulic pump that was run by an undefined fluid flowing through the nervous system. Second, that every disease was the result of overstimulation or inability to respond to stimulation. Treatment was then either a depressant or a stimulant (e.g., opium and alcohol). Third, that direct clinical observation should be used to define and categorize diseases. (This led to the absurd description of 2400 different diseases, as the same diseases were listed many times, just because the symptoms varied slightly between cases.)
	Surgery became a respected form of treatment in France after the court physician successfully repaired an anal fistula for King Louis XIV.	Surgery was upgraded from a craft to an experimental science. Procedures were developed that could cure problems that were treatable only through surgery.
	In 1761, Giovanni Battista Morgagni of Padua published a comprehensive book titled *On the Sites and Causes of Disease*.	Emphasis changed from concentration on general conditions and humors to specific changes in organs.
	Techniques for measuring blood pressure and temperature were developed.	Measurements of vital signs were used to monitor patient status.
	Science of chemistry came of age.	Digestion now seen as chemical process, rather than a purely mechanical process or one of putrefaction.
	The philosophy of "enlightenment" was developed, which stressed the rational approach to problems and dissemination of knowledge for others to read.	Numerous studies and experiments added rapidly to the expanding base of knowledge. Sharing of knowledge with others added to the increasing pace of progress.
	Focus went from belief in the devil and "possession" to recognition of mental illness as a disease. Previously, patients were locked up in filthy conditions, as mental illness was thought to be due to possession, sin, crime, or vice.	Mentally ill patients were released from their chains and treated in a more humane way.
	Preventive health came to the forefront in the form of public health.	Sanitary reform was initiated in hospitals, prisons, and military. Personal hygiene also improved dramatically.
	Interest in child health increased.	Decreased the appalling rate of deaths in infants and children.
	Edward Jenner (1749–1823) demonstrated that vaccination with cowpox provides immunity for smallpox.	Countless lives were saved. It opened the door into investigation for other vaccines to be developed.

Table 2.1 History of Health Care—cont'd

Time Frame	Event	Impact
19th Century	Industrial Revolution created growth of city population as peasants flooded into the city. Hospitals were built that could hold many patients.	Large hospital populations allowed for the clinical observation of many cases, followed by autopsy when patient died.
	Advances in physiology continued.	Emphasis moved from individual organs to the identification of the more specific tissues. For example, inflammation of the heart was now stated as endocarditis, pericarditis, or myocarditis (inflammation of one of the three layers of the heart).
	Tremendous increase in medical knowledge was acquired and documented. Physicians and surgeons were united into one profession.	Many first-time surgical operations were performed, such as tracheostomy and removal of thyroid and uterus. Medical profession started to develop specialty areas, such as pediatrics, psychiatry, dermatology (skin), public health, and preventive medicine.
	Medicine based on observation and autopsies had offered all it could to the field. Further advances would need the study and application of the sciences.	Study shifted from practicing physicians to full-time scientific researchers.
	More powerful microscopes were developed.	Human tissue could now be seen at the cellular level.
	Advances were made in chemistry.	Laboratory tests for diagnostic purposes became common. Metabolism and dietetics came under scientific study. Pharmacology was established as a new science.
	Dentists introduced anesthesia, and this practice expanded to major surgical procedures.	Large-scale surgery could now be done. Death rate fell as anesthesia decreased shock and the need for speed in surgery.
	Elizabeth Blackwell (1821–1910) was the first woman MD in the United States. She opened the first nursing school in the United States in 1860.	Medical education opened for the first time to a female. Nursing was established as a profession in the United States.
	Louis Pasteur (1822–1895), a chemist, proved that specific microorganisms called bacteria are the cause of specific diseases in both humans and animals.	The results of his work created the development of the germ theory.
	It was discovered that infectious microorganisms are carried by various means (e.g., humans, animals, mosquitoes, food). Specific identification of microorganisms led to the development of vaccines for prevention.	Revolutionized the ability to prevent, diagnose, and treat infectious diseases. Then in 1864, Lord Joseph Lister, MD, applied the germ theory to his surgical practice by reasoning that microorganisms could also fall into open surgical wounds.
	Anesthesia, asepsis, and invention of a variety of surgical instruments changed the face of medicine forever.	Previously the public viewed hospitals as a place one went to die. Now there was hope of recovery for the first time. Many more advanced surgeries could be performed (e.g., on joints, abdomen, head, spinal column).
	Psychiatry had come to a dead end as it eluded the scientific advances. No satisfactory explanation of mental illness could be given.	Sigmund Freud (1856–1939), an Austrian neurologist, and Joseph Breuer developed the theory of psychoanalysis and presented it to the public in their book on hysteria in 1893.

Continued.

Table 2.1   History of Health Care—cont'd

Time Frame	Event	Impact
		The theory was based on using hypnosis to allow patients to recall prior traumatic and repressed events. Freud later discarded hypnosis and based his new theory on repression of sexual urges as the central theme of psychological illnesses.
	Preventive medicine made great strides as pasteurization, vaccination, asepsis, and sanitation were implemented.	Life span increased from 40 years in 1850 to 70 years in 1950 due primarily to preventive, not curative, measures.
20th Century	In 1921, Karl Landsteiner of Vienna discovered blood groups.	Made transfusion of blood products safe for the first time in history.
	F. G. Banting of Toronto identified insulin in 1921 for treatment of diabetes.	Diabetes was no longer considered a fatal disease, but could be managed with injections of insulin.
	Large-scale vaccination programs were conducted.	Many commonly feared infectious diseases were eradicated. But the influenza epidemic of 1918 that killed 20 million brought reality back after the euphoria of success.
	New diagnostic and therapeutic techniques were developed. The field of biomedical engineering was advanced with the invention of the computer.	X-rays, electrocardiograph (ECG), electroencephalograph (EEG), ultrasound, pacemakers, dialysis, and tomography provided physicians with more diagnostic and therapeutic tools.
	Vitamins were discovered; the United States took the leadership role in this research.	The belief that all diseases were caused by microbes was disproved when lack of certain vitamins was linked to various diseases (e.g., scurvy, beriberi).
	New synthetic drugs were developed to treat specific problems.	Chemotherapy was used to fight cancer. Antibiotics were developed to fight various infections caused by bacteria. Medications for treating allergies were developed.
	Life span was 70–80 years.	Geriatrics became a specialty. Chronic illnesses were very common.
	Mental illness became an increasing problem in modern society.	Shock treatment and psychosurgery were replaced with new drugs and psychotherapy. Tranquilizers used to calm patients changed the approach to and assessment of mental patients.
	The end of the 19th and beginning of the 20th centuries were so laboratory and science based, with increasing specialization, that the patient focus was lost. It has always been known that mental processes can profoundly affect bodily illnesses and symptoms or even cause them, but this was lost in the science of medicine.	The increasing specialization continued to cloud this issue as specialization broke the individual into various parts rather than treating the patient as a holistic being (i.e., different physicians are seen for cardiac, intestinal, and neurological conditions; one physician may diagnose the problem and another do the surgery).
	Other health care specialties developed as the knowledge base increased (e.g., physical therapy, occupational therapy, speech therapy).	Increased number of people who came in contact with the patient and who viewed the concerns from a specialty focus versus holistic perspective.

Table 2.1 History of Health Care—cont'd

Time Frame	Event	Impact
	Health care costs increased due to increased specialization of knowledge and cost of technological advancements, which made health care services beyond the reach of many.	This social issue has been present for· many centuries, but the increased literacy of people and availability of information from a more global awareness increased the dissatisfaction of those unable to access health care. The question was raised, "Does everyone have an equal right to health care?"
	Surgical techniques and anesthesia methods made great advancements. Transplantation of organs was now possible.	Heart, brain, and prosthetic joint replacements were performed. Definition of death was changed from cessation of heart and lung function to demonstration of brain death by EEG.
	People could be kept alive by mechanical means beyond the point of having any quality of life.	Emphasis placed on people having written living wills to specify what they do and do not want done to prolong their lives. In 1975, the New Jersey Supreme Court ruled that the parents of a comatose woman could authorize the removal of life support systems.
	Patients with terminal illnesses wish to die with dignity.	England opened first hospice in 1967. Dr. Jack Kevorkian argued that patients should be allowed to request assistance to end their lives. Between 1990 and 1998, he participated in a number of physician-assisted suicides.
	Development of new and faster machines (e.g., automobiles, airplanes, various recreational vehicles) caused many accidental injuries.	Trauma medicine became a specialty.
	Mass media available to public (e.g., television, radio, newspapers, Internet). Medical physicians often seen as cold and uncaring as they focus on trying to find a diagnosis.	Quackery medicine had greater access to public for generation of huge sales of products. Outrageous claims of quick-acting results and complete cures requiring very little effort were a strong draw compared with other forms of health care.
	Scientific approach was used almost exclusively. Traditional medicine primarily based on diagnosis and then treatment with synthetic medications and surgical procedures. Rejection of herbal and alternative therapies by many traditional medical practitioners.	Practitioners of traditional medicine reject the "old methods" that had been useful in the past, but have not been scientifically proven. People flock to herbalists and alternative therapists in a search for more natural therapies, but lack of regulation in these areas results in many abuses.
	Genetic research into cause of certain diseases and conditions.	Identification of specific genes related to certain conditions, but how to alter to prevent condition has not been discovered.
	In 1978, the first "test tube" baby was born in England.	Opened up opportunity for couples previously unable to have children.
	In 1981, acquired immunodeficiency syndrome (AIDS) identified as a disease.	Huge challenge to medical research that resulted in medications that prolong life, but no cure available.
	First successful cloning of sheep in 1997.	Opened door for human cloning and growth of organs for transplantation.

Continued.

Table 2.1 History of Health Care—cont'd

Time Frame	Event	Impact
21st Century and Beyond— What Is Possible?	Some of the hopes for the new millennium: ■ Vaccine to prevent human immuno deficiency virus (HIV) ■ Cure for AIDS ■ Cure for obesity ■ Cloning of organs for transplantation to overcome extreme difficulty in finding suitable organ donors ■ Cures for heart disease, hypertension, and cancer ■ More effective treatment and cure for mental illnesses ■ Preventive health and alternative therapies used in complementary way with practice of traditional medicine ■ Life span of healthy living expanded to 100 + years ■ Less invasive diagnostic and therapeutic treatments and medications with less harmful side effects	When health care professionals several centuries into the future look back at the 20th century, they will be astounded. This reaction would be similar to when we look back to the previous centuries and are mystified by the ignorance and resulting unnecessary human suffering.

Modern discoveries and inventions build upon one another, increasing the rate of growth of new developments. There are now an amazing number of treatments, including organ transplants, microscopic and robotic surgery, **gene therapy,** and **targeted drug therapy.** Keeping informed about these changes and learning to use and apply new equipment and techniques will be a continual and interesting challenge for the health care professional of the 21st century.

Specialization

Another significant trend in health care over the last 30 years has been the specialization of medicine (Williams, 2005). This has had several important effects on health care delivery:

■ Diagnosis and treatment are improving as physicians and other practitioners concentrate on specific areas of expertise, such as endocrinology and cardiology.
■ Medical practice is more technical and fragmented, because specialists treat one aspect, rather than the patient as a whole.
■ The cost of providing health care has increased.

Fascinating Facts

It seems incredible that the importance of handwashing to prevent the spread of infection, a basic health care practice now taken for granted, was discovered less than 200 years ago. Ignaz Semmelweis, working in a hospital maternity ward in Vienna, became concerned about the high death rate of new mothers. He observed that it occurred most often among women who were assisted in childbirth by physicians who came directly from performing autopsies. Amazingly, his beliefs were rejected by colleagues. This is an example of how new ideas are often met with resistance and how being open to change can improve—and even save—the lives of many.

■ Long-term relationships between physicians and their patients are breaking down because one physician no longer provides all or most of the needed care.

Specialization has created many employment opportunities for health care professionals. At the same time, it has increased the need for caring attitudes and effective communication with patients. Lifelong relationships developed between physicians and their patients are rare today. Much of the care is provided by professionals whom the patient does not know. Therefore, health care professionals play an important part in helping patients understand and have confidence in the care they are receiving.

Aging Population

Improvements in medical care, especially the development of new drugs and surgical techniques, have lengthened the average life span. Life expectancy for a male born in 1900 was 46 years, and 48 years for a female. This increased dramatically to over 75 years for a male and 80 years for a female born in 2005 (Arias, Rostron, & Tejada-Vera, 2010).

A second reason for the growing number of seniors is the aging of the group known as the **"baby boomers."** An unusually large number of births occurred during the years following the end of World War II, starting in 1946 and lasting until 1964. These individuals have started and will continue entering their period of heaviest use of the health care system over the next 20 years.

Older persons are the heaviest users of health care services. The tremendous growth of this segment of the population is putting increased demands on all types of services, including the following:

- Facilities that provide long-term care for older persons unable to live in their own homes
- Treatment and care devoted to chronic (persisting for a long time, not cured quickly) problems that develop in people who live longer
- Home care services ranging from housekeeping duties to high-level nursing care

Increasing Costs

The cost of providing· health care has increased dramatically over the past few decades. While every product and service has steadily increased in price over the years, health care costs have grown at a faster rate than almost anything else. This is due to several factors:

- Technological advances, resulting in the use of very expensive equipment and supplies
- Increasing number of elderly citizens, resulting in higher number of patients seeking services

Thinking It Through

Joseph Appleton's primary care physician has referred him to Dr. Nester, an oncologist (physician who specializes in diagnosis and treatment of cancer). Preliminary tests show that Mr. Appleton may have colon cancer. Mr. Appleton, age 77, is uncomfortable about visiting a specialist he has never met. He is especially distraught about the possibility of having a life-threatening illness and doesn't understand why the doctor he has seen for many years can't take care of the· problem. Carmen Rodriguez, Dr. Nester's medical assistant, greets Mr. Appleton on his first visit to the office.
1. Discuss the changes in health care delivery that have led to the referral of patients to specialists.
2. What can Carmen do to help Mr. Appleton feel more comfortable?

- Rising prices of pharmaceutical products, which make up the most widely used methods of treatment
- Increasing number of diagnostic tests and treatment options available
- Increasing number of medical malpractice lawsuits, which results in higher liability insurance costs to physicians who must pass these costs on to patients
- Extensive use of diagnostic tests to protect physicians against the growing number of malpractice lawsuits
- Lack of competition that would encourage increased efficiency and provide incentives to lower costs
- Rising expectations of patients that health care should provide more effective solutions
- More effective treatments that encourage increasing numbers of patients to seek medical care
- Poor distribution of physicians and other health care providers
  (*Source:* Adapted from *Introduction to Health Services* [7th ed.], by S. J. Williams and P. R. Torrens, 2008, Clifton Park, NY: Delmar Cengage Learning.)

In response to skyrocketing health care costs, new methods have been and continue to be developed to deliver and pay for health care. At the same time, efforts are being made to control costs.

HEALTH CARE FACILITIES AND SERVICES

A wide variety of health care facilities are available that offer many services for patients with all types of needs. They range in size from a private physician's office to nationwide health care systems that include hospitals, clinics, and long-term care facilities. Health care facilities offer many kinds of services, ranging from preventive care to emergency treatment; from routine physical exams to in-home assistance for dying patients. There are many kinds of employment settings for today's health care professional.

Hospitals

Hospitals are the traditional facilities for the care of the ill and injured. The following conditions account for the majority of hospital admissions: heart problems, cancer, mental illness, stroke, respiratory conditions, and fractures caused by osteoporosis (Williams & Torrens, 2008). In the past, most patients remained in the hospital for all care needed until they were able to return home. The cost of hospital care has increased so dramatically that other means of patient care have been developed to limit the number and length of patient stays. Hospitals are now just one of many facilities that provide patient care.

The trend is for hospitals to be high-tech facilities that specialize in serving patients who need sophisticated treatment and 24-hour nursing care. The various levels of care offered by hospitals include the following:

- Trauma center: Offers comprehensive services for life-threatening injuries. Specific criteria must be met to quality as a trauma center, such as having certain sophisticated diagnostic equipment and trauma surgeons available.
- Emergency room: Treats conditions that occur suddenly and require immediate attention. Examples include serious injuries from accidents and heart attacks.
- Intensive care unit (ICU): Provides specialized equipment and continuous care and monitoring for patients with serious illnesses or injuries.
- Cardiac care unit (CCU): Provides specialized equipment and continuous care and monitoring for patients with serious heart conditions.

- General unit: Provides care for patients who are seriously ill but do not need a high level of specialized equipment and continuous nursing care.
- Transitional care unit (TCU): Provides lower-level care while patients' needs are assessed and arrangements made to release patients to return home or enter another care facility.

Some hospitals also have rehabilitation units, which provide treatment for musculoskeletal, neurological, and orthopedic conditions. Rehabilitation focuses on helping patients regain as high a level of normal function as possible.

Other hospitals offer specialized care for certain populations, such as children, or specific conditions, such as burns or psychiatric conditions. **Psychiatric hospitals** offer treatment to individuals with psychiatric and behavioral disorders, including assistance with crises, medication management, counseling, and monitoring of activities of daily living. Patients may be treated on an outpatient or **inpatient** (hospitalized) basis, depending on their needs.

The modern hospital faces the challenge of controlling expenses and at the same time maintaining a certain occupancy rate (number of patients) in order to meet its operating costs. A variety of approaches have been developed to resolve this conflict:

- Diversification of services. Examples include offering rehabilitation, outpatient surgery, and long-term care in lower-tech wings or separate buildings.
- Elimination of services that duplicate those offered at nearby hospitals.
- Merging with other hospitals to share expenses and avoid duplication of services.
- Joining a large health care system that also operates clinics, nursing homes, diagnostic centers, home health agencies, and so on.
- Being purchased by a national corporation that owns and manages many hospitals.

A serious problem faced by many hospitals is the number of uninsured individuals who use emergency rooms to provide care that could be provided by a clinic, physician, or other less costly provider. By law, emergency rooms must give basic, needed care. In many cases, patients who cannot afford routine care wait until their condition is critical before seeking help. What might be a $150 visit to a physician becomes a $1500 emergency-room expense for which the hospital is not reimbursed. Some hospitals, unable to afford the burden of providing free care, have closed their emergency rooms. Others have set up hospital clinics that offer basic care to walk-in patients.

Changes will continue to be made as hospitals seek ways to control costs and at the same time provide adequate services for the communities they serve. Maintaining quality of care is another concern, and many hospitals seek voluntary accreditation from **The Joint Commission,** a private, nonprofit organization whose purpose is to encourage the attainment of high standards of institutional medical care. It establishes guidelines for the operation of hospitals and other facilities, such as ambulatory surgery centers, long-term care facilities, and laboratories, and conducts inspections to ensure that standards are being met.

Health care professionals who are employed· at approved facilities by The Joint Commission should become familiar with the standards that regulate the duties and areas for which they are responsible. Being accredited is very important because Medicare and many insurance companies will not pay for services provided at nonaccredited facilities.

Ambulatory Services

Ambulatory services are those that do not require hospitalization. Also known as **outpatient services,** they are provided by the many diagnostic, treatment, and rehabilitation facilities that account for most patient care activities. Many procedures that were previously performed in hospitals are now done on an outpatient basis. For example, a growing number of surgeries are now performed in ambulatory surgery centers with some patients being discharged one to three hours after surgery (Williams & Torrens, 2008).

The physician's office is the location of the majority of ambulatory services. Ambulatory care is also provided by comprehensive facilities that offer a variety of services. A large clinic, for example, may have on-site radiographic and laboratory services. Other facilities are freestanding and offer one type of specialized service, such as an imaging center that only performs X-rays and ultrasound procedures. These facilities accept patients on a referral basis from professionals throughout the area. Table 2.2 lists common ambulatory settings and their services.

Table 2.2 Ambulatory Facilities

Facility	Services Offered
Adult Day Care	Activities, meals, and supervision for adults who need assistance, such as older persons and developmentally disabled persons
Dental Offices	Prevention, diagnosis, and treatment of problems with the teeth
Diagnostic Centers	Procedures, such as radiography, to determine the cause and nature of diseases and injuries
Emergency and Urgent Care Centers	Care for conditions that need immediate attention
Health Care Services in Companies, Schools, and Prisons	Basic and preventive care for employees, students, and prisoners
Laboratories	Clinical labs draw blood and collect urine and other samples, and perform tests that provide information needed to diagnose, treat, or prevent disease. Dental labs make false teeth, crowns, and corrective devices for the mouth.
Medical Offices	Prevention, diagnosis, and treatment of all types of health conditions
Rehabilitation Centers	Therapies to help patients regain maximum physical and mental function; types include physical, occupational, speech, and hearing. Specialized centers help patients overcome problems with substance abuse.
Specialty Clinics and Offices	Treatment for specific conditions such as cancer and venereal disease; rehabilitative services such as hand therapy, psychological counseling, and many others
Surgical Centers	Outpatient surgeries that do not require hospitalization
Wellness Centers	Routine physicals; preventive measures such as immunizations; educational programs about nutrition, exercise, and so on

Long-Term Care Facilities

Various forms of long-term care are available for people who do not need to be hospitalized but are unable to live at home. This is one of the fastest growing areas in health care and offers an increasing number of services for patients and employment opportunities for health care professionals. There are many types of long-term care:

- **Nursing homes:** There are two types of facilities commonly referred to as nursing homes:
  - **Skilled nursing facility (SNF):** Provides nursing and rehabilitation services on a 24-hour basis. Includes regular medical care for patients with long-term illnesses and those recovering from illness, injury, or surgery.
  - **Intermediate nursing care facility (INCF):** Provides personal care, social services, and regular nursing care for individuals who do not require 24-hour nursing but are unable to care for themselves.
- **Adult foster home:** Provides 24-hour personal care and supervision for a small number of residents (five is typically allowed by state regulations) in a family-type home or similar setting.
- **Assisted living residence:** Provides housing, meals, and personal care to individuals who need help with daily living activities but do not need daily nursing care. The level of assistance provided depends on individual needs. This type of residence is also known by other names, such as supportive housing, residential long-term care facilities, adult residential care facilities, board-and-care, and rest homes.
- **Continuing care community:** Provides a variety of living arrangements that support lifestyles as they change from independent living to the need for regular medical and nursing care. Additional services, such as meals and daily nurse visits, can be contracted for as required.

Providing quality care for an aging population will be one of society's biggest challenges in the coming decades. The expense of such care is not covered by Medicare, except for short periods of time under certain conditions. The burden on individuals can be heavy, as the average cost of a skilled nursing home ranges from $4000–$9000 per month. Long-term care insurance policies are available, but many people do not purchase these because of their relatively high cost. Other challenges include improving and maintaining the quality of care in long-term care facilities so that older Americans can live out their lives in a supportive, non-warehousing environment.

Home Health Care Providers

The provision of home health services is growing rapidly with various levels of services and care being provided to patients in their homes. Several factors have caused this trend:

- Shorter hospital stays
- Increase in the older population
- Advances in equipment that allow more technical procedures to be carried out in the home
- Desire of individuals to remain in their homes as they age

A wide range of professionals deliver care to patients in their homes:

- Registered and practical/licensed vocational nurses: Educate patients about self-care; administer medications, including intravenous (IV) therapy (administered through the veins); check progress; and change dressings, check the healing of wounds, and remove sutures following surgery.
- Physical therapists and physical therapist assistants: Recommend and teach physical exercises, work to increase physical stamina and movement, monitor progress following injury or surgery.
- Occupational therapists and occupational therapy assistants: Assist patients in attaining maximum function and performing activities of daily living (ADLs) as independently as possible.
- Speech therapists: Help patients recover speech and ability to swallow.
- Medical social workers: Assist with financial planning and arranging for in-home help or placement in the appropriate facility.
- Certified nursing assistants/home health aides: Provide personal care such as bathing and grooming, and follow care plans developed and monitored by a registered nurse or other designated professional.

Medicare pays for home health services only when it is expected that the person who is homebound will improve and recover. Although nonmedical services are also available to help individuals with shopping,

Table 2.3 Health-Related Agencies of the Federal Government

National Institutes of Health (NIH)	Centers for Disease Control and Prevention (CDC)
Twenty-seven institutes and centers that conduct and support all types of medical research.	Research ways to control the spread of diseases that are contagious, caused by environmental conditions, or spread by animals and insects.
U.S. Department of Labor Occupational Safety and Health Administration (OSHA)	**Food and Drug Administration (FDA)**
Develops and enforces minimum health and safety standards (which employers must follow) for all of America's workers.	Ensures that foods are safe, pure, and wholesome; that therapeutic drugs are safe and effective; and that cosmetics are harmless.

cooking, cleaning, and other housekeeping tasks, these are not considered medical in nature and are not usually covered by health insurance plans.

Some of the occupations showing the largest numerical increase in employment involve home health care (Bureau of Labor Statistics, 2010–11). At the same time, quality of care becomes a concern when health care providers work in off-site locations without direct supervision. In response to these concerns, states require the licensing of home health agencies. The types of care that may be performed in the home by various health care personnel are strictly regulated by both state law and insurance reimbursement guidelines. Medicare and most insurance companies will cover only those services provided by specific personnel.

Hospice

The hospice movement began in England and is growing in the United States as more people learn about its benefits. **Hospice** provides **palliative** (relieves but does not cure) care and support given to dying patients and their families. It involves a team of professionals and volunteers who provide medical, emotional, and spiritual assistance. The emphasis of hospice is to make the patient's last days as pain-free and meaningful as possible. Care may be provided in a special facility, known as a hospice, or in the patient's home. After the patient dies, continuing support is available for the family.

Consolidation of Health Care Services

Mainly due to efforts to control costs, many health care facilities are combining under the same ownership. In this way they enjoy a number of advantages:

- Buy supplies in large quantities, thus negotiating for better prices
- Share expensive equipment
- Avoid duplication of laboratory and diagnostic services
- Share knowledge and management expertise
- Consolidate services and prevent duplication

Multiservice systems offer patients more coordinated health care, a sort of "one-stop shopping." For example, following a hospital stay, a patient can be transferred to the system's skilled nursing facility and at the same time be referred to its rehabilitation services. Some systems include a home health division.

An advantage of consolidation for patients is that they may experience more consistent care and better follow-through when dealing with one system. A disadvantage to consolidation is that there are fewer choices for health care consumers. There is the danger, too, that the lack of competition will result in higher prices and lower quality. Government regulation and patient demands help prevent these problems and ensure that large health care systems are accountable and maintain good patient care as their first priority.

Government Health Services

Federal, state, and local governments provide a variety of important services to protect the health of the American public. Supported by taxpayers, agencies have been created that concentrate on conducting research, creating and enforcing regulations, and providing educational materials and activities. Four of the major federal health-related agencies are shown in Table 2.3. Other U.S. Department of Health and Human Services agencies include the

Administration on Aging, the Agency for Toxic Substances and Disease, the Indian Health Service, and the Substance Abuse & Mental Health Services Administration.

State and local health departments receive monetary and administrative support from the federal government. The following lists include examples of typical services offered:

State Health Departments

- License health care personnel, hospitals, and nursing homes
- Monitor chronic and communicable (contagious) diseases
- Provide laboratory services
- Provide emergency medical services
- Establish health data systems
- Conduct public health planning

Local Health Departments

- Collect **vital statistics** (births and deaths)
- Conduct sanitation inspections
- Provide health education
- Screen for diseases such as cancer and diabetes
- Carry out insect control measures
- Supervise water and sewage systems
- Provide immunizations
- Operate venereal disease clinics
- Provide mental health and substance abuse counseling (Adapted from Williams, 2005)

Government services provide a variety of employment opportunities for health care professionals. Everyone who works in health care, whether public or private, must understand the regulations of these agencies and how they affect their occupation. For example, the Centers for Disease Control and Prevention (CDC) has developed standard precautions for the safe handling of body fluids.

NEW APPROACHES TO HEALTH CARE

Many new approaches to health care are being explored today. This is due to several factors:

- Access to information about the health care practices of other cultures

- Search for less invasive and less costly alternatives to surgery and drugs
- Growing interest in the use of natural products
- Belief that the mind and body are more closely connected than previously thought
- Emphasis on preventing rather than simply curing disease
- Increasing number of patients who want to assume more responsibility for their health by participating in preventive and self-care practices
- More patients conducting their own research and taking an active role in making decisions about their treatment and care through access to web sites such as http://medlineplus.gov and www.mayoclinic.com
- Desire for increased humanization of medicine through touch, massage, and other hands-on methods
- Increased direct-to-consumer advertising of drugs and medical supplies and services

Wellness

Wellness is the promotion of health through preventive measures and the practice of good health habits. There are a growing number of people who believe that more emphasis should be placed in health care on the maximization of good health. This goes beyond the traditional view of health as the absence of disease. Wellness centers have been established to offer services such as routine physicals, immunizations, nutrition and exercise classes, and educational programs on disease prevention.

An important part of the wellness concept is the emphasis on the need for patients to take responsibility for their own health. Encouraging patients and teaching them about the basic principles of health promotion and self-care are increasingly important tasks of today's health care professionals. This is especially important today as we find ourselves in a

Fascinating Facts

Public health agencies were established early in our country's history, at the time of the colonies. Plymouth Colony collected vital statistics such as births and deaths. And Paul Revere, famous for his midnight ride at the beginning of the Revolutionary War, was the head of Boston's board of health in the late 1700s (Williams, 2005).

contradictory situation: we understand the importance of personal habits on health, but at the same time, are experiencing increasing rates of health risks such as obesity and lack of physical exercise. Stephen Williams, a professor of public health, states it very well: "We cannot expect to be rescued from every source of morbidity [being diseased] and mortality [death] by the nation's health care system if we do not individually and collectively emphasize prevention of disease and illness in the first place" (Williams, 2005).

Some traditional health care providers are becoming more interested in extending the definition of health to mean more than the absence of disease. Margaret Newman, RN, developed a theory she calls **expanding consciousness.** She realized that many of her patients would never be "well" in the traditional sense. They would be living with a noncurable disease or the results of an injury for the rest of their lives. Newman developed a nursing approach to assist patients in making their lives as meaningful as possible by focusing on their possibilities rather than on their limitations (Newman, 2010).

Complementary and Alternative Medicine

Complementary and alternative medicine (CAM) refers to health care systems, practices, and products that have not traditionally been performed by conventional medical practitioners. They cover a wide range and include practices such as using herbs and plants to treat symptoms, teaching patients meditation as a way to promote healing, and acknowledging the influence of the mind on physical symptoms. Although many health care providers do not accept the claims made for these techniques, a growing number of traditionally trained physicians, nurses, and others are conducting studies and adopting methods that were once considered to be unscientific and ineffective.

Complementary medicine is used together with conventional medicine. One example is using meditation, along with medication, to help patients lower their blood pressure. **Integrative medicine** combines treatments from conventional medicine with CAM for which there is high quality scientific evidence of safety and effectiveness (National Center for Complementary and Alternative Medicine, 2007). **Alternative medicine** refers to practices used instead of conventional medicine. One example is the use of acupuncture rather than surgery to treat back pain.

There is a wide range of complementary and alternative therapies. The National Center for Complementary and Alternative Medicine has divided CAM practices into five categories, which are listed in Table 2.4 along with examples of each.

Complementary and alternative medicine is becoming increasingly popular among patients. In 2007, just over 38 percent of Americans over the age of 18 used some form of complementary medicine (National Center for Complementary and Alternative Medicine, 2008). Health care professionals are likely to come into contact with one or more forms of complementary or alternative medicine. Patients may ask opinions about something they have heard about; a friend or family member may seek these services; or their employer may be exploring the use of integrative medicine. Because the effectiveness and safety of many popular nontraditional therapies have not been proven, it is important for health care professionals to be aware of the various forms of complementary therapies so they can make intelligent decisions and direct patients to reliable sources of information where they can learn more for themselves. It is recommended that they inform themselves through reading, attending workshops and seminars, and asking questions. The National Center for Complementary and Alternative Medicine, part of the National Institutes of Health, is a reliable source of information and can be accessed at http://nccam.nih.gov.

CAM is susceptible to health fraud, the deceptive sale or advertising of services and products that claim to be effective against various health conditions. The U.S. Food and Drug Administration considers the following to be signs a product may be fraudulent:

- Claims product is quick, effective cure for wide variety of health problems
- Suggests that product is based on a "scientific breakthrough," "miraculous cure," or "secret ingredient"
- Uses text with impressive sounding terms that you can't find defined elsewhere
- Provides undocumented case histories of amazing results
- Has limited availability and requires you to pay in advance

Certain diseases and conditions are reportedly often the targets of false remedies. These include cancer, AIDS, arthritis, obesity and overweight, sexual dysfunction, and diabetes. Patients should be warned to

Table 2.4   Complementary and Alternative Medicine

Category	Examples
Whole Medical Systems *Complete systems of theory and practice*	■ Homeopathic medicine: assists body to heal itself of symptoms by giving very small quantities of a substance that produces the symptoms ("like cures like"). ■ Naturopathic medicine: assists the body to use its own healing power with methods such as exercise and medicinal plants. ■ Traditional Chinese medicine: ancient system based on balancing and maintaining the body's vital energy flow ("qi," pronounced "chee"); treatments include acupuncture and herbs. ■ Ayurveda: 5000-year-old system practiced in India; treatments include herbs, massage, and yoga.
Mind-Body Medicine *Enhance the mind's influence on the body*	■ Patient support groups ■ Meditation ■ Prayer ■ Creative outlets, such as art and music
Biologically-Based Practices *Use substances found in nature*	■ Aromatherapy: scent of essential oils from plants is inhaled ■ Herbs ■ Dietary supplements ■ Use of natural products, such as shark cartilage
Manipulative and Body-Based Practices *Move parts of the body to regain health and function* *(Manipulation: controlled force to a joint beyond its normal range of motion)*	■ Chiropractic manipulation ■ Osteopathic manipulation ■ Massage ■ Reflexology: application of pressure to parts of the feet believed to be connected to specific parts of the body

Energy Therapies
Involve the use of energy fields and pathways
	■ Biofield therapies: manipulate the fields of energy believed to surround and penetrate the body; practitioners use their hands to channel and balance this energy. Therapies include:
	  ■ qi gong: combines movement, meditation, and controlled breathing
	  ■ Reiki: practitioners attempt to transmit universal energy to a person to heal the spirit and thus the body
	  ■ therapeutic touch: patient's energy field is altered when energy is passed from the practitioner's hands to the patient
	■ Bioelectromagnetic-based therapies: unconventional use of electromagnetic fields such as using magnets to relieve arthritis pain

Source: "What Is CAM?" National Center for Complementary and Alternative Medicine, 2007. Available at http://nccam.nih.gov/health/whatiscam/overview.htm

check with their health care provider and to research the advice of government agencies, such as the Food and Drug Administration, before purchasing remedies online.

Holistic Medicine

Holistic medicine is a general term to designate the belief that the traditional view of medicine must be expanded. All aspects of the individual—physical, mental, emotional, and spiritual—contribute to states of health and disease. The entire person must be considered when making therapeutic decisions.

Also, the causes and prevention of disease, rather than simply the relief of symptoms, are emphasized. There is a growing interest in holistic medicine today as evidence mounts that the mind has a powerful effect on physical health. Disorders caused by mental or emotional factors are known as **psychosomatic.** Researchers now know that these illnesses are not "all in one's head" but that physical symptoms can be the result of what is happening in the mind. It is believed that as many as 85 percent of visits to doctors' offices are due to psychosomatic disorders. This is explained by the fact that the emotions influence the functioning of the internal organs (Milliken & Honeycutt, 2004).

Holistic medicine providers tend to combine traditional and nontraditional treatments and emphasize that:

- Patients must accept responsibility for their own health.
- Stress is an important factor in health and should be reduced.
- Proper nutrition and exercise are essential.
- Attitude has a powerful effect, both positive and negative, on the body and its functioning.

Osteopathy and Chiropractic

Osteopathy and chiropractic health care practices have become so widely accepted that they are no longer generally considered to be alternative. **Osteopathy** is based on the belief that the body can protect itself against disease if the musculoskeletal system, especially the spine, is in good order. The importance of good nutrition and favorable environmental conditions is also emphasized. Osteopathic physicians receive training that is similar to that of traditional doctors of medicine (MDs). They can prescribe drugs, perform surgeries, and have staff privileges at most hospitals. Osteopaths take the same state licensing examinations as MDs.

Chiropractic is based on the belief that pressure on the nerves leaving the spinal column causes pain or dysfunction of the body part served by that nerve. Treatment involves manipulation of the spine to correct misalignments. Chiropractors are not allowed to prescribe drugs but may recommend nutritional and herbal remedies. Every state has licensure requirements for chiropractors.

Massage Therapy

Massage therapy is widely recognized, when administered by a trained practitioner, as a beneficial health practice. It involves using pressure or friction on the body. By enabling the muscles to relax, massage therapy promotes better blood circulation, faster healing of injuries, and pain relief. It is often recommended to supplement other forms of therapy and to provide an effective method of stress relief. Many types of formal training programs are available for people who wish to practice massage therapy. Most states and localities require therapists to be licensed.

Naturopathy

Naturopathic medicine is based on the belief that the human body has its own natural healing ability. Naturopathic doctors (NDs) teach their patients to use diet, exercise, lifestyle changes and cutting-edge natural therapies to enhance their bodies' ability to ward off and combat disease. They combine traditional medicine and natural remedies when developing treatment plans for their patients (American Association of Naturopathic Physicians, 2010). Naturopathic physicians seek the causes of symptoms and believe the whole person, not just the symptoms, must be treated. As of the end of 2009, 15 states, the District of Columbia, and the United States territories of Puerto Rico and the United States Virgin Islands have licensing laws for naturopathic doctors.

Homeopathy

Homeopathy is a method of treatment developed by a German physician in the early 1800s based on the idea of stimulating the body's own healing responses. Disorders are treated with very small amounts of the natural substances that cause the symptoms of the disorder in healthy people. For example, exposure to onions causes the same runny nose and eyes as are experienced with a head cold. Therefore, very diluted amounts of plants in the onion family are administered to treat cold symptoms (Milliken & Honeycutt, 2004). Belladonna, secured from a poisonous European plant, is widely used in homeopathy to treat a variety of symptoms, including pain. It has been used in traditional medicine to dilate the pupils to facilitate examination of the eyes. Homeopathy has been practiced in Europe and India for more than 200 years. It is gaining popularity in the United States among people who believe that these remedies are safer than prescription drugs. It is important to understand that any substance, including those that are "natural," can be harmful if taken improperly. Only three states, Arizona, Connecticut, and Nevada, license homeopathic physicians.

Energy Theories

Theories about the existence and importance of body energy developed in Asia thousands of years ago. There is growing interest today in therapies that claim to encourage the free flow of energy throughout the body. This flow, it is believed, is necessary to promote and maintain good health. **Acupuncture** may be the oldest application of this theory. Developed by the Chinese more than 5000 years ago, it involves the insertion of tiny needles into specific points in the body to relieve energy blocks. This treatment is becoming accepted in the United States as people who receive it find relief from various health problems.

CHALLENGES IN HEALTH CARE TODAY

The tremendous medical progress made during the last century continues into the new millennium. At the same time, our country faces many challenges in effectively delivering the results of this progress to all who need it. These challenges represent complex problems that affect millions of people. Problems of this size are not easy to solve. Finding solutions that satisfy the needs of everyone is very difficult.

It is important for the health care professional to be aware of major health care issues. They will affect where and how you perform your job, as well as influence your relationships with patients and other members of the health care team.

Access to Health Care

Millions of Americans do not have health insurance, cannot afford needed medical care, or have inadequate insurance coverage. These people belong to three major groups:

- The unemployed: Group insurance plans provided by employers are the most common source of insurance coverage. Many unemployed persons cannot afford to buy private medical insurance or do not qualify for **Medicaid,** a program funded by federal and state governments for individuals below certain income levels.
- The "working poor": These are people who are employed but do not have the opportunity to participate in group coverage. The employer may not offer health insurance, or the employee may work on a part-time or temporary basis and does not qualify. These workers usually do not earn enough to purchase medical insurance on their own.
- People with preexisting conditions: Many insurance companies will not accept applicants who already have health problems.

It is often the case that individuals who most need health care services are the ones least likely to have access to it. As this book is being written, the U.S. Congress has passed sweeping health care reform legislation that will enable most Americans to access health care. At the same time, opponents of the legislation are concerned about possible overregulation of the health care industry, the inability of the government to efficiently oversee health care, a shortage of trained health care providers to handle increased numbers of patients, and the need to ration (limit) services because of cost or lack of personnel. Another problem with government programs is that when not enough taxes can be collected to support the costs, services must be cut. This is an especially serious concern when the economy is poor and unemployment is high, which results in decreased tax revenues. It is hoped that cutting fraudulent claims for Medicare reimbursement, raising taxes, and promoting efficiencies in the delivery of health care will support the costs of the new legislation.

Many economists have warned that Medicare, a government-run insurance program for persons age 65 and older and the disabled, is in danger of running out of funding within the next 20 years. The problem is worsened by fraudulent claims paid out by Medicare. During the 2008–2009 budget year, fraud cost the government an estimated $47 million. Some sources report the figure to be $60 million. The system is so large—4.4 million claims are

---

Thinking It Through

Craig Oakley is a physical therapy assistant who does home visits for a rehabilitation service. One of his patients, Mr. Singh, suffers from rheumatoid arthritis and has asked Craig's opinion about taking Chinese herbal remedies that he has read help restore joint health.
1. How should Craig respond?
2. What are resources he can consult in order to find out more about the treatment?
3. What precautions should Craig follow when speaking with Mr. Singh about complementary and alternative therapies?

processed daily—that only about 3 percent of claims are reviewed before they are paid (Terhune, 2009).

Social Conditions

Many social problems affect the country's health care delivery systems, as well as the health of the nation as a whole. An example is the return of tuberculosis as a public health concern. This contagious disease was nearly eliminated by the mid-1900s. The people who are most susceptible to tuberculosis live in crowded, unsanitary conditions and suffer from malnutrition, drug abuse, alcoholism, and general poor health. Unfortunately, these are the conditions in which many Americans live today. The standard treatment for tuberculosis is medication taken over an extended period, sometimes up to 1 year. Most patients remain at home during treatment. A problem that has developed is the number of patients who require continual monitoring by social workers or nurses to ensure that they take their medicine as prescribed. This care is provided at public expense, if necessary, because of the highly contagious nature of the disease. Table 2.5 lists a number of social conditions that can produce negative consequences for individual health, as well as for health care delivery systems.

The sad result of poverty and other social problems is that those who most need health care services are the least able to pay for them. People who cannot afford preventive care are more likely to develop serious conditions. They eventually seek care in emergency rooms, one of the most expensive providers of health care. Preventive care, had it been available, would have spared both patient suffering and the need for expensive emergency care.

Maintaining the Quality of Care

The skyrocketing costs of health care have prompted all levels of government, as well as providers of health care, to initiate cost controls. This has caused widespread concern that quality of care is being sacrificed to cut expenses. For example, patients are given drugs following certain types of surgery to prevent blood clots from forming and moving into vital organs, such as the lungs or brain. A provider may choose to give a drug that has proven to be less effective than another because it costs much less. A related area of concern is that for-profit insurance and health care organizations may emphasize profits more than providing high-quality patient care. Complaints reported by residents in nursing homes may be related to the growth of for-profit facilities.

Some current methods of paying physicians and other providers for their services encourage them to provide less rather than more care. Reviewers who work on behalf of insurance companies make many decisions about patient care. The purpose is to determine whether the proposed procedures are medically necessary and whether lower cost alternatives are available. Permission is required in advance for

Table 2.5 Social Conditions That Affect Health and Health Care Systems

Condition	Impact on Health and Health Care System
Breakdown of Family Unit and Children Born to Single Women	Poverty among women and children. Lack of access to prenatal care, immunizations for children, and other preventive measures.
Homelessness	Lack of access to medical care. Malnutrition and poor hygiene. Difficult to contact patient for follow-up care. An increasing number of families and children now number among the homeless.
Violence	Use of emergency and other health care services. Inability of many victims to pay.
Substance Abuse	Increased violence and susceptibility to disease. Inability to care for self and family.
Spousal and Child Abuse	Need for health and protective services. Use of emergency room services for injuries.
Poverty and Malnutrition	Poor health and inability to access health care. Lack of prenatal care.
26% of Americans Live Alone	Need outside assistance when ill or injured. Lack of emotional support.

Sources: Adapted from *Essentials of Health Services*, by S. J. Williams, 2005, Clifton Park, NY: Delmar Cengage Learning. U.S. Census Bureau, www.census.gov/Press-Release/www/releases/archives/families_households/006840.html

certain procedures, a process called "preauthorization." For example, nonemergency hospital admissions and surgeries commonly require approval.

Reviewers may or may not have extensive medical training. Their decisions are based on what is known about the "average patient" under the same or similar circumstances. Reviewers can make a variety of decisions. For example, they can:

- Approve the procedure as recommended by the physician
- Deny the procedure
- Require surgery to be performed as an outpatient service (patient does not occupy a bed in the facility, such as a hospital)
- Approve a different, usually less-costly method
- Approve a limited number of treatments

Many physicians feel they have lost control of the practice of medicine to business interests. Accustomed to having the authority to make decisions about the best care for their patients, they are frustrated by what they see as interference from nonmedical personnel.

Patients, in turn, believe the decisions of their physicians are being questioned and have concerns about the resulting quality of care. They worry that they are being denied needed procedures and treatments and that their health is being sacrificed for the sake of increasing profits.

At the same time, other health care experts point out that the number of unnecessary surgeries and other procedures, especially those used for diagnosis, have decreased. They believe that patient care has not suffered but has actually been improved by efforts to prevent the overuse of available techniques.

Restoring confidence in the system while at the same time controlling costs is a major challenge to ensuring continued quality of care. As a health care professional, you can help restore this confidence by providing the best care possible and supporting the decisions of the professional for whom you work.

Public Health Concerns

The United States faces challenges in its efforts to safeguard the health of the public. Monitoring and researching health issues must be ongoing. For example, although most infectious diseases are under control in this country, there are increasing concerns about a **pandemic** occurring in the near future. The global out-break in 2009 of influenza caused by the H1N1 virus demonstrated how difficult it can be to respond quickly as the United States encountered slow-downs in its efforts to develop an effective vaccine. Research must also continue to find effective immunizations and treatments for diseases such as cancer, which ranks as one of the three top causes of death in the United States.

An important indicator of the effectiveness of a nation's health care system is its infant mortality rate. This is the number of infants who die in the first year of life per 1000 live births. In 2009, estimated infant mortality statistics had the United States ranked 44th in a list of 224 countries. The United States rate of 6.26 deaths per thousand was almost triple Singapore's rate of 2.31 per thousand (Central Intelligence Agency, 2009). The U.S. statistic is due to many factors, including poverty, unhealthy behaviors such as drug abuse, and lack of access to prenatal care. These factors not only affect infant mortality rates but also contribute to physical and mental development problems in many children who do survive.

Antibiotic Resistance

Antibiotics are drugs that fight infections caused by bacterial infections. They are not effective against viruses, the microorganisms that cause colds and flu as well as other illnesses. Antibiotic resistance occurs when the bacteria the drugs target change in ways that reduce the effectiveness of antibiotics in destroying them. According to the Centers for Disease Control and Prevention, antibiotic resistance "has been called one the world's most pressing public health problems" (Centers for Disease Control and Prevention, June 30, 2009). This is because as bacteria become resistant, they become increasingly difficult or even impossible to treat.

Personal Responsibility for Health

The three leading causes of death in the United States—heart disease, cancer, and stroke—are often influenced by lifestyle choices. Individuals have control over the habits that contribute to the state of their health. The following behaviors have been identified as contributing to healthier and longer lives:

- Not smoking
- Getting enough sleep
- Eating moderately and maintaining a balanced diet and normal weight
- Exercising regularly
- Avoiding alcohol or drinking in moderation
- Practicing preventive measures such as getting immunizations and wearing seat belts
- Using stress reduction techniques
  (*Source:* Adapted from *Understanding Human Behavior* [7th ed.], by M. E. Milliken & A. Honeycutt, 2004, Clifton Park, NY: Delmar Cengage Learning.)

Individuals must also realize that modern medicine has limitations and that new technological advances do not guarantee that every disease can be cured and every injury repaired. On the other hand, nearly everyone can improve his or her own health and quality of life by making positive lifestyle choices.

IMPLICATIONS FOR HEALTH CARE PROFESSIONALS

Meeting the challenges that face our health care system is everyone's responsibility. Health care professionals are in the fortunate position of being able to positively influence this important area of life. Some steps they can take to help meet these challenges are to:

- Keep informed of important issues by reviewing appropriate websites, attending workshops, and participating in professional organizations.
- Contribute to the delivery of high-quality service by pledging to perform duties to the best of their ability.
- Model good health habits and learn to provide effective patient education.

CHAPTER 3

Professions and Professionalism

Professionalism and Ethics in the Workplace

Learning Objectives

- Identify appropriate professional behaviors and attitudes.
- Describe professional attire.
- Identify attributes that are used to measure a professional.
- Discuss the use of cell phones and technology in the workplace.

Key Terms

Customers	Ethics	Professionalism
Decorum	Professional behavior	Timeliness

INTRODUCTION

Although Chapter 3 is written for students going into pharmacy technician, please realize that almost everything discussed as professionalism for a pharmacy technician is applicable to all allied health professionals. As you are reading through this chapter evaluate the information for how it applies to your chosen profession.

Being professional and being ethical are important to maintaining the confidence that the public has in pharmacists and people who work in pharmacies. Public relations is often thought of as the key to business success. Every employee working in a pharmacy is perceived by the public as an ambassador of that business. A good impression is equivalent to a single advertisement, but a poor image is almost impossible to shed. Therefore, all employees, no matter what their positions in the company's hierarchy, must understand that if any of the positions were not important, they would have been eliminated. In addition, all actions that employees take while at work create the overall perception the public has of the business.

Professionalism is determined by how we look and how we act. Like it or not, we make decisions about whether we want to associate with someone by how they appear. After the first impression and once people get to know one another, "company dress" is less important. Although friends and family may know you and appreciate your distinctive personality and many virtues, in the business world some level of conformity is expected. Clients and patients choose services from businesses that they perceive as maintaining certain standards. The first way to convey business competence is through your image, and image is determined by your appearance and your actions.

Put a different way, how appetizing would a restaurant be if the hostess had dirty fingernails, the waitress constantly scratched her arm, and the busboy looked like he had just finished changing the oil in his car? How much confidence would you have in a banker who wore a torn T-shirt and cutoffs and had a stale half-eaten bagel on his desk? Would you hire an attorney who had a small basketball hoop in his office and "shot a few" while he listened to your case?

The answer is obvious. Now think about the fact that you are working in an environment where people trust you with one of their most valuable assets—their health. They want to know that they can trust what you say, what you do, and what you prepare for them. Developing this confidence in an impersonal world is done by living up to or exceeding the image patients have for the person doing the job. In pharmacy, confidence is built by looking like a professional and acting like one.

The first rule of professionalism is fundamental cleanliness and presentation. It is important to be well groomed and relatively conservative in dress. Coming to work looking disheveled sends a message to your boss that you don't value your position. It also sends a message to patients and other customers that you don't care and, by association, neither does the business.

Cleanliness and modest makeup are preferred business grooming. Makeup should be worn to enhance features, not to make a statement. Remember, you are working close to people, so heavy makeup will appear overdone. Conservative tones are more businesslike than bright colors. The same is true of hair tones. Hair should be styled in a manner that allows your eyes to be seen and that gives you freedom of movement without it becoming untidy or "coming down" if you bend down. If you tend to fidget with your hair, find a way to keep it back so you are not tempted to play with it while talking with a patient or pharmacist.

A daily shower or bath, as well as deodorant, is standard. Being malodorous disturbs your fellow technicians and pharmacists, offends patients, and makes for an uncomfortable conversation with your supervisor. In most cases, light or no perfume should be used, since many people are allergic to scents. Moreover, strong scents are not perceived the same way by all noses. What appeals to one person may smell like a moldy attic to another. In a small area, a strong, sweet scent can become unpleasant over time. A rule of thumb regarding perfume is that if you can smell your own, it's too much.

Standard pharmacy dress for men is slacks—not jeans—and a shirt. Many businesses prefer button shirts, but in some places, golf shirts are allowed. Some venues require ties as well. These may be colorful and creative, but they should not serve as billboards for political agendas of any sort. T-shirts of any kind should not be worn in a pharmacy unless it is a nonpublic compounding type of pharmacy. Unless issued by the organization in which you are working, logo wear is inappropriate. Even when you work in a compounding or sterile-product area where you change into scrubs, if you need to walk through public areas of the building or hospital before and after work, it is preferable that you blend in with the clientele or the business image.

Similarly, women should be presentable when walking in public places whether or not a uniform is required at work. For nonuniform positions, slacks or skirts and business tops are appropriate. Dresses may also be worn, keeping in mind that you will frequently be bending and moving about. Therefore, a skirt of modest length that affords flexibility without being revealing is preferred. Shirts or blouses that show the midriff are not acceptable in a business environment. Neither are low-cut, sheer, or otherwise provocative tops. Again, like men, you are not a human billboard, so logo wear of any business other than the one you work in is inappropriate. Suits may be worn by either sex, although in most patient-care pharmacy areas, suits are considered a little too formal.

Hose or socks should be worn with closed-toe and closed-back shoes. A heel height that allows you to stand comfortably for long periods is also helpful. Jewelry should be tasteful and not get in the way of job function. Shoes for either male or female employees should be clean, polished, and in good repair.

Hands and nails are an important part of grooming too. Because a handshake is still the conventional business greeting, hands are often on display. They should be smooth and clean. Nails should be relatively short, since long nails can harbor germs. Although you will wear gloves in most sterile manufacturing and compounding areas, jobs involving a lot of sterile compounding may require that you not have any type of artificial nails. This is a direct outcome from the Centers for Disease Control and Prevention's recommendations published in 2002.[1] No subsequent guidelines have been published. In addition, there are no data to refute or support the necessity of not having artificial nails in light of the use of gloves for patient care and for sterile manufacturing. Washing your hands between patients and before regloving is a good hygiene and safety practice. Such a great amount of hand washing can leave hands rough, so applying a good lotion is often essential.

Like the overall first impression, a handshake is often a bond builder or deal breaker. If you wear polish, it should not be chipped. A handshake should be

Table 3.1 Do's and Don'ts of Professional Attire

- Do wear wrinkle-free or neatly pressed slacks, skirts, and blouse or shirts.
- Do wear closed-toe shoes.
- Do wear hose without holes and in a color that complements the outfit.
- Do have a neatly styled haircut that is easy to maintain during the workday.
- Do shower or bathe before the start of each workday.
- Do wear a conservative amount of makeup in relatively natural-looking colors.
- Don't wear clothing that allows undergarments to show.
- Don't assume that a lab coat will cover a wrinkled or unclean, casual appearance.
- Don't wear dramatic makeup.
- Do wear clothing that allows you to bend, stand on your toes, and move comfortably.
- Don't wear flip-flops.
- Don't wear fabrics that are too clingy or too sheer.
- Don't wear logo attire unless it is issued by the operation where you work.

Table 3.2 Who Are Pharmacy Customers?

- Patients
- Nurses
- Doctors
- Patients' families and friends
- Insurance company personnel
- Hospital administrators
- Pharmacy CEOs
- Businesses

firm, not too long, and not too tight. Offering your hand first is a gesture of friendliness and should be accompanied by making eye contact.

You may also use your hand to reassure a patient or family member. You can offer your hands to support a patient or to steady someone getting up. Your hands also are on display when you give someone a medication, take in a prescription, lend a pen, or direct someone to another area.

Whether you wear a smock or lab coat depends on the supervisor of your pharmacy. In some practice sites, a lab coat signifies a professional, such as a pharmacist or doctor. In some institutions, short coats signify interns or trainees, and fingertip-length coats are reserved for degreed and licensed personnel. If your place of practice puts ranks on the coats, then it is inappropriate for you to wear one. But if technicians wear short coats and pharmacists wear long ones, then the norm would be appropriate.

Table 3.1 summarizes the do's and don'ts of attire in the workplace.

WHO ARE YOUR CUSTOMERS?

When we talk about professionalism, does that mean being professional only with other professionals? Whose respect are we trying to cultivate anyway?

Let's consider who the customers are in any line of pharmacy work. **Customers** are people interacting with you and the pharmacists during the course of the business day. In general, a business considers those who are in a position to form an opinion that can affect the business to be customers.

Obviously, patients and their families are customers. Whoever comes to pick up a prescription, inquire about over-the-counter medications, accompany a patient, or shop in the store where the pharmacy is located is a customer. Everybody who makes contact is a potential pharmacy patron even if the immediate visit has nothing to do with a personal need for pharmacy services. Who knows who may be sick or need preventative medications in the future? In addition, doctors, nurses, and other health care providers are customers in the sense that the pharmacy provides a service to them. The service could be answering a question, sharing a patient, providing a medication, or giving advice.

Depending on who your employer is, pharmacists may be your customers. If you are working in a warehouse of some sort or in an outsourced pharmacy that provides services such as sterile-product admixtures or nuclear pharmaceuticals to pharmacies, pharmacists are certainly your customers. Technicians working in a pharmacy benefit management business also have pharmacists as customers. Technicians working in the business aspect of any pharmacy may have business executives, managers, accountants, clerks, insurance adjusters, and pharmacy benefit managers as customers. People working in a hospital setting or for a chain drugstore may have corporate office employees as customers. Table 3.2 lists some of the many categories of people who are pharmacy customers.

Whether someone is a patient or not, your interaction should always be at a professional level. At work, **decorum** is important, and how you handle yourself with everyone—patient, client, customer, or anyone else—is likely to be witnessed and to make an impression on others. For this reason, it is essential that you handle yourself with each patient or customer as though you were interacting with the most important person you can imagine.

In addition to dress, demeanor is another measure of your professionalism. Have you ever entered a business only to be ignored by someone catching up on last night's gossip via the company phone? Do you remember feeling invisible to a service provider who seemed more interested in stocking shelves than in giving assistance? Have you ever overheard two employees complaining about a customer or describing someone in negative terms? These are all examples of unprofessional behavior.

Professional conduct shows observers that you respect your surroundings and you respect your patients and customers. You can easily reinforce your professional image in a couple of ways.

Posture is important. If possible, stand and sit straight. Your mother was right when she suggested that sitting slumped in a chair makes you look like a tired piece of cloth, not an energetic, helpful person. Good posture conveys a sense of self-respect. It also conveys a sense of openness and a willingness to assist people.

Making yourself aware of your surroundings and particularly the people in it is another way to support a professional image. Scanning your pharmacy environment at frequent intervals provides you with the opportunity to greet newcomers soon after their arrival with at least a friendly, "Hello, I'll be right with you." Everyone is busy in today's understaffed, overworked world. (It's not entirely true, but we've all had "those days" often enough.) Even so, unless you just engaged in activity with another patient, excuse yourself from the first conversation to acknowledge a newcomer. If you can predict about how long the wait might be, it is appropriate to mention that as well.

Managing your interaction with customers is also important. When a long-winded and frequent patient or customer comes to your pharmacy on a busy day, place a limit on your conversation ahead of time. You can do this through a comment such as, "Hi, Mrs. Bloom. It's good to see you. It's awfully busy today. What can I do for you?" This communicates in advance that you won't have a lot of time for conversation. If others start to line up or you simply must get back to the work at hand, ask permission to move on after you've finished the business part of the visit. You might say, "I'd love to hear more about

Table 3.3 How to Measure a Professional

- Dress
- Cleanliness
- Attitude
- Voice tone
- Work ethic
- Attention to detail
- Persistence to the task at hand

that, but right now, I should help the gentleman behind you," or, "It's good to see you. You won't mind if I get back to filling these orders [or finishing this report] before I fall further behind, will you?"

Table 3.3 summarizes some key elements for evaluating professionalism.

GREETING PATIENTS

The welcome is an important step in engaging a patient or pharmacy customer. People should be acknowledged as soon as they enter the space in which you can reasonably interact with them. Even if you are on the phone with a patient or customer, nodding your head to newcomers goes a long way toward calming them and assuring them that you will get to them as soon as possible.

You can also convey a welcome with a smile, the words *welcome* or *hello*, or a question such as, "How may I assist you?" The question "Whaddaya want?" is not a professional greeting. Neither is a grunt disguised as a greeting. Continuing to bow your head and work on a task convinces no one that you did not see the newest customer, doctor, nurse, or other co-worker.

Once you greet people, it is important to address their concerns as soon as possible. If you see a newcomer to the operation near the area where you are, you might volunteer to help out if possible. This can easily be done in a small satellite pharmacy, since nurses and doctors come sporadically. In a larger retail pharmacy, patients arrive in a more constant flow, so allowing a small line to develop is not unreasonable. Even in such a setting, however, if one patient or client is taking up an inordinate amount of time, it would not be unreasonable for another staff member to take care of the waiters and then resume normal chores. If a second staff member is not available to help, it is also not unreasonable to ask the patient if you could be excused to help the "quickies"— but only if the transaction is exceptionally lengthy.

What is most important to remember as a professional is that the customers, patients, and clients *are* the reason you are there. They are *not* the interruptions that interfere with getting your work done. Were it not for the human beings in need of every order you fill or every prescription you take in, you would have no work to get done. As an employee, you must develop the skill to work efficiently and in such a way as to finish routine tasks in between taking care of "live" or "walk-up" customers. It is up to the manager to employ enough staff to take care of routine business efficiently and maintain and service the customers and patients. It is also up to the manager to work out a schedule that puts enough people in the pharmacy at times when it is busiest.

EMPATHY, SYMPATHY, AND OTHER EXPRESSIONS

Professionalism is also how you say things and your non-verbal communication. Conducting yourself as a professional means being empathetic and sympathetic, as well as being a coach who may deliver information that the patient does not want to hear. Sympathy and empathy entail listening attentively to stories that may not interest you. It also means recognizing when a person may need extra reassurance. Sometimes it means giving someone space. In the pharmacy world, people often share things that are personal. It is important to listen when appropriate and to learn how to graciously end a conversation that is either inappropriate or that is taking up too much of your time.

PROFESSIONALISM AND PATIENT CONFIDENTIALITY

People tell health care providers all kinds of stories. Sometimes they share something because they are lonely. Other times, they have no one else to turn to. Sometimes they are scared or confused. It's your job to help reassure, educate, and console. Some of these emotions can be eased by an understanding technician, but other times the patient needs to be referred to a pharmacist because the pharmacist is best able to handle the patient's concern or because the patient is requesting advice. Regardless of how entertaining the story might be, tales from the trenches should not be shared at parties, with close friends, or at dinner. The adage "You never know who knows who" particularly applies in these situations.

ANSWERING DIFFICULT QUESTIONS

One of the signs of being a professional is recognizing that you do not know everything. It is perfectly acceptable to say that you need to consult someone else or check the facts. Make sure, however, that you get back to the person even if it is to say you need more time. You can also refer someone to a better resource, such as a pharmacist.

It is unprofessional to lie or make up an answer to appear knowledgeable. It is also unacceptable to tell patients or customers that you don't know and not follow up with a resource to find out. Besides referring patients to a pharmacist, you can direct them to employees in other departments. For instance, if a person asks about visiting hours and you don't know, you might send or take the person to the information desk. If someone is having an issue with a third-party payer, you might offer to dial the insurance claims department. If a person is looking for a location in the building that is unfamiliar to you, you might provide a map or offer to make a phone call.

Professional conduct involves problem solving. Although technicians perform tasks that do not involve professional judgment, acting like a professional is an asset to the organization and to yourself. When you deal with patients, ask yourself, "How would I like to be treated if I were in their workplace and needed assistance with a problem?" or, "If I needed this answer myself, how would I go about getting it?" This type of problem solving may sound a bit creative. The more information you accumulate as a result of experience, however, the better able you are to help people directly, and even if you can't, you are still better equipped to use your knowledge and skills to direct people to the correct source of the information.

PROFESSIONAL IMAGE AND THE OFFICE PARTY

Everyone wants to have fun. Many organizations have holiday parties or seasonal get-togethers that allow people to mingle and get to know one another outside the formality of the work environment. Nothing ruins more careers than poor behavior at an office get-together.

Remember that although it is a party, it is a work party. If the event takes place at your place of business and includes patients or customers, it is especially important that you maintain a work image, albeit a relaxed one. Even if the owner is telling off-color jokes or a key customer is drinking too much, the wise employee exercises restraint.

The saying "Loose lips sink ships" is particularly true in the work environment. Nothing loosens lips faster than alcohol. In social situations involving work, limit alcohol consumption to one less drink an hour than you know you can easily tolerate. If drinking excessively is a problem you have encountered before, then it is prudent to avoid alcohol altogether.

Like drinking excessively, telling crude and off-color stories is unacceptable. And gossip is not party conversation. Develop some topics you can offer as conversation starters. These might include vacations you have enjoyed or those someone else is going on, movies or other entertainment events, accomplishments of your colleagues you'd like to know more about, or current events. Avoid topics that can become emotional, and change subjects if someone is getting upset. While discussion of an issue is healthy, a fight is not what a party is all about.

PROFESSIONALISM AND MANNERS FOR THE WORKPLACE

Today, the term *rude* often refers to an attitude, not to an action. Traditional manners are often thought of as stuffy, and yet most of them have been developed to provide comfort to all individuals involved. Manners dictate expectations and allow people interacting with one another to anticipate what comes next. Despite the evolution of manners, there are some rules that need to be followed in the business setting.

CELL PHONES AND PAGERS

Today, most people have cell phones, and inconsiderate behavior is often an unfortunate consequence. At work, a personal cell phone should be turned off or in the silent position. In most cases, keeping it in your locker or car is best. Unless you have some pressing need, calls should be received and returned after work. After all, you have been hired because the organization needs you to devote your attention and skills to it.

A pressing need is something that immediately affects health or quality of life—for example, a call about the outcome of a relative's surgery or a call from a physician about your health. In rare cases, it may involve a household emergency. Pressing issues do not include notification from your best friend about a sale at a favorite store or an announcement that concert tickets are available. It is most inappropriate to shout during a call taken at a business, whether it is a happy scream or one directed at misbehaving children.

For calls that you expect, it is best to let your supervisor know ahead of time. When a call comes, excuse yourself from the work area for a short period of time to answer it. If you are attending a meeting during which you expect a call, it is appropriate to let the other attendees know that you may be called away during the meeting.

For business-issued pagers, the protocol is different. Pagers are used by those in fields such as medicine who need to be contacted immediately about critical issues. Pages should be returned as soon as possible. Alpha pagers make returning calls easier because they can give you preliminary information about the matter and allow you to retrieve necessary files or other materials before returning the call. When you page others, using the alpha page option also allows them to be prepared. With alpha pagers, you can communicate whether or not immediate attention is necessary. For instance, you could page a doctor with a request such as, "Please confirm dose of propranolol on patient Morgan."

TAKING RESPONSIBILITY IS PART OF PROFESSIONALISM

Everyone makes mistakes. Professionals take responsibility for their actions. It is also a professional responsibility to try to make things work better and to work things out when they don't go as planned.

Mistakes occur for many reasons, but primarily they are "accidental"—that is, the people making them did so unintentionally. Although they are accidents, some errors are preventable. Sometimes an error is made because there is a flaw in the system. Errors of this nature can be prevented by adjusting the system in some way. For example, a double-check system might be put in place, adding another person or another step to a process. Sometimes errors occur because of insufficient training. For example, a lack of knowledge might lead a technician to mistake a new drug for a familiar one that looks and sounds similar. Some errors result from poor management. They are committed by staff but are really caused by understaffing or unreal expectations by management in terms of what can be done in a specified time frame. Finally, though, some mistakes occur no matter what anyone does.

When an error occurs, it is everyone's responsibility to learn from the mistake so that it does not get repeated. In some operations, near misses are reported so that teams can figure out ways to prevent even these from occurring. In the pharmacy world, a near miss is an error that is caught before it gets to the patient.

Besides figuring out how to prevent an error from recurring, errors that get to patients need to be reported to them. This allows patients to stop taking a medication that could cause damage. It can also inform them about what effects to watch for from an incorrect drug.

In the outpatient setting, patients may call to ask about the physical appearance of a medication. Nowadays, a description of the medication is required on the container in many states, although the print is small and difficult for some to read. When brands of generic drugs are switched, the computer is updated so that the description printed on the container is accurate. Nonetheless, when a patient calls about the accuracy of a prescription, it is always prudent to double-check in case an error has occurred. Even if the description on the container matches what is in it, an error may have been made in what was ordered or what was used to fill the prescription. It is better to be interrupted a hundred times and be right than it is to assume you are right and be wrong, especially if there are major ramifications. Always thank a person who calls to confirm a product, even when you are correct.

In the inpatient setting, patients are less likely to question medications. Still, patients are entitled to the five rights of medication: the right drug to the right patient at the right time in the right dosage form and dose.

If you make an error, apologize for it. Don't make excuses, and don't blame someone else for an error you made. Try to fix it as soon as possible. If you can think of ways to prevent the error in the future, share them with your boss. Finding better ways

to do things is not the same as making excuses for an error because the fixes were not in place.

Some mistakes in the pharmacy setting do not involve medications. Sometimes errors in judgment or errors of omission occur. An error in judgment, for example, is holding rigorously to a policy where there is room for flexibility. Or a staff member might oversleep or get confused about a shift, inadvertently causing staffing problems. If the problem is an error in judgment or a recurring issue, the supervisor should discuss it with the staff member. Errors of omission include forgetting to schedule someone, not placing an order when asked to, or forgetting to reconcile something. Correct the situation as soon as you are notified. If this means going in to work as soon as you are called, give a realistic time for when you can be there and make it happen.

TIMELINESS

Like taking responsibility for fixing errors, maintaining a commitment to **timeliness** reflects positively on your professionalism. Being at work on time is one aspect of this. If you get caught in traffic, admit it and try to determine alternate routes to work. If you are regularly late, promise to leave earlier in the future and do it. Empty promises and repeated excuses cause others to lose respect for you.

Similarly, timeliness is an issue with work assignments. Often when assigning reports or project work, a supervisor asks for a time frame in which to expect the finished product. In other cases, a deadline is given. When asked to estimate a time frame, consider what needs to be accomplished and give a realistic date for completion. Once you have estimated the time, do everything you can to meet the deadline or finish early. Regardless of how significant missing a deadline is, the inability to meet the deadline, self-imposed or otherwise, should be brought to the supervisor's attention as soon as it is known. This allows the supervisor to change the priorities, assign more staff to the project, or extend the deadline. Not mentioning it with the hope that no one will notice is unprofessional and often disappoints the boss who is expecting the work. Your project may be part of a larger project that depends on your work to move forward. In some cases, missed deadlines have financial consequences that you may not be aware of. Keeping the boss informed of progress avoids surprises and shows that you are responsible.

MEETING MANNERS

Another misstep that many people make in business is regularly showing up late to meetings. This is acceptable only if you work in direct patient care—and only once in a while. Keeping others waiting so you can catch up on something else is unacceptable. Asking people to repeat what occurred in your absence shows others that you value your time more than theirs.

If you are running a meeting, the most professional approach is to print an agenda ahead of time. An agenda informs participants about what is to be discussed and allows them to prepare. Including on the agenda an estimate of the amount of time that will be devoted to each topic is helpful. For example, updating everyone on work in progress should require less time than discussing a proposition that needs approval to go forward. Don't waste time reading something to participants that they can read themselves, but don't assume that everyone is up to speed on an important issue that has not been discussed.

Meetings should occur only when everyone's input is necessary or an announcement needs to be made in a way that ensures everyone hears it at the same time and understands it. Meetings can be run with one-way communication—that is, when the chairperson does most of the talking. It is then akin to a briefing session. Other meetings invite input and have multiple participants sharing ideas.

Regularly occurring meetings held with no purpose promote disrespect. If staff members are made to come to such meetings, they may tune out and miss an important issue. They may also start to plan conflicting appointments to avoid the meetings. Canceling too many routine meetings, however, invites mistrust as well. Why schedule a meeting if you have no intention of holding it? A good manager holds formal or informal staff meetings regularly so that both the manager and the staff are kept abreast of what is occurring in the organization. A manager has made a critical mistake if the staff must hear about important information from sources outside the department.

ETHICS

While professionalism has specific attributes, ethics are much more personal. Professional behavior is in part judged by others, and their perceptions—right or wrong—determine the acceptability of you as a technician or health care worker. A lack of acceptance can result in a business losing patients. The personal principles of ethics people adopt reflect who they are—their upbringing, religious affiliation, and core values—but cannot be easily identified from the outside. In addition to personal ethics, widely accepted professional ethics often guide workplace behavior. In the pharmacy world, for example, many organizations have developed codes of ethics for pharmacists and technicians. Like acting in an unprofessional manner, exhibiting questionable personal and professional ethics can lead to a loss of business.

Ethical behavior is shaped by basic values such as not stealing, treating others in an honest and respectful fashion, recognizing and respecting property that is not yours, and not being envious of the accomplishments and property of others. In some situations, the right path is obvious, but there are many situations where it is less certain. In ethics, sometimes there are no right or wrong answers, just better options than others. Slight variations in situations may completely change how they are resolved. Let's look at how some of these values translate into ethical business practices.

Situation 1

You and a colleague started working at the pharmacy on the same day. Several years have passed, and the two of you do similar work with a similar level of accuracy. Because you are friends, you have shared your evaluations and raises with each other, and you both have progressed at about the same rate.

A position that would be a small promotion is going to open at a new location. Only one of you can get it.

- The position would be a closer drive for you than for your friend, so you arrange for an opportunity to tell the boss. Is this ethical? Why or why not?
- The pharmacist working at the new location went out with your colleague many years ago. The relationship ended badly. Both went on to new relationships, however, and are married to other people. You tell the decision maker that this previous relationship may be a problem if the two are going to work together. Is this ethical? Why or why not?

- Your colleague once called in sick to go skiing. You know that the decision maker disapproves of lying. Since you want the job badly, you tell the decision maker, hoping this information will sway the job in your favor. Is this ethical? Why or why not?
- You find out that the job will be awarded in two weeks. You make an appointment with the decision maker and explain why you think you should get the job. Is this ethical? Why or why not? What if your colleague is away on vacation and can't make an appointment as well?

Situation 2

The pharmacist is going on a vacation and tells you that she can't sleep on planes. You notice that she writes a prescription for herself for five sleeping pills and uses the name of a doctor you know is her friend as the prescriber. The pharmacist asks you to type the prescription. She notes it as a verbal prescription, but you know there were no phone calls to the pharmacy. After the prescription is filled, the pharmacist pays for the medication.

- Is the pharmacist's conduct ethical? Why or why not? What action, if any, should you take?
- Would the situation be different if the sleeping pills are a controlled substance?
- What if the doctor wants to prescribe medication for himself, but because it is a controlled substance, he calls and asks the pharmacist to use her name as the patient. Is this ethical? Why or why not?
- Suppose the prescription is for a medication for someone with no insurance. The pharmacist uses her name because she has insurance. The patient pays the co-pay, and the rest is billed to the third party. Is this ethical? Why or why not?

Situation 3

You work in a pharmacy. Other employees expect the pharmacist to give them free medication when they forget to take their own at home or when they develop a symptom at work.

- The pharmacy is owned by a sole proprietor. Business is falling, but the pharmacist still wants to be a nice guy. Is this ethical? Why or why not?

- The pharmacy is in a large hospital. Volume is high, and the census is always near capacity. A few tablets will not be missed. Is this ethical? Why or why not?
- The person asking is a doctor who asks for medications at least once a week. She tells you that she could get samples anyway. Is this doctor being ethical? Why or why not? Is giving her a few doses ethical?
- An employee who never asks for free medication is suffering from an awful headache. If the pharmacist doesn't give him something for the symptoms, he will have to go home, leaving the operation short-staffed and increasing the workload of the rest of the staff. Is this ethical? Why or why not?

Situation 4

You work in a pharmacy that you like. Everyone is fun to work with. You know, however, that the prices are better down the street. You wonder if you should tell the patients.

- Some of your customers have limited resources. You send them to the other pharmacy when nobody can hear you. Is this ethical? Why or why not?
- An affluent patient complains about the prices. You send her to the other pharmacy. Is this ethical? Why or why not?
- A patient complains about the prices. You suggest he shop around. Is this ethical? Why or why not?
- You figure if people were concerned enough about the prices, they would shop around. You keep the information to yourself and assume it's the service or location that keeps the patients coming back. Is this ethical? Why or why not?
- People start transferring their prescriptions to the other pharmacy. The boss is concerned. You mention that the prices are better down the street and suggest that your pharmacy try to match them. Is this ethical? Why or why not?

Situation 5

Someone who doesn't use your pharmacy or hospital calls repeatedly to ask the pharmacist questions. Most of the time, the questions are complex and take at least 5 minutes to answer.

- Is the patient's conduct ethical? Why or why not?
- Does it matter if your pharmacy doesn't take the patient's health insurance?
- What if the person used to be a patient of your pharmacy?
- What, if anything, should the pharmacist say?

Situation 6

You have heard about an efficient pharmacy operation not too far away from your pharmacy. The pharmacist-in-charge at your pharmacy wants to find out how the other pharmacy is run.

- You get a part-time job at the other pharmacy with the intention of leaving in a few months after you learn about the operation. After all, you think, who couldn't use a little extra cash? Is this ethical? Why or why not?
- You call the other pharmacy pretending to be a patient. Is this ethical? Why or why not?
- You visit the other pharmacy and ask to speak with the person in charge. Then you explain what you want to know and ask if you can talk with him. Is this ethical? Why or why not?

Situation 7

Your friend gets tickets to a hot concert. You are scheduled to work the next day. The concert is several hours away, and the likelihood of your returning in time to get adequate rest is slim.

- The last time you asked a colleague to trade shifts with you, she couldn't do it. You decide to call in sick. After all, you think, you've earned it. Is this ethical? Why or why not?
- You explain the situation to the boss and promise to come in as soon as you wake up. Is this ethical? Why or why not?
- You ask to have the next day off. The boss explains that he can't give it to you, so you call in sick. Is this ethical? Why or why not?

Ethics determine the respectability of a business, but ethical behavior is governed by personal values of right and wrong. One gold standard is, can you look yourself in the mirror tomorrow if you do what you are doing today? The Golden Rule—Do unto others as you would have them do unto you—is another standard of ethical behavior. These principles are similar, but are they practical? In a business setting, questions to think about include the following: Is the time you are asking someone to spend with you taking away from his or her productivity? Will tangible losses be sustained if the request is granted? Is the action going to increase the pharmacy's business or reputation in the long run even though it is going to cost now?

Ethics differs from law. Although law is based on ethical standards, illegal actions lead to consequences. Law has definite rights and wrongs—it is black and white. With ethics, rights and wrongs are gray. Even in the situations above, there may be exceptions to the standard "right" answers. In other words, in ethics there are no hard and fast rules. In similar situations, different circumstances may lead you to completely different answers.

What would happen if a person decided how to act solely by answering the question, "Why not do it, since I can and if I did, it wouldn't bother me?" Is it still the right thing to do if that individual is OK with the act? Sometimes it is, and sometimes it is not. What about a situation where the act would have undesirable consequences if someone found out, but the likelihood of it being discovered is slim? Ethics consider not only the person acting but also the good of the whole. Ethical behavior is governed by the belief that if something were found out, it would pass the decency test. Another way to refer to this is called the "sunshine rule"—if the action took place in broad daylight with everyone concerned around, would it appear to be ethical? If not, don't do it.

From the sunshine rule developed the disclosure rule. Many professionals felt that some speakers were subtly and not so subtly slanting their presentations toward particular drugs because they were funded by pharmaceutical companies. To address this ethical issue, the pharmaceutical industry, continuing-education providers, the American Medical Association, and pharmacy associations developed guidelines requiring disclosure of speakers' funding sources or sponsorships. The intent was to inform people about the possible biases of speakers and keep presentations open and informative.

Many pharmacy societies have developed their own codes of ethics for pharmacists and technicians.

SUMMARY

- **Professionalism** is a code of conduct that gives an outward appearance to observers and customers. **Professional behavior** gives an air of importance and a sense of trust to an operation.
- Honesty and accountability are two important attributes of professional demeanor.
- **Ethics** is a set of personal principles that guide a person in making decisions. These principles are based on religious teaching, community morals, and upbringing.

REFERENCE

Centers for Disease Control and Prevention. Guideline for hand hygiene in health-care settings: recommendations of the Healthcare Infection Control Practices Advisory Committee and the HICPAC/SHEA/APIC/IDSA Hand Hygiene Task Force. *MMWR Recomm Rep.* 2002;51(RR-16):1–45.

CHAPTER 4

Team Approach

Group Contexts

From *Contemporary Communication Theory* by Dominic Infante, Andrew Rancer, Theodore Avtgis. Copyright © 2010 by Kendall Hunt Publishing Company. Reprinted by permission.

Learning Objectives

- List the types of groups.
- List and define the various roles team members hold within a group.
- Define the different style of leadership that can be used within a group and the pros and cons of each.

Key Terms

Activity tracks	Difficulty	Public compliance
Argumentative minority	Disruptions	Relational activity track
Assertiveness training	Functional approach to	Small-group communication
Authoritarian style	leadership	Style approach to leadership
Breakpoints	Groupthink	Task activity track
Cohesiveness	Idea-generation group	Task-oriented groups
Conformity	Laissez-faired style	Therapy groups
Consciousness-raising groups	Learning groups	Topical activity tract
Coordination requirements	Multiple sequence model	Trait
Delays	Pacers	Trait approach to leadership
Democratic style	Problem-solving group	Unitary sequence model
Decision-making groups		

Important aspects of relationships (affection, trust, and attraction, for example) differ when they occur between two individuals and when they occur in a small group. The feeling of trusting one other person is not the same feeling as trusting a given group of people. Differences in communication between two individuals and the communication among several people necessitate identifying interpersonal and small group as two distinct contexts of communication. After clarifying certain aspects of groups, we will discuss several concepts that set communication in groups apart from communication in other contexts. Then we will examine some recent and significant developments in the communication field in terms of building group communication theories.

NATURE OF GROUPS

Group Size

Small-group communication refers to communication in gatherings that vary in size from three to about fifteen persons. A group is considered small if members are able to switch roles from receiver to source with relative ease (DeVito, 2002). When groups are composed of fifteen people or more, it becomes difficult to switch from receiver to source. In such a situation, the order of speaking is often assigned, and more formal rules of parliamentary procedure may be followed.

The size of a small group influences the likelihood that everyone will get along with one another. A group of four people involves six dyadic relationships, whereas a group of twelve has sixty-six. The greater the number of possible relationships, the more potential for individual dyads within the group to be incompatible. Group size affects satisfaction. The larger the group, the greater the probability that some members will not be able to talk as much as they would like. Size can also impair group performance, as implied in the adage "too many chefs spoil the broth." There may be an optimal number of people for solving a given problem; additional people may cause confusion and impede, rather than help, group progress.

Types of Groups

When you think of "groups," what comes to mind? You can probably identify quite a few reasons for people to gather together. A group's *purpose* provides perhaps the clearest way of distinguishing one type of group from another.

Task-oriented groups are those that have a job to do. Within this designation, we can make additional divisions. A problem-solving group attempts to discover a solution to a problem by analyzing it thoroughly. Typically, problem-solving groups use discussion to investigate a problem and examine possible solutions in terms of which solution best solves the problem. **Problem-solving groups** have received the most attention from researchers, and problem-solving discussion is also the most common assignment in group communication courses in communication departments. **Decision-making groups** are also concerned with problem solving. However, they have the added function of actually deciding which solution will be implemented, when and how it will be put into effect, how progress will be monitored, how changes in the solution will be handled, and how the program involving the solution will be evaluated. The **idea-generation group** is a third kind of task group. The purpose of idea-generation groups is to discover a variety of solutions, approaches, perspectives, or consequences for a topic. The ideas generated are not evaluated be-

cause value judgments tend to inhibit members. For example, a member might hesitate to express an idea if he or she fears a negative reaction. The idea-generation group is often called a "brainstorming" group.

A second type of group is the **therapy group.** The purpose of therapy groups is to help the individual solve personal problems. These groups are conducted by professionals such as clinical psychologists. There are many different kinds of therapy groups. Some of the most common are encounter groups, T-groups, and sensitivity groups, all of which hope to promote personal growth. Tactics to stimulate personal insights often include challenges, criticism, personal attacks, displays of strong emotions, and demonstrations of support. **Assertiveness training** involves the use of groups to help individuals learn to protect their rights, to resist group pressure, to assume leadership roles, and to approach social situations confidently. Other examples include groups to help people exercise regularly, lose weight, quit smoking, and stop drinking alcoholic beverages. The communication discipline has conducted little research and has had little experience with therapy groups because few communication scholars are trained therapists.

Consiousness-raising groups exist to increase members' awareness of shared characteristics or concerns. These commonalities can be a characteristic such as gender, nationality, or religion; a value such as respect for animal rights; an experience such as serving in the military; an ability such as intercollegiate athletics; or a profession. The purpose of consciousness-raising groups is to have members realize more vividly who they are, to be proud of what makes them unique, and to have members change their behavior so it is more in line with this new consciousness. For instance, a consciousness-raising group might help members realize various ways that women today are victims of discrimination and offer methods for dealing with each form of discrimination.

Learning groups constitute a fourth type of group. The purpose is for individuals and the group to acquire more information and understanding of a topic. This type of group is sometimes used in educational settings such as high schools and colleges. There are some advantages to group versus individual effort in learning. For example, group members can divide the work; each member adds his or her unique perspective to enrich what the group learns; members gain insight from discussing information that might not have been gained in the absence of such discussion; and motivation to continue learning can be enhanced.

Therapy, learning, and consciousness-raising groups have been studied generally by the fields of psychology, sociology, education, and counseling. As mentioned earlier, group communication theory and research in the communication field has focused primarily on problem-solving and decision-making groups. We will now examine several important elements in such groups.

Roles

The concept of roles is a very basic one in the study of group communication. Certain communicative behaviors in groups (such as using humor to get members to relax) are intended to accomplish certain goals (releasing group tension, for example). Someone enacting those behaviors can be described as playing or taking a given role. In 1948 Benne and Sheats provided an analysis of roles that has remained influential over the years. They said there are three main categories of roles enacted by group members. *Group task roles* pertain to group discussions aimed at selecting, defining, and solving problems. The specific task roles identified by Benne and Sheats are

1. **Initiator-Contributor**—proposes new ideas, changes, procedures.
2. **Information Seeker**—asks questions about information and others' suggestions.
3. **Opinion Seeker**—asks questions about the values guiding the group.
4. **Information Giver**—presents evidence relevant to the group problem.
5. **Opinion Giver**—states his or her position on issues.
6. **Elaborator**—clarifies what is being considered, extends the analysis of an issue.
7. **Coordinator**—gets people to function together, puts information together
8. **Orienter**—keeps group focused on goals, points out departures from goals.
9. **Evaluator-Critic**—argues the evidence and reasoning pertaining to issues.
10. **Energizer**—motivates group toward a quality decision.
11. **Procedural Technician**—performs routine tasks, busywork.
12. **Recorder**—writes group proceedings so a record exists.

These roles are often performed by more than one person in a group. One person might perform several of the twelve task roles during the course of a discussion. In fact, a single incident of communication might involve several roles: a member offers an opinion, follows that with a question, and then tries to energize the group so it will not "drag its heels."

The second category of roles is termed *group building and maintenance*. These roles are concerned with the socioemotional climate in the group. That is, the feelings that group members have for one another and the task are recognized as very important in terms of the group achieving its task goals. These roles are

1. **Encourager**—provides positive feedback to members, shows warmth.
2. **Harmonizer**—reduces tension between members and mediates conflict.
3. **Compromiser**—attempts to have each party in a conflict gain something.
4. **Gatekeeper**—promotes open channels of communication and participation by everyone.
5. **Standard Setter**—suggests and uses standards to evaluate the group.
6. **Group Commentator**—describes the processes operating in the group to change or reinforce the group climate.
7. **Follower**—conforms to group ideas, acts as a good listener.

These seven roles and the first twelve roles are all concerned with the group achieving its purpose. Thus, each of these nineteen roles is very group centered. However, not all behavior in a group conforms to this selfless behavior. Sometimes a person tries to satisfy individual needs, which may be totally irrelevant to the group's task. Such behavior can be counterproductive to the group achieving its goals. These behaviors are termed *individual roles*.

1. **Aggressor**—attacks self-concepts of others to assert dominance.
2. **Blocker**—is hostile by being negative and opposing things unreasonably.
3. **Recognition-Seeker**—offends members by calling too much attention to self.
4. **Self-Confessor**—works personal problems into the discussion in hope of gaining insight.

5. **Playboy**—indicates a desire to be somewhere else, preferably having fun.
6. **Dominator**—interrupts, manipulates, and tries to control others.
7. **Help-Seeker**—wants sympathy, acts insecure, confused, and helpless.
8. **Special Interest Pleader**—argues for a "pet" idea, often based on prejudice.

Leadership

It is not difficult to imagine how chaotic our institutions, corporations, organizations, clubs, and political parties would be if they had little leadership. However, such speculation is a moot point. Without leadership, the groups would never have formed in the first place! The many fields studying leadership have produced an enormous body of literature. In his classic analysis of leadership, Ralph Stogdill (1974; Stogdill & Bass, 1981; see also Bass & Stogdill, 1990) identified forty major topics and examined over 3,000 books and articles. He found that most topics were organized around seven main categories: leadership theory, leader personality and behavior, leadership stability and change, leadership emergence, leadership and social power, leader-follower interactions, and leadership and group performance.

The communication field has taken four approaches to leadership: trait, functional, style, and situational. A **trait approach to leadership** is based on the idea that leaders have traits that distinguish them from followers. A **trait** is a characteristic of an individual that is generally consistent from one situation to the next. Trait research suggests leaders are more likely than followers to be high on traits such as self-esteem, extroversion, open-mindedness, aggression, achievement motivation, analytical thought, sociability, and argumentativeness.

A **functional approach to leadership** focuses on the leadership behaviors needed by a group to accomplish its goals (Barnlund & Haiman, 1960), not on the individual as in the trait approach. The leadership behaviors that are essential to the success of a group do not have to be performed by a single person. Instead, leadership can be enacted by any number of group members. Two types of leadership behaviors are task and group maintenance. One person in a problem-solving group might provide leadership for the task, another person for group maintenance, while a third person might provide some help in both areas. Task leadership behaviors include initiating ideas and procedures, coordinating members' contributions, summarizing to let the group know its progress, and elaborating on ideas; group maintenance behaviors involve releasing tension that builds to an unproductive level, regulating the amount of talk by each member, improving group morale, and mediating group conflict (Beebe & Masterson, 2003).

John Cragan and David Wright (1999) provided a useful analysis of the leadership behaviors needed in a problem-solving or decision-making small group. Leadership communication behaviors in the *task area* are contributing ideas, seeking ideas, evaluating ideas, asking others to evaluate ideas, and fostering understanding of ideas. The leadership behaviors in the *procedural area* are setting goals for the group, preparing an agenda or outline for the group to follow, clarifying ideas, summarizing at various points in the discussion, and verbalizing when the group is in complete agreement on something. There also are several leadership communication behaviors in the *interpersonal relations area*: regulating participation so no one feels "left out," creating a positive emotional climate, promoting group self-analysis, resolving conflict in the discussion, and instigating conflict to stimulate a more thorough examination of issues.

The **style approach** has identified three major types of leadership: authoritarian, democratic, and laissez-faire (White & Lippett, 1968). Each style represents a unique set of leadership behaviors. In contrast to individual traits or functions any group members can perform, the emphasis is on different ways of leading.

The **authoritarian style** involves the leader being very directive in terms of the group goals and procedures, the division of work, and deciding the outcome of conflict. Group members do not feel free to argue with the leader on these matters. Research suggests that groups can be quite productive with an authoritarian leader; however, members' satisfaction with their experience in the group tends to be lower than with other leadership styles. The authoritarian style is said to be most appropriate in situations that are highly stressful or dangerous (emergencies, for instance) or highly competitive (such as an athletic contest). The belief is that argument in such situations can be counter-productive; what works best is a strong, competent central figure who guides the group forcefully down an efficient and productive path.

In contrast, the **democratic style** views all issues (including goals, procedures, and work assignments) as matters to be discussed by the group. The actual decision on the issues can be made in one of three ways. A *majority decision* is produced when members vote. The agreed-upon percentage (for example, 51 percent, 67 percent) of votes must be obtained for an idea to pass. *Consensus* occurs when the group tries to find a resolution to the given issue that everyone in the group can support. This can be difficult to achieve. If such a solution can be found, it will enjoy significant group support. A *participative* decision involves members contributing ideas and the leader then being guided by the expressed preferences in making the decision. On a more macro level, of course, this is a central feature of our representative form of government. The democratic style of leadership tends to produce the most member satisfaction, even if the group is not as productive as those operating under another leadership style.

The **laissez-faire style** of leadership involves a minimum of involvement by the leader in group activity. Basically, the leader provides as much information as needed, and then the group members are left to make decisions as a group, to act as individuals, or as subgroups. This lack of direction from a leader can be counterproductive, especially in groups with low motivation for a task. However, this style can work very well with people who are highly motivated, experienced self-starters who work well together. The leader says in essence, "You don't need me to tell you what to do."

Conflict

The term *conflict* has unfavorable connotations for some people. Certainly, there are types of conflict that are destructive. However, not all forms of conflict are necessarily bad. In fact, certain kinds of conflict are essential to the success of a problem-solving or decision-making group. The theory of groupthink discussed later in this chapter illustrates rather vividly what happens when there is too little conflict in important decision-making groups.

Conflict exists in a small group when proponents of differing positions on an issue are motivated to defend their positions. Overt disagreement in a group is another way to think of conflict. According to B. Aubrey Fisher (1970), problem-solving and decision-making groups typically go through four stages: orientation to the task, conflict over

what the group should do, the emergence of a group position, and group reinforcement of the decision. The conflict stage is especially important in determining what will be the final group product.

The influence of conflict on the group product was clearly illustrated in research by Charlan Nemeth (1986). She discovered that conflict in a small, problem-solving group improved the quality of the group's process in making decisions. The conflict she studied took the form of an **argumentative minority** that opposed the majority opinion. Nemeth found that having a vocal minority view did not necessarily persuade the majority away from their initial position. Instead, an argumentative minority tended to stimulate the majority toward a more careful, thoughtful, and thorough decision. This illustrates an important function of conflict in small groups. The conflict does not have to result in the proponents of one position "converting" the believers of another position. Instead, conflict can lead to a more carefully considered decision—one that looks at a number of advantages and disadvantages before reaching a conclusion.

Conflict in small groups can be viewed in terms of argument. That is, the interaction in problem-solving groups can be analyzed according to the issues over which there was disagreement, the positions taken and defended by the various group members, the attempts to refute the positions, and whether these aspects of argument help explain the group outcome, especially the quality of the group decision. An argumentative approach to studying small group communication holds considerable promise. Randy Hirokawa's functional theory (discussed later in this chapter) reveals that certain kinds of communication in small groups, including argument, distinguish effective from ineffective problem-solving groups.

Following the principles of argumentation theory (careful analysis of issues, emphasis on evidence, use of rigorous forms of reasoning, avoiding fallacies in reasoning, etc.) can produce constructive conflict; other forms of disagreement or competition can be very destructive. For instance, conflict over scarce resources with individuals who are concerned only with "getting their share" can result in long-lasting bitter feelings. Another destructive type of conflict involves personal disagreements between people that result in the use of verbal aggression. A verbally aggressive message attacks the self-concept of the receiver to deliver psychological pain. This tactic used in conflicts between people makes it very difficult for them to work together on a problem-solving task.

A central premise in the belief that conflict can be constructive is the idea that argumentation is a tool for discovering which ideas are valid and which are not. Whenever there is concern over whether something is right or wrong, valuable or worthless, exists or not, and especially whenever there is a solution to be selected, conflict is an asset rather than something to be avoided. The solution that survives the rigors of argumentation is the one that is most likely to be effective. This is "trial by fire" or a "survival of the fittest" test as applied to ideas.

Conformity

Conformity is sometimes a product of group communication. Conformity can be defined as: "*A change in behavior or belief toward a group as a result of real or imagined group pressure*" (Kiesler & Kiesler, 1969, p. 2). Conformity is a type of group influence, a change in the individual brought about by pressure (real or imagined) for the person to behave in a manner advocated by the group. For example, some students in a study group might say, "Let's take a break and finish this job tomorrow." One member might dissent and say he or she wants to continue and to finish the job today. After all the other members of the group express dissatisfaction with continuing, the lone dissenter says, "Well, OK, let's call it quits for now." The person was not able to resist the pressure to conform to the wishes of other members. This experience is generally a universal one. All of us at times decide to conform to what the group wants to do rather than to resist. Often we conclude that to resist would be too costly. It would create many more problems than it would solve, so we decide resistance is not worth it, and we "go along to get along."

One type of conformity is **public compliance;** the individual behaves in the way desired by the group only when being observed by group members, because the person does not really believe in the behavior. Thus, a person might speak favorably about a given political candidate because of pressure from a group. However, in the privacy of the voting booth the person might vote for someone else. This type of conformity recognizes that our behavior is not always consistent with our beliefs and attitudes. Sometimes we believe one way but behave in another manner because of group pressure. *Private acceptance* is a second kind of conformity. Here the person behaves

as suggested by the group because the group produces a change in the person's beliefs and attitudes. Thus, the person is not "pretending" when behaving in a particular manner (Kiesler & Kiesler, 1969).

In our study group example, one of the members in the majority might say to the lone dissenter, "You are suggesting that we make this a marathon session. However, I recently read some research that showed the quality of performance for a group with a task such as ours falls off sharply right about where we are now in the number of nonstop hours worked." Our lone dissenter might then say, "I didn't realize that, but it certainly is plausible given other things that I've read about achievement. OK, let's finish tomorrow." Conformity in this instance is different because it is based not only on group pressure but also on an internal change in the individual.

There also is the possibility that one does not have to change a behavior to conform. A group can essentially reinforce the individual's ideas by pressuring him or her to remain a certain way, to continue a certain behavior and not to change. For instance, a physical fitness club might take a strong stance against the use of anabolic steroid drugs as performance enhancers. One of the members might be tempted to try steroids. However, the group pressure might keep the person from experimenting with the drug. In this case, the group influenced the person by strengthening or reinforcing previous beliefs (for example, the knowledge that steroids cause liver damage) and patterns of behavior (following a routine to build muscles gradually and safely, for instance). This reinforcement can be viewed as a type of conformity—one that has received little attention from researchers, but one that could have some useful applications, especially in preventing destructive influences on children and adolescents.

There are several reasons for our compliance with group pressure. Being a member of a given group partially satisfies our *need to belong,* to be included. Thus, if the group threatens to exclude us because we do not want to go along, our feelings of belonging are endangered. The group is also influential because it serves a valuable *reference function* by informing members on what is and what is not acceptable behavior. The group provides a basis for comparison so that individuals can evaluate their behavior. "I must be dressing OK; everyone in the group dresses just like me." *Group attractiveness* is a third reason for being influenced by group pressure. Generally, the more attractive a group is to us, the more we are likely to be influenced by it. If we are attracted to a group, we have strong feelings of liking, and it is difficult to go against those feelings unless the issue is very important. Moreover, because we usually evaluate a group as attractive because its members express liking for us, we find it difficult to resist pressure from the group because we fear members will stop liking us. This is a powerful incentive to yield to group pressure because we have a need for affection and generally deplore losing the respect of others. Such a loss could threaten our need to belong (the first reason). Finally, *group maintenance* sometimes is a reason for conforming. We realize that the group needs to put on a united front. If one member behaves differently, it will weaken the image of the group. Thus, we may conform for the good of the group.

FUNCTIONAL THEORY OF GROUP DECISION QUALITY

Groups—and researchers who study them—want to know whether decisions reached were good or bad. In a problem-solving discussion, can you distinguish high- from low-quality decisions by what is said? Do certain types of communication lead to an effective decision, whereas others predict that the decision will be defective? This issue of group decision quality is the focus of Hirokawa's functional theory. The principles of the theory involve the communication characteristics of group interaction that lead to quality decisions. Stating such principles in probability terms constitutes a law: if a group does A, B, and C, it is highly likely that they will make a quality decision.

One study analyzed videotaped discussions of various groups who were judged to have reached an effective or an ineffective decision (Hirokawa & Pace, 1983). Four communication characteristics distinguished effective from ineffective groups. The first was that effective groups rigorously evaluated the validity of opinions and assumptions made by the individuals in the group. Ineffective groups, however, glossed over the evaluation procedure and accepted opinions and assumptions as facts without critical analysis. A second difference in communication pertained to how groups evaluated alternatives. Effective groups analyzed possible solutions thoroughly with very critical attention paid to consequences—what would happen if the solution were adopted. Ineffective groups were superficial. Usually they simply said a given solution did or did not meet the criteria for a

good solution; they did not argue why. Third, effective groups based their decisions on reasonable premises (assumptions); ineffective groups based their decisions on inaccurate, highly questionable premises. No member of the ineffective groups made an effort to correct these mistakes. The fourth communication characteristic was the quality of leadership. In effective groups, the leaders encouraged *constructive argumentation* by introducing issues, challenging other positions, and identifying fallacies in reasoning. The leaders of ineffective groups exerted a negative effect on the quality of the group's decision by influencing the group to accept faulty ideas, introducing ridiculous ideas, or leading the group on a tangent.

Interestingly, this study also identified communication characteristics that did *not* distinguish effective from ineffective groups: participating equally, trying to identify important information, attempting to generate a number of possible solutions to a problem, and using a set of criteria in evaluating the various possible solutions. These characteristics were found in both effective and ineffective groups.

Hirokawa's functional theory maintains that a group needs to fulfill four critical functions to reach an effective, high-quality decision:

1. Achieving a thorough understanding of the problem that requires a decision
2. Discovering a range of realistic and acceptable possible solutions
3. Identifying the criteria for an effective, high-quality solution
4. Assessing the positive and negative consequences of possible solutions to select the solution with the most desirable consequences

Hirokawa (1985) conducted a study that examined the communication behavior of groups and found that the more the four functions were satisfied, the higher the quality of the group's decision. Statistical analysis revealed that understanding the problem and recognizing the possible negative consequences of each potential solution best differentiated the groups that reached effective decisions from those which were ineffective. In a later study Hirokawa (1988) found the amount of time spent talking about the four functions did not predict decision quality. Instead, it was the quality of talk that mattered.

Hirokawa and Scheerhorn (1986) identified factors that contribute to a group making a faulty decision. Their basic idea is "that group members influence the quality of a group's decision by facilitating or inhibiting the occurrence of errors (for example, faulty interpretations and conclusions) during various stages of the decision-making process." The five factors are:

1. Inadequate assessment of the problem (failing to recognize signs of the problem, its full extent, seriousness; not identifying the causes of the problem)
2. Inappropriate goals and objectives for dealing with the problem (not identifying objectives that will correct the problem; selecting unnecessary objectives that burden the group)
3. Improper assessment of consequences (ignoring or underestimating the positive and/or negative consequences of a possible solution; overestimating the positive and/or negative consequences)
4. Establishment of an inadequate information base (flawed information, group rejecting valid information, group collecting too little or too much information)
5. Invalid reasoning from the information base (making mistakes in reasoning; using only the information that supports a preferred but flawed choice)

These five sources of faulty decisions result from the communication of the group members. A group member facilitates the errors through social influence by convincing members to accept an invalid inference. Group members can also prevent these five factors from contributing to a bad decision. This too is accomplished through communication, as when a member corrects a fallacious conclusion by another group member.

Dennis Gouran and Randy Hirokawa (1986) termed this kind of corrective communicative behavior counteractive influence. It counteracts by neutralizing or negating faulty communication. In doing so, the group is then able to make progress toward an effective decision. This type of influence is very important in getting a group back on track. Both effective and ineffective groups make mistakes. However, a characteristic of effective groups is that counteractive influence is prevalent, and uncorrected mistakes are rare in comparison to ineffective groups. Counteractive influence is another illustration of the positive role of argument in group decision making.

Hirokawa's theory, and the one by Janis discussed next, represent the laws perspective for the-

ory building. The emphasis is on discovering conditions that lead to certain outcomes; this probabilistic reasoning takes an "if this, then that" form. There is a direct interest in what happens to groups and the antecedent conditions that lead to an outcome, such as decision quality. Hirokawa's theory represents an important step in understanding the communicative conditions that need to exist for a group to reach a quality decision. Future research will build on that foundation and further our understanding of the type of communication necessary for effective decision making in groups.

THEORY OF GROUPTHINK

Social psychologist Irving Janis's (1982) theory of groupthink is also concerned with the quality of decisions reached in groups. However, whereas functional theory centered on explaining superior group decisions, the theory of groupthink is about group failures—decisions that in hindsight seem incredibly poor, ill advised, and generally incompetent. The basic problem Janis tried to solve is how a group of persons, who individually are quite competent, can make a collective decision that is utterly incompetent. The theory was based on historical analyses of national fiascoes such as the Bay of Pigs invasion, inactivated defenses at Pearl Harbor, and escalation of the Vietnam War. The theory of groupthink was offered as an explanation of such failures.

Groupthink is a communication process that sometimes develops when members of a group begin thinking similarly, greatly reducing the probability that the group will reach an effective decision. To explain groupthink, we will first say what it is *not*. Groupthink is not critical thinking, where decisions are based on thorough discussions of the problem and the possible good and bad consequences of potential solutions. Groupthink does not involve group argumentation where ideas are tested for validity; remember, superior ideas are those that survive the argumentation process. Groupthink is not an attitude that says, "I am going to present this objection to what the group favors even if it means some people will be a little upset with me for not going along."

The definition by negation, then, suggests several features of groupthink. When groupthink develops, there is a high level of cohesiveness among members and a great deal of reluctance to deviate from the group position. **Cohesiveness** is the feeling of "oneness" in a group, being "close-knit," bound to

Facilitating Conditions	Symptoms of Groupthink	Defective Decision Making	
Cohesive group	Overestimation of power and importance a. illusion of invulnerability b. belief in the inherent morality of the group	Inadequate analysis of problem Limited range of solutions No rigorous assessment of consequences of preferred solution Failure to reconsider initially rejected solutions	Successful Solution Unlikely
Group structure a. too isolated b. biased leadership c. lack of procedure	Closed-mindedness a. collective rationalizations b. stereotypes of out-groups	Inadequate research Biased processing	
Environment a. external pressure b. lack of alternatives c. low self-esteem	Great pressure toward consensus a. self-censorship b. illusion of unanimity c. direct pressure on dissenters d. self-appointed mindguards	Lack of contingency plans	

Figure 4.1 The theory of groupthink.
Adapted from Janis (1982). p. 244.

one another, and united, as members of a team. Cohesiveness is normally a desirable condition in groups. It is undesirable when members place such a priority on solidarity that they do not analyze problems thoroughly and reach decisions without adequately considering the consequences of proposed solutions. As a result, groups reach consensus on a course of action prematurely. This can cause a group of superior individuals to make a very inferior decision and to select the wrong solution. The communication in a group that is operating under groupthink lacks argumentation and has little rigorous clash of positions on issues. Figure 4.1 presents a summary of the theory of groupthink.

According to the theory, groupthink is more likely when three conditions are present in decision-making groups. The first is a necessary condition but not a sufficient one. For groupthink to develop, *the group must be cohesive* with a strong desire for the group to remain that way. However, just because a decision-making group is cohesive is not sufficient for groupthink to develop. At least two other conditions are necessary: group structure that promotes groupthink and an environment where groupthink flourishes.

The *structure of a decision-making group* can lead to groupthink. For example, if a group is isolated from

information and from other persons in a larger organization, the structure can preclude exposure to differing opinions. A biased leader, one who clearly establishes very early the solution he or she prefers, creates a group structure conducive to groupthink. Group members may not advance other possible solutions and may be reluctant to question critically the leader's preferred solution. Another structural factor occurs when the group does not have established procedures for making decisions. Having a set of rigorous procedures (such as bringing in outside experts before the final decision is reached) can reduce the chance of a disastrous decision. Without a tradition of rigorous decision-making procedures, a group can more easily succumb to pressure toward uniformity and thus agree to a very flawed course of action.

The *nature of the situation* represents another facilitating condition for groupthink. Stress nurtures groupthink, especially when the group feels pressure from outside sources to solve a particular problem. A group can make a very bad decision because they feel pressure to present a united front and not to "rock the boat." If the group fails to consider and evaluate a number of solutions, perhaps because they don't have sufficient resources or time, they may agree to one solution without considering other possibilities. If a group feels low in esteem because of recent failures, they will also be more susceptible to pressure toward consensus.

Three major symptoms indicate the groupthink syndrome. First, the *group tends to overestimate its power and importance*—believing strongly that "right" is on its side and that opposing forces are "evil." This creates a false sense of confidence that entices groups to take greater risks than they otherwise would. A second symptom is that the *group becomes very closed-minded*. In selecting a risky course of action, they discount clear warnings and avoid considering information that refutes their choice. In the case of foreign policy decisions, enemy leaders are viewed as too weak or too stupid to find any flaws in the group's selected course of action, so success seems assured. The third symptom of groupthink is *great pressure in the group to reach consensus*. Individuals minimize the importance of their doubts to preserve unanimity. Pressure is exerted against any group member who expresses a strong argument against the group's positions. When these symptoms occur, the process of groupthink is probably operating.

Groupthink impairs decision making, greatly increasing the probability of a blunder. Of course, pure luck can "save" a group in such circumstances; the solution selected by a flawed procedure could serendipitously turn out to be the best of all possible solutions. However, the likelihood of that happening is low because the process by which a decision is reached through group think will have several major defects. First, the pressure of cohesiveness results in faulty analysis. The problem is not understood thoroughly; thus, its causes are not well known. Because a solution should deal with a problem's cause, this defect is indeed serious. There are also other deficiencies. Other possible solutions are ignored or dismissed because there is an early preference for a particular solution. The consequences of the preferred solution are not examined rigorously. This is perhaps the most fatal flaw in the process. Also, there is not enough reanalysis of solutions that were initially rejected. When groupthink operates, there is typically a lack of research and thus a shortage of necessary information. Because there is an early preference for a particular solution, information is processed in a biased fashion. For instance, information that suggests the preferred solution will cause economic hardship may be viewed as outdated despite its accuracy in the past. A final defect is that groups tend not to make contingency plans when they fall into the trap of groupthink because of the unjustified confidence they have in their solution. For example, if a decision was made by a company to save labor costs by moving its manufacturing plant to a developing country, a necessary contingency plan would deal with possible political instability in that country.

Although groupthink can be a serious problem in decision-making groups, Janis pointed out that several strategies can avoid groupthink. All the procedures are designed to prevent a group from reaching premature consensus and to keep feelings of cohesiveness from turning into group pressure for uniformity.

- The leader of a decision-making group should encourage group members to voice doubts, concerns, or objections.
- The leader should be impartial in presenting the task to the group by using unbiased language and being careful not to show a preference for a particular solution.
- The organization or larger group should set up more than one group with different leaders to work on the same problem.
- The decision-making group should at times divide into two or more subgroups that work separately and then meet together to debate differences.
- Each member should get the reactions of someone outside the group and report concerns back to the group.
- Trusted members of the organization who are not members of the actual decision-making group should be brought into some meetings to challenge the positions of the group.
- To stimulate debate, one member of the group should be assigned the role of devil's advocate when solutions are being evaluated.
- When the decision involves rivals, such as a competing organization, scenarios of the rival's possible reactions should be created. Emphasis should be placed on the potential risks of the various solutions.
- Once preliminary agreement is reached on a solution, a "last chance" meeting should be held for members to present lingering doubts and to rethink the issue before making the final decision.

It is apparent that the groupthink remedies involve communication that is argumentative in nature. The prevention of groupthink involves encouraging group members to engage in vigorous debate. The idea is that confidence in a solution is warranted if it survives in a competition of intense debate with other possible solutions.

Although the theory of groupthink has been used mainly to study historical accounts of bad decisions, one study demonstrated that groupthink can be examined in a laboratory setting (Courtright, 1978). The results supported the theory of groupthink. This support is important for a laws theory. Remember that a basic goal of laws theories is to identify the antecedent conditions that lead to the prediction.

MULTIPLE SEQUENCE MODEL OF GROUP DECISIONS

There have been two distinctive approaches to how groups reach decisions in discussions concerned with problem solving. The **unitary sequence model** suggests groups pass through certain stages as they move toward a decision. For instance, a problem-solving group first determines the nature of the problem to be solved, the standards that a solution should meet, which of the available solutions best meet the standards, and how the solution selected should be implemented and evaluated. According to Marshall Scott Poole (1981) the unitary sequence model represents a logical ideal of how groups should move toward a decision. Groups do not often follow this ideal.

One study looked at forty-seven group decisions to determine the paths taken in reaching decisions (Poole & Roth, 1989). Only eleven of the forty-seven decisions followed the unitary sequence. Fourteen of the decisions followed a solution-oriented path because almost none of the communication pertained to the problem. Twenty-two of the decisions involved complex paths in which the group followed from two to seven problem-solution cycles.

Research such as this suggests a second approach to how groups reach decisions. The **multiple sequence model** (Poole 1981, 1983a, 1983b) contends groups can have different patterns of sequences because they can take various paths to a decision, depending on the contingencies in the situation. This model uses a systems perspective; the emphasis is on patterns of interaction and situational contingencies. The multiple sequence model identifies three separate tracks of group communication activity: *task, relational,* and *topical.* The three **activity tracks,** in a given decision-making group, develop simultaneously but usually at uneven rates.

The development of the tracks is influenced by break-points that tend to interrupt the development of the activity tracks. There are three kinds of **break-points:** *pacers, delays,* and *disruptions.*

The **task activity track** includes the processes in which the group engages to accomplish its task. Some of these are deciding how to proceed, gathering information, analyzing the problem, establishing standards for solutions, and selecting a solution. Imagine a group responsible for acquiring football players for a professional football team. They begin meeting well before the National Football League collegiate player draft in April. Their task is to decide which eligible collegiate players they should draft to strengthen their team. One of the tasks the director of player personnel would introduce early is a problem analysis. Specifically, what positions were weakest this past season; where is the need for new talent greatest? If it is decided the need is most apparent at defensive tackle, another task process will be to establish the standards for a solution. For instance, what should the player's time be in the 40-yard dash, what height and weight are ideal, does he have to be a proven pass-rusher, etc.? The process of selecting a solution would involve strategies such as: in the first round of the player draft, if our first choice for defensive tackle has been selected, we will go to our second; if the second has also been selected, we will switch to our first, second, and third choices for free safety (our second greatest need).

The **relational activity track** involves the activities that emphasize the relationships among the group members that pertain to how the group works together. These include how ideas are introduced and criticized, how conflict is managed, and how roles are defined and reinforced. In our pro football example, the director of player personnel might specify how scouts will work together to evaluate players. At meetings where prospective players are evaluated, one person in the group might be asked to give an overview of a player's strengths and weaknesses, and then the other members are invited to argue for or against drafting the player. When traveling to evaluate players, hotel room assignments might be made so that good friends room together.

The **topical activity track** is made up of the content of the issues and arguments of concern to the group at various times in the discussion. The distinction between the first two tracks and the topical track is process versus content. The first two tracks concern the paths the group follows in discussing content. An example of the topical process track in our pro football example might be: player A has the size and speed that we are looking for but he only had three quarterback sacks last season; player B managed fifteen sacks, but he is not quite big enough for us. This topic could be considered while a group is selecting a solution (task track) or while managing a conflict (relational track).

Breakpoints influence how decisions develop. There are three types. **Pacers,** or normal breakpoints, determine how a discussion moves along. A topic shift is the most common breakpoint influencing pacing. Other normal or expected breakpoints are adjournments, planning periods, or getting away to reflect on topics. **Delays** occurs when the group cycles back to rework an issue. The group might go back through the very same analysis several times to solve a problem. For instance, an argument might be repeated several times. This may be a difficult period for the group, but it can also stimulate great creativity if the group rises to meet the challenge. **Disruptions** are a type of breakpoint that occurs in at least two different forms. The first is a major disagreement. When this happens, all three activity tracks could be disrupted. Even after the disagreement is settled, it may take the group a while to get back on track. For example, relational difficulties might be created by conflict that hinders task and topical activities. In our example, two scouts who dislike each other (a relational difficulty) may argue about a particular player, slowing down the decision-making procedure (a task activity). Further, they might distort the player's strengths and weaknesses (topic track), which makes it difficult for the group to get back to a productive discussion. A second type of disruption occurs when a process adopted by the group fails. This could occur when the work is divided among group members, but one assignment turns out to be many times more difficult than the others. Another example is a group selecting the wrong criteria for a solution. In our pro football example, this could involve emphasizing the size of a player when, instead, the number of quarterback sacks should have been the major consideration.

The activity tracks and the breakpoints in Poole's model identify what goes on when a group meets to solve a problem. The objective of all the activities is to accumulate what is needed to complete the task. What is needed to solve a problem might be thought of as *prerequisites* for decision making. Sometimes a group will begin a problem-solving discussion with some of the prerequisites already satisfied.

For a decision-making group, the prerequisites include recognition of the need to make a good decision, analysis of the problem to be solved, determining the criteria for a good solution, discovering the possible solutions, adapting the solutions to the needs of the group, selecting a solution, planning to implement and also to evaluate the solution.

Groups can vary greatly on how ready they are to satisfy each of these prerequisites for a decision. If a group has completed most of the prerequisites, the path to a decision could be relatively simple. On the other hand, if a group has satisfied none of the prerequisites, the path to a decision could be very complex; there could be several problem-solutions cycles.

The decisions resulting from a given path or cycle are governed by several contingencies. Poole's model emphasizes two. The first is the nature of the task. Two dimensions are important. **Difficulty** refers to the amount of effort necessary to complete the task. **Coordination requirements** pertain to the degree that members must integrate their actions and work together. The likelihood of a group accomplishing its task is influenced by these factors. That is, the likelihood of task accomplishment is lower when task difficulty and coordination requirements are higher.

A second contingency of decision development is *group history*. What happened earlier in a group creates expectations about what will happen in the future. Such expectations influence current progress toward an effective decision. Poole (1983b) identified three aspects of a group's history that affect how decisions develop. One aspect pertains to how *involved* members are in the group. Low levels of involvement indicate an individualistic, competitive climate. Higher levels of involvement indicate that members are more dependent on one another. This is typified by a more cooperative climate of decision making. A second factor of a group's history relates to their beliefs about *leadership*. Who the leader is, whether leadership changes over time, and the functions of the leader are relevant concerns. The third factor involves *procedural norms*. A group develops rules, procedures, and roles for guiding its work.

Poole's multiple sequence model of group decisions has emerged as an elaborate and sophisticated explanation of communication and group decision making. The idea that there are three interlocking tracks of activity involved in group decision making is a powerful concept, especially when combined with the concepts of breakpoints and prerequisites.

SUMMARY

This chapter examined communication in the small-group context—discussions involving three to approximately fifteen members. The problem-solving group is the one studied most by communication scholars. The kinds of roles that people take in groups are task roles, group building/maintenance roles, and individual roles. Leadership behaviors needed in problem-solving groups include task behaviors, procedural behaviors, and interpersonal relationship behaviors. Conflict in group communication can be either constructive or destructive; argumentation is essential for constructive conflict. Conformity is a frequent outcome of group communication; two types of conformity are public compliance and private acceptance. Group pressure creates conformity because of the need to belong, the reference function of groups, the influence of group attractiveness, and the desire for group maintenance.

Three theories of group communication were discussed in some detail. Hirokawa's functional theory of group decision quality attempts to explain effective and ineffective group decisions according to the communication that takes place in the group. The theory posits critical functions groups need to fulfill to reach a quality decision. Janis's theory of groupthink also addresses decision quality. The theory identifies the conditions that encourage groupthink, its symptoms, and consequences; it also suggests methods for controlling groupthink. Poole's multiple sequence model of group decisions explores the paths groups take in reaching decisions. Activity tracks are identified along with breakpoints and discussed in terms of how they develop in problem-solving discussions.

CHAPTER 5

Communication in Healthcare

The Process and Components of Human Communication

Communication is one of the most commonly used words in the English language. In our culture, there are four certainties: death, taxes, changes, and communication. Of the four, *only* changes and communication enhance our lives.

Humans must communicate with each other to survive, yet communication can be potentially harmful. If you express the wrong idea or the right idea the wrong way, it might be better not to try to communicate at all. It's unfortunate that many individuals do not know how to communicate *competently*.

Ineptness in communication is rooted in a lack of understanding of what communication *is* and how it *works*. This chapter considers the foundation for developing an understanding of communication. First, *communication versus communications* will be defined. Second, the three types of communication will be discussed. And third, the two models of communication will be considered.

From *Applied Communication for Health Professionals* by E. Phillips Polack, Virginia P. Richmond, James C. McCroskey. Copyright © 2008 by Kendall Hunt Publishing Company. Reprinted by permission.

DEFINITIONS OF COMMUNICATION

Communication has different meanings for different people. "Communicate" means whatever people who use it think it means. Most people define "communication" in two different ways:

1. Communication is defined by McCroskey and Richmond in their book *Fundamentals of Human Communication: An Interpersonal Perspective* (1996) as "a *process* of a source stimulating meaning in the mind of a receiver by means of verbal and nonverbal messages." For the purposes of this book, this will be our definition of communication. Furthermore, **medical communication** in this text refers to communication between health provider and patient or colleague (an interpersonal perspective). Among the many things that increased communication competency will do are the following:
   - Increase your personal job satisfaction
   - Let patients know that you care

- Reduce costs
- Reduce liability
- Increase efficiency

2. **Communications** is the *technology* of moving messages over time and distance, such as by radio, television, print journalism, and the Internet. The plural "s" in "communications" refers to technology. Communications emphasizes the *exchange of messages*.

This section concerns communication, and communication emphasizes meaning. McCroskey and Richmond (1996) identify four critical components of communication:

1. *Process*—something that is ongoing. Here's an example: If you were to get into an argument with your friend and you stop the verbal communication but go out of the room and slam the door, the words stop but the process continues.
2. *Meaning*—the ideas or intents of the communication. Ideas or intents occur in the brain, and the words that express the ideas or intents are symbols. The symbols will have different meanings for different individuals. For instance, you might use the word "nice" to tell another that you approve of how he looks, or you might say, "Nice," after your friend spills her coffee. Your sarcastic tone of voice in the second example gives the word a completely different meaning.
3. *Verbal communication*—the words (speech that we use) are organized according to syntax (a connected or orderly system—the *sequence*) and grammar (word functions and relationships in the sentence—the *rules*).
4. *Nonverbal communication* (eliminates words)—all other facets of the communication process after eliminating words. In his book *Kinesics in Context* (1970), Birdwhistell has estimated that the percentage of the message transfer can be as high as 95% of the message, depending on source and receiver. In the example of the word "nice," attaching a pleasant or sarcastic smile to the message greatly changes the meaning. **Gestures** (nonverbal messages) generally do not carry across cultures. In cross-cultural communication, the probability of nonverbal failure is high. In a famous example from the 1950s, then—Vice President Richard Nixon, debarking from a plane in Latin America, was asked by a reporter about his flight. Mr. Nixon gave the nonverbal okay sign, making a circle with his thumb and index finger.

The gesture, unfortunately, is the Latin American equivalent to an extended middle finger in the United States. This caused great turmoil at the time, generating front-page newspaper coverage worldwide.

In the 20th century, scholars began the study of dyads (two people) as well as small group dynamics. Prior to the mid-20th century, public speaking (speaking to a mass audience of 25 or more) and classical rhetoric (communication intended to persuade based on the teachings of Aristotle and Plato) were the major thrusts of communication education.

David Berlo of Michigan State University, author of *The Process of Communication* (1960), founded the first Communication Arts Department in the early 1950s. This department was established out of the disciplines of classical rhetoric (qualitative) and social psychology (quantitative). The term "communicator" is attributable to the media. The first person referred to as "the communicator" was Dave Garroway, host of NBC's *Today* show, which first aired in 1952. In the 1980s, President Ronald Reagan was lauded as "the Great Communicator" for his public speaking ability and his talent at getting people to understand his political messages.

THE THREE MAJOR TYPES OF COMMUNICATION

Accidental Communication

Accidental or unintentional communication happens when you do not know or realize that you are communicating. With accidental communication, other people attribute meaning to our communication. Here's an example of accidental communication: Imagine that you developed a nosebleed in church and had to leave during the sermon. Some churchgoers might think you took issue with the preacher's words, when in fact you were just leaving in search of first aid.

Our body language can communicate powerfully. Standing too close or too far away from another person can send signals of aggression or disinterest. In *The Silent Language* (1959), E. T. Hall refers to the importance of the nonverbal dimension of space. In Latin America, the established conversational distance is about 18 inches, whereas most people in North America consider 4 feet a comfortable distance. Thus, were you to talk to a Latin American at the 4-foot distance, he or she may *accidentally* perceive this as coldness and unfriendliness on your part, whereas you *accidentally* might perceive the Latin American standing 18 inches from your face as pushy and aggressive. What seems natural to one culture may be unnatural to another culture.

Expressive Communication

The second type of communication is **expressive,** and it is defined by McCroskey and Richmond (1996) as "characterized by messages that express how the sender feels at 'a given time.'" Expressive communication may have either a positive or negative affect. For instance, if you miss when drawing blood, you might say, "Whoops." In expressive communication, we can either reword our comment or regulate our voice and movements to convey another emotional state. Watzlawick, Beavin, and Jackson (1967) divide this type of message into two levels: content and relational. The content level of the message is what we have said. It is the words that compose the message. The rational level of the message is the emotional expression of how we feel about the other person or our relationship with that other person.

Rhetorical Communication

McCroskey and Richmond (1996) define **rhetorical communication** as having a specific goal in mind. It is the most common type of communication and represents the majority of our interactions. A familiar example is the State of the Union message given each year by the President of the United States in an effort to influence and/or persuade. "Influence" and "persuasion" are very different terms. When you influence someone, you cause the person to alter his or her thinking or behavior. This may occur because of accidental, expressive, or rhetorical communication. On the other hand, when you persuade someone, this is done with *conscious* intent and always involves rhetorical communication in an effort to alter thinking or behavior.

McCroskey and Richmond (1996) further advise that people from birth to age 5 years get information through their parents and child care providers. From ages 5 through 8 years, the majority of information comes from teachers, television, and the Internet, and beyond 8 years of age, the majority of information comes from peers.

MODEL OF COMMUNICATION

The Rhetorical (One-Way) Communication Model

The rhetorical (one-way) model of communication (McCroskey, 1993) illustrates intentional communication. This model includes three elements: source, channel, and receiver. The source and receiver are constant, not interchangeable.

Prior to initiating communication, a source carries on what is known as **"encoding"** this is the process of conceiving an idea, determining your intent, and selecting the meaning you wish to express. This encoded message is then transferred through a channel. The channel is any of the five senses (hearing, sight, smell, taste, and touch). This encoded message must be designed such that it can create a message that is adaptable to the receiver. The receiver then decodes the message, interpreting and evaluating the source's message. In fact, the subsequent thoughts and actions of the receiver are the meaning (**decoding**) that the source wished to create.

One relevant element in rhetorical (one-way) communication and interpersonal (two-way) communication is **noise.** This is defined (McCroskey & Richmond, 1996) as any physical or psychological stimulus that distracts the receiver from focusing on the communication process. For example, noise can be as literal as a dog barking in the background while you are speaking to another. Noise can also be psychological. For instance, if your significant other speaks to you while you are watching a football game, you may be psychologically distracted by the game.

In summary, rhetorical communication is a one-way process whereby the source encodes a message that is sent through a channel (any of the five senses) to a receiver, who listens to the verbal or nonverbal message; the receiver is responsible for decoding the message. All of this can be derailed or distracted predicated on the principle of noise.

The Interpersonal (Two-Way) Model of Communication

The interpersonal (two-way) model of communication was first depicted by McCroskey, Larson, and Knapp (1971). **Interpersonal communication** is communication that occurs between two people.

The most important element of this type of communication is that it is two-way, with the source (sender) becoming the receiver and vice versa. The same components of encoding, transmitting through a channel, and decoding occur, but the process is perpetually cyclical. This means the person who starts out as the receiver is unlikely to remain only a receiver in the communication; at some point, he or she will become a source (sender).

Face-to-face communication (FTF) is the preferred form of human communication. In any communication scenario, group size affects the communication. In a dyad (two people), communication is quite simple, so we frequently use the interpersonal model of communication. The source and receiver are interchangeable. In a larger group, the number of channels is multiplied, and the individual tends to become more of a receiver than a source. The less the source time involved, the greater the receiver time. As the size of a conversational group enlarges, either the group divides into dyads or someone assumes a position as group leader.

REFERENCES

Berlo, D. K. (1960). *The process of communication.* New York: Holt, Rinehart & Winston.

Birdwhistell, R. (1970). *Kinesics in context.* Philadelphia: University of Pennsylvania Press.

Hall, E. T. (1959). *The Silent Language.* Greenwich, CT: Fawcett Publications.

McCroskey, J. C. (1993). *An introduction to rhetorical communication* (6th ed.). Englewood Cliffs, NJ: Prentice Hall.

McCroskey, J. C., Larson, C. E., & Knapp, M. L. (1971). *An introduction to interpersonal communication.* Englewood Cliffs, NJ: Prentice Hall.

McCroey, J. C., & Richmond, V. P. (1996). *Fundamentals of human communication: An interpersonal perspective.* Prospect Heights, IL: Waveland Press, Inc.

Watzlawick, P., Beavin, J., & Jackson, D. D. (1967). *Pragmatics of human communication.* New York: W. W. Norton & Co.

Communication Skills

INTRODUCTION

When companies expand overseas and convert their slogans from English to the local language or vice versa, it can be downright hilarious. For example, Electrolux, which is a Scandinavian vacuum manufacturer, used the following in an American ad campaign: "Nothing sucks like Electrolux." Needless to say, it was pulled after two days. In Taiwan, the translation of the Pepsi slogan "Come alive with the Pepsi generation" came out "Pepsi will bring your ancestors back from the dead." In Chinese, the Kentucky Fried Chicken slogan, "Finger lickin' good" translated as "Eat your fingers off." When General Motors introduced the Chevy Nova in South America, it was unaware that *no va* means "It won't go" in Spanish. After the company figured out why the car wasn't selling, it changed the name to "Caribe" for its Spanish-language markets. Ford had

a similar problem when the Pinto flopped. The company found out that *Pinto* was Brazilian slang for "Tiny male genitals."

Communication, or rather miscommunication, can be a great source of stress. It's estimated that the average person spends three-quarters or approximately 75 percent of his or her waking day communicating in some way. Over a lifetime, communicating with others takes up a huge portion of our lives. Yet, how many of us receive some type of education or training on how to communicate effectively and how to resolve conflict effectively? Fortunately or unfortunately, we learn communication skills from our parents and the environment in which we were raised. For many people, these environments were not conducive to learning effective communication skills.

Similarly, our patterns of communication are influenced by our culture. It's thought that Americans tend to be indirect. Obviously, differences in communication patterns exist throughout various regions of the United States. For example, those on the East Coast may be more direct than those on the West

From *Stress Management for Healthy Living* by Kristine Fish. Copyright © 2010 by Kristine Fish. Reprinted by permission.

Coast. But generally speaking, it's thought that Americans need to be more direct. **Miscommunication** results when people are indirect. Even within the same culture or the same region, people grow up in different homes with different families with different ways of communicating and resolving conflict, which often result in miscommunications and misunderstandings, which result in stress.

What percentage of your stress stems from other people? It may vary at different points in your life with different people in your life. But my guess is that because we spend so much of our lives communicating in some way with other people, it's inevitable that stress resulting from miscommunication will comprise a somewhat significant portion of the total stress that we experience in our lifetime. Also, the importance of learning and practicing good communication skills is illustrated by the fact that lack of conflict resolution skills is cited as the most common reason for violence and divorce.

Results of one study indicate that one out of every five messages is not completely or accurately understood, even among good communicators. Operation of a nuclear submarine requires zero tolerance for mistakes. As a result, every instruction that the captain gives is repeated verbatim. Although we don't live on a nuclear submarine and risk catastrophic consequences if we don't communicate effectively, significant problems can result when we don't communicate and/or receive messages accurately.

Even though other people may play a role in your level of stress, having people in your life is not only inevitable, but it's actually healthy. Lack of social contacts was found to be a stronger risk factor for colds than was smoking, low vitamin C intake, or even elevated stress hormones. Researchers say that interacting with a broad array of individuals likely tempers a person's physical response to stressful situations. So it's good to have people in your life—but sometimes it can be frustrating.

NONVERBAL COMMUNICATION

It's thought that 90 percent of communication is nonverbal. Studies have shown that when a contradiction occurs between verbal and nonverbal messages, people are more inclined to believe nonverbal cues. Nonverbal communication wins just about every time. For example, if you ask someone, "How are you?" and the other person responds with "Fine!" in a rough, abrasive tone, you're probably not going

to believe the person is fine. Verbal communication refers only to the actual words spoken, but nonverbal communication includes the following:

- *Touch*—any type of physical contact such as touching someone's arm as you express concern for him or her.
- *Adaptors*—body language such as crossing your arms.
- *Regulators*—body movements used to regulate or manipulate conversation such as eye movements, head movements, or shifting your weight from foot to foot.
- *Affect displays*—facial expressions.
- *Paralanguage*—the pitch, tone, and volume of your voice and the rate at which you speak.

Of these five types of nonverbal communication, paralanguage is perhaps the most influential. Have you ever been offended by someone not because of what was said but how he or she said it? The very same words can have very different meanings. For example, think of how many different ways the sentence "I'm going to the store" can be said. You can express anger, excitement, depression, and other emotions by saying the exact same words. Paralanguage, more so than the other types of nonverbal communication, can easily cause offense and be a source of stress. Someone once recommended that we always keep our words soft and sweet, just in case we have to eat them.

LISTENING SKILLS

In addition to paralanguage, lack of effective listening skills can cause misunderstanding and be a source of stress. It's thought that the average person has terrible listening skills. Most of us are thinking of what we're going to say back to the person who is talking to us, which impedes our ability to listen. Here's a list of just a few recommendations for improving your listening skills:

- *Assume the role of the listener:* See it as a role; you are not the speaker, you are the listener. Your job is to listen.
- *Maintain eye contact:* Have you ever tried to talk with someone who is looking off in the distance or over your shoulder? It's frustrating.
- *Avoid prejudice:* Be careful of forming opinions and judgments about what the person is saying. Just listen .

- *Use "minimal encouragers"*: This refers to saying "really, ahh, huh, mmm." Have you ever talked to someone on the phone and you haven't heard anything in a while, so in the middle of your sentence, you ask, "Are you there?" Females typically tend to use more minimal encouragers than males.
- *Be prepared to paraphrase*: Listen to someone as if you were going to paraphrase what was said when he or she is done talking. It's amazing how much better you listen.

GENDER AND COMMUNICATION

Another source of stress pertaining to communication is the major differences in the way males and females typically communicate. All or some of these differences may be considered stereotypes. Nevertheless, studies have shown that differences in the way that males and females are socialized result in differences in the way the genders communicate. However, everyone is different. You may know people who don't exhibit typical characteristics that match their gender. But again, studies have shown that most males and females tend to communicate differently.

Communication styles differ between men and women in three ways: content or what they talk about, body language, and vocal characteristics.

Females

Studies have shown that females speak to generate involvement, have more direct eye contact, and tend to face the person head on. Their hand movements when they talk are smaller and closer to their body. They tend to talk faster than males, but they have excellent articulation. Obviously, females have a higher pitch, and they also tend to use rich descriptive language and provide empathy when they hear someone complain. The way females feel closer to another person or feel more emotionally intimate with others is to talk about their feelings or to disclose their thoughts and emotions.

Males

Predominant themes in conversations among males are sports, mechanical things, and inanimate objects. They have more of a tendency to interrupt, change the topic, and ask more questions. Males tend to dominate in a group setting such as a business meeting. They talk more slowly but are less articulate. They have less eye contact and provide less verbal and nonverbal encouragement, and they tend to want to provide solutions when someone complains to them. Males feel closer to others by doing something with them, such as biking.

CONFLICT RESOLUTION STYLES

There are a variety of conflict resolution styles. Some of you may use a combination of them, depending on the type of conflict or the person with whom you're having a conflict. But most of us have a predominant style that we typically use.

Withdrawal refers to the style in which a person avoids conflict altogether. Any hint of conflict or confrontation and he or she is out of there. This conflict resolution style is most similar to the anger mismanagement style of a somatizer.

Surrender, somewhat similar to withdrawal, refers to someone who just gives in to avoid conflict: "Okay, whatever you say." People who surrender just want to do whatever they have to do to keep the peace.

Persuasion refers to the style in which people do whatever is needed to get a point across and to persuade the other person to agree with them.

Hostile aggression refers to the style in which a person uses intimidation to get his or her point across. An exploder, a person who uses the type of anger mismanagement in which he or she loses his or her temper, probably uses hostile aggression to resolve conflict.

Dialogue refers to the style in which a person exchanges opinions, attitudes, facts, and ideas. The person is open minded and willing to see both sides and detaches him- or herself from emotions that might result in becoming defensive. He or she looks at the situation from the outside and is completely objective. The person looks at what needs to be done to resolve the conflict. He or she doesn't take things personally. This is a healthy way of resolving conflict.

CONFLICT RESOLUTION RECOMMENDATIONS

There are differences in communication styles between males and females, between individuals among different cultures, between individuals who grew up in different environments, and between individuals with different personalities. What do we do about these differences, especially during conflicts? Probably the greatest source of stress pertaining to communication is ineffective skills for resolving conflict. John Lund, a professor of marriage and family therapy at Brigham Young University, offers the following recommendations whenever you have a criticism to make.

- *Say at least one positive for every negative:* Some experts recommend two positives for every negative or the use of the sandwich approach in which you start off with something positive, which represents a piece of bread, then provide the constructive feedback, which represents the meat, and then end with another positive or piece of bread. Lund relayed a story of a woman who had almost lost her children and husband in a divorce because the judge heard a recording that her husband had taped of her screaming. The judge determined that she was an unfit mother after listening to only a few minutes of the recording because her words were considered to be emotional abuse. Lund challenged her to refrain from saying anything critical for one week.

    After a week, she came to him crying because she had nothing to say. For the entire week, she was silent. She didn't realize how much criticizing she was used to doing. She admitted after this week's experiment that she didn't know how to love. The marriage was salvaged because she learned to stop criticizing.

- *Bring at least one solution for every criticism:* Don't just complain and criticize. Offer a suggestion or possible solution. When I served as department chair, I was amazed at how many complaints I received on a daily basis. Complaints from everyone: students, staff, faculty, and part-time instructors. I quickly realized that I would go crazy if I had to come up with a solution to every complaint. So I began asking people to provide at least two possible scenarios that would resolve the problem or the source of their complaint. It was interesting that some didn't want to come up with solutions themselves. They just wanted to complain. Before bringing any type of criticism or complaint to your roommate, significant other, professor, or anyone else, it's always a good idea to offer a possible solution rather than just complain.

- *Begin with "May I offer a suggestion?"* If your partner knows that this phrase means you'd like to offer a bit of constructive feedback, then your partner can decide if this is a good time to hear it and vice versa. If you are not in the mood to hear any type of criticism at the moment and you know you'd just get defensive, then feel free to say "not right now," but make sure you offer a suggested alternate time. Respect boundaries. Timing is important. But starting out with "May I make a suggestion" is much less offensive than "You need to . . ."

- *Use the language of "request and respect":* Don't say "you should" or "you need to." Instead, use "I would really appreciate it if you would . . . ." Communication should be respectful but very clear. Being disrespectful in any way impedes resolution of the problem. If you truly want to resolve the problem, then you have to refrain from being disrespectful, as difficult as that might be at times. Many people think that to get their point across, they have to be aggressive, rude, or abrasive. This is completely false. You can most definitely get your point across and be very clear without being rude. If your partner, whether it be your friend, boss, co-worker, or significant other, does not use the language of request and respect and acts and communicates in a rude manner, you still have the choice to respond in the language of request and respect. By being respectful, you maintain your level of credibility, and oftentimes the person will feel bad and see that he or she was inappropriate, especially if you keep your cool. You have 100 percent control in 50 percent of a relationship.

- *Take a time out and a time in:* If you don't feel that you're able to maintain control of your emotions, it may be better to take a time out and talk about it later. However, you don't see a basketball team take a time-out without the clock ticking, indicating how much time is left. Can you imagine if there were no time limits on those time outs during games? If you need to take a time out and you really don't want to discuss an issue at the moment, you need to let the person know when you will be ready to discuss it: "I'm sorry but I can't talk about this right now. It's a bad time for me. How about after dinner tonight?" Make sure that you're specific and clear as to when you'd like the time in to occur.

- *Use the mirror technique:* As noted, it's estimated that one in five messages that you communicate is not completely or accurately understood. There is a technique that has been shown to result in only

1.5 errors on average out of 100 communication messages and involves paraphrasing what the other person said. The mirror technique is basically paraphrasing what your partner is saying in a conflict situation. A large percentage of the frustration that comes from arguing with someone is feeling as if he or she is not listening, which results in your not feeling validated. People often repeat what they've said multiple times during an argument because they feel as if the other person isn't listening. And actually the other person probably isn't listening if he or she is not using the mirror technique. But if you and the other person know that you're going to have to paraphrase back what each of you has said, you're both going to listen better. Having someone paraphrase back to you what you said without including his or her own personal opinions and vice versa can be incredibly validating and provides a more conducive environment for resolving conflict. Here's how it works.

1. You express your complaint or concern for 30 to 60 seconds to your partner, definitely no more than one minute at a time or else it's difficult for the person to paraphrase what you've said because he or she can't remember everything. If you're not able to get everything out in 60 seconds, you can speak again in a minute. But it's important to speak for no more than one minute at a time to prevent the other person from tuning you out. Sometimes it takes much less than a minute. For example, "I'm really frustrated because you ate all of my ice cream."

2. Then the other person paraphrases back to you what you said, includes his or her interpretation of your feelings, and ends with "Is that right?" "So what I heard you say is you don't like it when I eat your ice cream. And you seem pretty irritated when I do this. Is that right?" If you need to clarify, do so at this point. "Yes, I'm frustrated that you ate my ice cream, but I want to make sure you understand that the real reason that I'm so frustrated is that this is the fifth time you've done this and I've asked you not to do this several times now. I feel like you disregard and disrespect my feelings."

3. Then your partner needs to *paraphrase again until he or she gets it right*. It's important that the paraphraser does not include any of his or her opinions while in the paraphaser's role. "So

what I heard you say is you don't like it when I eat your ice cream. And you seem pretty irritated when I do this. *But you ate my ice cream before and I didn't get mad at you.*" As soon as the paraphraser includes his or her opinion while in the paraphraser role, it invalidates and defeats the purpose of the mirror technique. The paraphraser will have a chance to get out of the paraphraser's role and express his or her opinions. But it's essential that the paraphraser's primary responsibility is to understand the other person's opinion and not express his or her opinion while in the paraphraser's role.

4. Then, if necessary, *explore mutually acceptable solutions*. This technique may sound complicated, but it really works as long as both people are willing to incorporate the technique. Understanding and agreement are not necessarily synonymous terms. Understanding does not necessarily result in agreement. You can disagree with something, but it's important that you understand the other person's perception. Agree to disagree without being disagreeable. Many people forget that last part—without being disagreeable. They don't know how to agree to disagree.

- *Be a **content communicator**:* A couple was on a road trip together out in the middle of the desert with the windows rolled down. The woman says to the man, "It's really hot, dear" because she wanted him to turn on the air conditioning. The man, thinking he was being an empathetic listener, says, "It really is." And they drive on. She was horrified that he didn't turn the air conditioner on. She thought she'd give him one more chance. They were driving out in the middle of nowhere when the woman sees a convenience store up ahead. She says to the man "Honey, I'm really thirsty." In her mind, if he doesn't stop, she thinks, "he doesn't love me; he never cared." He was tried and convicted in the court of her mind. She thinks that she shouldn't have to tell him. He should know her well enough to read her mind. She believes if you have to ask, it doesn't count. A content communicator would say, "Can we stop so that I can get a drink at the store up ahead?" Being a content communicator means that you say what you mean and mean what you say. There are no expectations of someone being able to read your mind. I'm amazed at the number of women who dig their heels into their ground and still believe that their partner should be able to read their mind. Remember, women tend to rely on nonverbal communication more so than men. Expecting another woman to read your mind might work, but it's really not fair to expect a man, who has been socialized and therefore wired completely differently. And it doesn't take that much more time and energy to simply say, "Let's stop at the convenience store up ahead so that I can get a drink," instead of "Honey, I'm really thirsty."

REFERENCES

Burley-Allen, M. *Listening: The Forgotten Skill.* New York: John Wiley & Sons, 1995.

Seaward, B. L. *Managing Stress: Principles and Strategies for Health and Well-Being,* 5th ed. Sudbury, MA: Jones & Bartlett, 2006.

Tannen, D. *You Just Don't Understand: Women and Men in Conversation.* New York: Quill. 2001.

CHAPTER 6

Problem Solving Strategies in Healthcare

Critical Thinking

DEVELOPING CRITICAL SKILLS FOR THE TWENTY-FIRST CENTURY

What are we to believe? What should we accept with reservations, and what should we dismiss outright? As we gather information about the world via the media (e.g., television, radio, the Internet, and newspapers and magazines), we tend to take much of the information at face value, ignoring the fact that the information has been selected and organized (shaped and edited) by the person or organization presenting it. People are often lulled into a false sense of security, believing that the sources of information they are basing their decisions on are objective and truthful (Chaffee, 1998). Discovering the answers to the six important questions that reporters are trained to answer near the beginning of every news article—who, what, where, when, why, and how—is not enough to allow us to think critically about complex and sometimes controversial topics. To engage in thinking at this higher level, one needs to know how to ask questions and think independently.

The authors of this chapter view critical thinking developmentally as a set of complex thinking skills that can be improved through knowledge and guided practice. Thinking skills are categorized in the problem-solving/decision-making set of life-skills necessary for information seeking. These skills include information assessment and analysis; problem identification, solution, implementation, and evaluation; goal setting; systematic planning and forecasting; and conflict resolution. Presented in this chapter are developmental thinking models, critical thinking and problem-solving models, and information about the construction and evaluation of an argument.

THINKING AS A DEVELOPMENTAL PROCESS

Cognitive psychologists study the development and organization of knowledge and the role it plays in various mental activities (e.g., reading, writing, decision making, and problem solving). What is knowledge? Where it is stored? How do you construct mental representations of your world? The personal answers to these and other questions are often found for the first time in college when students focus their attention on what they know and how they know it.

Models of Knowledge

Different forms of knowledge interact when you reason and construct a mental representation of the situation before you. Joanne Kurfiss (1988) wrote about the following three kinds of knowledge.

- **Declarative knowledge** is knowing facts and concepts. Kurfiss recognizes the considerable amount of declarative knowledge that students acquire through their college courses. To move students to a higher level of thinking, instructors generally ask students to write analytical essays, instead of mere summaries, to explain the knowledge they have acquired in the course.
- **Procedural knowledge,** or **strategic knowledge** is knowing how to use declarative knowledge to do something (e.g., interpret textbooks, study, navigate the Internet, and find a major).

- **Metacognition** is knowing what knowledge to use to control one's situation (e.g., how to make plans, ask questions, analyze the effectiveness of learning strategies, initiate change). If students' metacognitive skills are not well developed, students may not be able to use the full potential of their knowledge when studying in college.

William Perry

You may have read about the developmental theorist William Perry. In his research on college-age students, Perry distinguished a series of stages that students pass through as they move from simple to complex levels of thinking. Basically, they move from **dualism,** the simplest stage, where knowledge is viewed as a factual quality dispensed by authorities (professors), to **multiplicity** in which the student recognizes the complexity of knowledge (e.g., he or she understands that there is more than one perspective of the bombing of Hiroshima or the role of the United States in the Vietnam war) and believes knowledge to be subjective, to **relativism** where the student reaches an understanding that some views make greater sense than other views. Relativism is reflected in situations where a student has made a commitment to the particular view they have constructed of the world, also known as *Weltanschauung.* Constructing a personal *critical epistemology* is an essential developmental task for undergraduates, according to Perry (Chaffee, 1998).

Bloom's Taxonomy of Thinking and Learning

Benjamin Bloom (1956) and his associates at the University of Chicago developed a classification system, or taxonomy, to explain how we think and learn (see Figure 6.1). The taxonomy consists of six levels of thinking arranged in a hierarchy, beginning with simple cognitive tasks (knowledge) and moving up to more complex thinking (evaluation). Thinking at each level is dependent on thinking skills at lower levels.

One of the reasons that college students often experience difficulty learning and studying during their first semester is that the learning and study strategies from high school are not necessarily effective in the new setting. In high school you are gener-

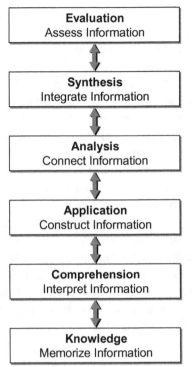

Figure 6.1   Bloom's Hierarchy of Thinking

ally asked to memorize, comprehend, and interpret information. In college you are asked to do all that and more. To be successful in a college setting, you need to learn how to apply, analyze, synthesize, and evaluate information. Let's look at Bloom's six: levels of learning and thinking.

Knowledge Level.   If you are cramming for a test, chances are good that you are thinking at the knowledge level, the lowest level of thinking. You are basically attempting to memorize a lot of information in a short amount of time. If you are asked on the test to identify, name, select, define, or list particular bits of information, you might do okay, but you will most likely forget most of the information soon after taking the test.

Comprehension Level.   When you are classifying, describing, discussing, explaining, and recognizing information, you are in the process of interpreting information. At the bottom of your lecture notes for the day, see if you can summarize your notes using your own words. In doing so, you can develop a deeper understanding of the material just covered in class.

Application Level.   At this third level of thinking, you are constructing knowledge by taking previously learned information and applying it in a new and different way to solve problems. Whenever you use a formula or a theory to solve a problem, you are thinking at the application level. Some words used to describe how you process information at this level are *illustrate, demonstrate,* and *apply*. To increase thinking at the application level, develop the habit of thinking of examples to illustrate concepts presented in class or during reading. Be sure to include the examples in your notations in your books and notes.

Analysis Level.   When you analyze information, you break the information down into parts and then look at the relationships among the parts. In your literature class, if you read two plays from different time periods and then compare and contrast them in terms of style and form, you are analyzing. When you analyze, you connect pieces of information. You *discriminate, correlate, classify,* and *infer*.

Synthesis Level.   When you are synthesizing information, you are bringing together all the bits of information that you have analyzed to create a new pattern or whole. When you synthesize, you *hypothesize, predict, generate,* and *integrate*. Innovative ideas often emerge at the synthesis level of thinking.

Evaluation Level.   This is the highest level of thinking according to Bloom's taxonomy. When you evaluate, you judge the validity of the information. You may be evaluating opinions ("Is that person really an expert?") or biases.

Answer the following questions to test your understanding of Bloom's taxonomy. According to Bloom's taxonomy of thinking, which level of thinking would you be engaging in if you were asked to

- Read an article about an upcoming candidate in a local election and then summarize the candidate's characteristics?
- View a video about hate and prejudice and then write an essay about how you can confront hate and prejudice on a personal level?
- Determine the most effective way for you to study?
- Identify and define the parts of the forebrain?
- Judge a new campus parking policy created by your college's parking services?

MODELS OF CRITICAL THINKING/ PROBLEM SOLVING

Critical Thinking

One of the primary objectives of a college education is to develop the skills necessary to become an autonomous, independent learner. Critical thinking prepares you to be an independent thinker. To ensure that you are thinking critically, you can follow the CRITICAL model developed by the authors (Glauser & Ginter, 1995). This model identifies important steps and key ideas in critical thinking: construction, refocus, identify, think through, insight, conclusions, accuracy, and lens.

Construction.   Each of us constructs a unique view of the world. Our construction, or perception, of the world is based on our thoughts and beliefs. Our cultural background influences our perceptions, and they form the basis of our assumptions. For example, you might assume that a college education can help you to get a better job. How do you know this? Maybe you know this because a parent or teacher told you so. If this is the only bit of information on which you are basing your assumption about the value of a college education, you have not engaged in critical thinking. If you had engaged in critical thinking, you would have analyzed and synthesized information that you gathered about the benefits of a college education. If you have based your decision to attend this college on good critical thinking, then you will know why you are here and will more likely be motivated to graduate.

Perceptions of information, behaviors, and situations are often based on unexamined assumptions that are inaccurate and sketchy. The first step in this model is to investigate personal underlying biases that are inherent in your assumptions about any issue before you. For example, let us say that you are with some friends and the topic of surrogate motherhood comes up. Maybe you have already formed an opinion about the issue. This opinion could be based on strong critical thinking, but if not, then your opinion is merely a strong, personal feeling. If you choose to look at surrogate motherhood from a critical-thinking perspective, you would begin by examining your own thoughts and beliefs about motherhood and surrogacy. No matter what issue is before you (e.g., racism, abortion, euthanasia, genetic engineering), the process is the same; begin by examining your own assumptions. As you do this,

look for biases and other patterns of thinking that have become cemented over time and are influencing the way you view the issue.

Refocus.   Once you have acknowledged some of your own biases, refocus your attention so you can hear alternative viewpoints. Refocus by reading additional information, talking to people with opposing viewpoints, or maybe watching a movie or a video. You are trying to see other people's perspectives. Read carefully, and listen carefully with the intent to learn. Can you think of any books that you have read or movies that have influenced the way you see a particular issue?

To illustrate the effect of refocusing, list three sources of additional information (e.g., book, movie, another person, newspaper, or experience) that changed your mind about something important to you. Explain how it changed you.

1. _____
   _____
   _____
2. _____
   _____
   _____
3. _____
   _____
   _____

Identify.   Identifying core issues and information is the third step of critical thinking. After you have gathered all your additional information representing different viewpoints, think over the information carefully. Are there any themes that emerge? What does the terminology related to the issue tell you? Look at all the facts and details. We all try to make sense out of what we hear and see by arranging information into a pattern, a story that seems reasonable. There is a tendency to arrange the information to fit our perceptions and beliefs. When we engage in critical thinking, we are trying to make sense of all the pieces, not just the ones that happen to fit our own preconceived pattern.

Think Through.   The fourth step of critical thinking requires that you think through all the information gathered. The task is to distinguish between what is fact and what is fiction and what is relevant and not relevant. Examine premises and decide if they are logically valid. Look for misinformation. Maybe you have gathered inaccurate facts and figures. Check the sources for reliability. Asking questions is a large part of good critical thinking.

This step of the model is where you analyze and synthesize information. You are continually focusing your attention in and out, similar to the way you might focus a camera. This step of the critical-thinking process can be very creative. You are using both parts of the brain. The right brain is being speculative, suspending judgment, and challenging definitions. The left brain is analyzing the information received in a more traditional style, thinking logically and sequentially. While thinking critically, have you detected any over-generalizations (e.g., women are more emotional and less rational than men are) or over-simplifications (e.g., the high dropout rate at the local high school is due to an increase in single-parent families)?

Insight. Once key issues have been identified and analyzed, it is time to develop some insight into some of the various perspectives on the issue. Sometimes some of the best insights come when you can sit back and detach yourself from all the information you have just processed. Often new meanings will emerge that provide a new awareness. You might find that you have developed some empathy for others that may not have been there before.

When you hear the term "broken home," what images do you conjure up? How do you think a child who resides with a single parent or alternates between divorced parents' homes feels when hearing that term applied to his or her situation? A lot of assumptions are embedded in such concepts.

Conclusions. If you do not have sufficient evidence to support a decision, suspend judgment until you do. An important tenet of critical thinking is not to jump to conclusions. If you do, you may find that you have a fallacy in your reasoning. A **fallacy** is an instance of incorrect reasoning. Maybe you did not have sufficient evidence to support your decision to major in biology, or maybe your conclusions about the issue of euthanasia do not follow logically from your premise. Also look at the conclusions you have drawn, and ask yourself if they have any implications that you might need to rethink? Do you need to consider alternative interpretations of the evidence?

Accuracy. You are not through thinking! In addition to looking for fallacies in your reasoning, you also need to consider some other things.

- Know the difference between reasoning and rationalizing. Which thinking processes are your conclusions based on?
- Know the difference between what is true and what seems true based on the emotional attachment you have to your ideas and beliefs.
- Know the difference between opinion and fact. Facts can be proven; opinions cannot.

Lens. In this last step of critical thinking, you have reached the understanding that most issues can be viewed from multiple perspectives. These perspectives form a lens that offers a more encompassing view of the world around you. Remember that there are usually many solutions to a single issue.

Problem Solving

Problem solving involves critical thinking. Are problem solving and critical thinking the same? Not really. Problem solving is about having the ability and skills to apply knowledge to pragmatic problems encountered in all areas of your life. If you were trying to solve a financial problem or decide whether or not to change roommates, you probably would not need a model of thinking as extensive as the one previously described. The following steps offer an organized approach to solving less complex problems.

1. Identify the problem. Be specific and write it down.
2. Analyze the problem.
3. Identify alternative ways to solve the problem.
4. Examine alternatives.
5. Implement a solution.
6. Evaluate.

Identify the Problem. What exactly is the problem you wish to solve? Is it that your roommate is driving you crazy, or is it that you want to move into an apartment with your friend next semester? Be specific.

Analyze the Problem. Remember, analysis means looking at all the parts. It is the process by which we select and interpret information. Be careful not to be too selective or simplistic in your thinking. Look at all the facts and details. For example, suppose you want to move into an apartment with your friends. Do you need permission from anyone to do so? Can you afford to do this? Can you get a release from your dorm lease? Your answer to all the questions might be yes, with the exception of being able to afford it. You want to move, so now the problem is a financial one. You need to come up with the financial resources to follow through on your decision.

Identify Alternative Ways to Solve the Problem. Use convergent and divergent thinking. You are engaging in **convergent thinking** when you are narrowing choices to come up with the correct solution (e.g., picking the best idea out of three). You are engaging in **divergent thinking** when you are thinking in terms of multiple solutions. Mihaly Csikszentmihalyi (1996) says, "Divergent thinking leads to no agreed-upon solution. It involves fluency, or the ability to generate a great quantity of ideas; flexibility, or the ability to switch from one perspective to another; and originality in picking unusual associations of ideas" (1996, p. 60). He concludes that a person whose thinking has these qualities is likely to come up with more innovative ideas.

Brainstorming. This is a great way to generate alternative ways to solve problems. This creative problem-solving technique requires that you use both divergent and convergent thinking. Here are some steps to use if you decide to brainstorm.

- Describe the problem.
- Decide on the amount of time you want to spend brainstorming (e.g., 10 minutes).
- Relax (remember some of the best insights come in a relaxed state).
- Write down everything that comes to your mind (divergent thinking).
- Select your best ideas (convergent thinking).
- Try one out! (If it does not work, try one of the other ideas you selected.)

Students have successfully used the process of brainstorming to decide on a major, choose activities for spring break, develop topics for papers, and come up with ideas for part-time jobs. Being creative means coming up with atypical solutions to complex problems.

Examine Alternatives. Make judgments about the alternatives based on previous knowledge and the additional information you now have.

Implement a Solution. Choose one solution to your problem and eliminate the others for now. (If

this one fails, you may want to try another solution later.)

Evaluate. If the plan is not as effective as you had hoped, modify your plan or start the process over again. Also look at the criteria you used to judge your alternative solutions.

Think of a problem that you are currently dealing with. This is an opportunity to try to solve a problem using this six-step problem-solving model.

ARGUMENTS

Critical thinking involves the construction and evaluation of arguments. An **argument** is a form of thinking in which reasons (statements and facts) are given in support of a conclusion. The reasons of the argument are known as the premises. A good argument is one in which the **premises** are logical and support the conclusion. The **validity** of the argument is based on the relationship between the premises and the conclusion. If the premises are not credible or do not support the conclusion, or the conclusion does not follow from the premises, the argument is considered to be invalid or fallacious. Unsound arguments (based on fallacies) are often persuasive because they can appeal to our emotions and confirm what we want to believe to be true. Just look at commercials on television. Alcohol advertisements show that you can be rebellious, independent, and have lots of friends, fun, and excitement by drinking large quantities of alcohol—all without any negative consequences. Intelligence is reflected in the capacity to acquire and apply knowledge. Even sophisticated, intelligent people are influenced by fallacious advertising.

Invalid Arguments

It is human irrationality, not a lack of knowledge, that threatens human potential.
—Raymond Nickerson, in J. K. Kurfiss,
Critical Thinking

In the book *How to Think About Weird Things*. Theodore Schick and Lewis Vaughn (1999) suggest that you can avoid holding irrational beliefs by understanding the ways in which an argument can fail. First, an argument is fallacious if it contains **unacceptable premises** or premises that are as incredible as the claim they are supposed to support. Second, if they contain **irrelevant premises,** or premises that are not logically related to the conclusion, they are also fallacious. Third, they are fallacious if they contain **insufficient premises,** meaning that the premises do not eliminate reasonable grounds for doubt. Schick and Vaughn recommend that whenever someone presents an argument, you check to see if the premises are acceptable, relevant, and sufficient. If not, then the argument presented is not logically compelling, or valid.

Schick and Vaughn abstracted from the work of Ludwig F. Schlecht the following examples of fallacies based on illogical premises.

Unacceptable Premises

- **False dilemma** (also known as the either/or fallacy) presumes that there are only two alternatives from which to choose when in actuality there are more than two. For example: You are either with America or against us. You are not with America, therefore you are against us.
- **Begging the question** is also referred to as arguing in a circle. A conclusion is used as one of the premises. For example: "You should major in business, because my advisor says that if you do, you will be guaranteed a job." "How do you know this?" "My advisor told me that all business majors find jobs."

Irrelevant Premises

- **Equivocation** occurs when the conclusion does not follow from the premises due to using the same word to mean two different things. For example: Senator Dobbs has always been *patriotic* and shown a deep affection and respect for his country. Now, though, he is criticizing the government's foreign policy. This lack of *patriotism* makes him unworthy of reelection.
- **Appeal to the person** (ad hominem, or "to the man") occurs when a person offers a rebuttal to an argument by criticizing or denigrating its presenter rather than constructing a rebuttal based on the argument presented. As Schick and Vaughn note, "Crazy people can come up with perfectly sound arguments, and sane people can talk nonsense" (1999, p. 287).
- **Appeal to authority** is when we support our views by citing experts. If the person is truly an

expert in the field for which they are being cited, then the testimony is probably valid. How often do you see celebrities endorsing products? Is an argument valid just because someone cites an article from the *New York Times* or the *Wall Street Journal* for support?

- **Appeal to the masses** is a type of fallacy that occurs when support for the premise is offered in the form, "It must be right because everybody else does it." For example: It's okay to cheat. Every college student cheats sometime during their undergraduate years.
- **Appeal to tradition** used as an unsound premise when we argue that something is true based on an established tradition. For example: It's okay to drink large quantities of alcohol and go wild during Spring Break. It's what students have always done.
- **Appeal to ignorance** relies on claims that if no proof is offered that something is true, then it must be false, or conversely, that if no proof is offered that something is false, then it must be true. Many arguments associated with religions of the world are based on irrelevant premises that appeal to ignorance.
- **Appeal to fear** is based on a threat, or "swinging the big stick." For example: If you don't start studying now, you will never make it through college. Schick and Vaughn remind us, "Threats extort; they do not help us arrive at the truth" (1999, p. 289).

Insufficient Premises

- **Hasty generalizations** are often seen when people stereotype others. Have you noticed that most stereotypes are negative? When we describe an individual as pushy, cheap, aggressive, privileged, snobbish, or clannish and then generalize that attribute to the group we believe that person belongs to, we are committing a hasty generalization.
- **Faulty analogy** is the type of fallacy committed when there is a claim that things that have similar qualities in some respects will have similarities in other respects. For example: Dr. Smith and Dr. Wilson may both teach at the same college, but their individual philosophies about teaching and learning may be very different.
- **False cause** fallacies occur when a causal relationship is assumed despite a lack of evidence to

support the relationship. Do you have a special shirt or hat that you wear on game days to influence the odds that the team you are cheering for wins?

CLOSING REMARKS

Belgian physicist Ilya Prigogine was awarded the Nobel Prize for his theory of dissipative structures. Part of the theory "contends that friction is a fundamental property of nature and nothing grows without it—not mountains, not pearls, not people. It is precisely the quality of fragility, he says, the capacity for being shaken up, that is paradoxically the key to growth. Any structure—whether at the molecular, chemical, physical, social, or psychological level that is insulated from disturbance is also protected from change. It becomes stagnant. Any vision—or anything—that is true to life, to the imperatives of creation and evolution, will not be 'unshakable' (Levoy, 1997 p. 8).

In reference to education and learning, the philosopher Jiddu Krishnamurti said that there should be "an intent to bring about change in the mind which means you have to be extraordinarily critical. You have to learn never to accept anything which you yourself do not see clearly" (1974, p. 18). He said that education is always more than learning from books, or memorizing some facts, or the instructor transmitting information to the student. Education is about critical thinking, and critical thinking is the foundation of all learning.

Critical thinking is thinking that moves you beyond simple observations and passive reporting of those observations. It is an active, conscious, cognitive process in which there is always intent to learn. It is the process by which we analyze and evaluate information, and it is how we make good sense out of all the information that we are continually bombarded with.

Marcia Magolda believes that critical thinking fosters qualities such as maturity, responsibility, and citizenship. "Both the evolving nature of society and the student body has led to reconceptualizations of learning outcomes and processes. In a postmodern society, higher education must prepare students to

shoulder their moral and ethical responsibility to confront and wrestle with the complex problems they will encounter in today and tomorrow's world. Critical, reflective thinking skills, the ability to gather and evaluate evidence, and the ability to make one's own informed judgments are essential learning outcomes if students are to get beyond relativity to make informed judgments in a world in which multiple perspectives are increasingly interdependent and 'right action' is uncertain and often in dispute." (Magolda & Terenzini, 1999, p. 3)

REFERENCES

Bloom, B. (1956). *Taxonomy of educational objectives: The classification of educational goals. Handbook I: Cognitive domain.* London: Longmans.

Chaffee, J. (1998). *The thinker's way.* Boston: Little, Brown.

Csikszentmihalyi, M. (1996). *Creativity.* New York: Harper-Collins.

DiSpezio, M. (1998). *Challenging critical thinking puzzles.* New York: Sterling.

Glauser, A., & Ginter, E. J. (1995, October). *Beyond hate and intolerance.* Paper presented at the southeastern Conference of Counseling Center Personnel, Jekyll Island, GA.

Johnson, D., & Johnson, F. (2000). *Joining together.* Boston: Allyn and Bacon.

Krishnamurti, J. (1974). *Krishnamurti on education.* New York: Harper & Row.

Kurfiss, J. G. (1988). *Critical thinking: Theory, research, practice, and possibilities. Critical thinking, 2.* Washington, DC: ASHE-Eric Higher Education Reports.

Levoy, Gregg. (1997). *Callings.* New York: Three Rivers Press.

Magolda, M. B., & Terenzini, P. (1999). Learning and teaching in the twenty-first century: Trends and implications for practice. In C. S. Johnson & H. E. Cheatham (Eds.), *Higher education trends for the next century: A research agenda for student's success.* Retrieved November 30, 1999, from http://acpa.nche.edu/seniorscholars/trends/trends.htn

Perry, W. (1970). *Forms of intellectual and ethical development during the college years: A scheme.* New York: Holt, Rinehart and Winston.

Schick, T., & Vaughn, L. (1999). *How to Think About Weird Things: Critical Thinking for a New Age.* Mountain View, CA: Mayfield.

CHAPTER 7

Wellness/Illness

What Is "Health"?

Learning Objectives

- Define health.
- Compare healthy versus unhealthy lifestyles.
- Define quality of life.
- Compare health status globally.

Key Terms

Activities of daily living (ADLs)	Medical model	Quality of life
	Multidimensional concept	Rule-out definition
Health	Physical health	SF-36
Illness	Psychological model	Sociocultural model

HOW SHOULD WE DEFINE IT? HOW SHOULD WE MEASURE IT?

The United States fares relatively poorly when compared to other developed countries on measures of its population's health status such as life expectancy and infant mortality. On the other hand, we appear to have the best population health in the world when measured as the number of additional years someone who has reached the age of 80 can expect to live. It should be apparent that the health of a population relative to other populations in the world will be different based on which measure of "health" one uses.

The same principle holds when comparing the health of individuals. How "healthy" one person appears, or feels, relative to another person will depend on how health is defined and measured. Consider, for example, the following descriptions of six different people. Each is drawn from an actual person I have known in my years as a practicing physician and professor. As you read the descriptions, ask yourself the following two questions:

1. Who is the healthiest?
2. Who is the least healthy?

SIX PEOPLE—HEALTHY OR UNHEALTHY?

1. The CEO of a large company who has between six and 10 alcoholic drinks every 24 hours
2. A student at Stanford University in the middle of studying for final exams
3. A teenager born weighing two pounds who is now exhibiting problems with coordination and cognition

4. A paraplegic person (that is, someone with a spinal cord injury who is paralyzed from the waist down) who bikes to work each morning as an engineer at a major high-tech company (using a hand-crank bike)
5. A teenager who is 25 pounds overweight and is sad and discouraged because she has few friends
6. A 94-year-old who has lived in the same house for 20 years and who has the beginnings of kidney failure and is in the early stages of Alzheimer disease

When I present this list to my students at Stanford, there typically is little consensus on the answer to either question. The CEO is obviously successful and probably has a substantial income. He would be at the top of most social hierarchies. However, he is an alcoholic, exhibiting the characteristics of chronic alcohol abuse identified by the National Institute on Alcohol Abuse and Alcoholism. There are few outward signs that this person is unhealthy—no heart disease, with blood pressure within reasonable limits. Yet a physician who has accurate information about his alcohol consumption would have to view him as unhealthy.

Most Stanford students enjoy excellent physical health. Yet each year a few students develop potentially serious emotional problems when under the stress of final exams. Fortunately, the exams last only a few days, and with proper support and counseling the students who experience the emotional cost of the stress triggered by exams recover completely and are ready to resume classes after a short period of rest.

As we will see later in this chapter, there has been careful research on the health outcomes of babies born prematurely at extremely low birth weight (usually defined as weighing less than 1,000 grams at birth). A two-pound baby weighs less than 1,000 grams, and 10 to 20 years ago experienced fairly high levels of permanent disability as a result of prematurity. Some of these former preemies have significant problems with muscular coordination and mental ability. How should we view a teenager in this situation?

Rather than developing physical disabilities as a result of prematurity, many otherwise healthy individuals, at some time during their childhood or early adulthood, are involved in an accident that damages their spinal cord, leading to permanent paralysis from the waist down, known medically as paraplegia. How are we to view a person with this level of disability? Does it matter that this person graduated from a top university and has a successful career as a computer professional, or has superb cardiovascular health based on an excellent diet and regular, vigorous exercise?

A teenager who is 25 pounds overweight is probably obese (that is, the ratio of a person's height to weight exceeds the guidelines established by the National Institutes of Health). There are few abnormal signs or symptoms due to the obesity for this teenager. The health effects of obesity more typically show up in adulthood. However, this person, in addition to being obese, is consistently sad and discouraged and has few friends. (Having few friends and social contacts is associated with worse health outcomes independent of other factors.) I would be concerned about this person's health—her emotional health now and the long-term health consequences of obesity and social isolation later.

Finally, we have the 94-year-old. Clearly, she has chronic medical problems that will affect her daily life and may eventually lead to her death. Can we consider a person such as this to be healthy? When students pose this question, I respond: what would this woman say herself? Few 94-year-olds have the luxury of being able to stay in their own home until the end of their life. This particular 94-year-old had a regular circle of friends who visited her every day, took her to church every week, and helped her with shopping and going to the doctor. As 94-year-olds go, this one was fairly healthy—at least, she thought so.

It should by now be clear that there is a principle we must acknowledge in measuring health:

- How healthy or unhealthy a person is will depend on which definition of health we use.

There is an associated principle that we must also consider:

- How you define health will depend on the level at which you analyze health, with different measures used:
  - at the level of an individual
  - at the level of a community or neighborhood
  - at the level of a country or society

DEFINING HEALTH AT THE LEVEL OF AN INDIVIDUAL

The World Health Organization (WHO) attempted to define what "health" means for an individual anywhere in the world. The constitution of the WHO was first adopted at the International Health Conference held in New York in 1946. The preamble to that constitution states: "**Health** is a state of complete physical, mental and social well-being and not merely the absence of disease or infirmity."

The intent of the global community adopting this definition was to make it clear that the health of any individual is measured not simply by the presence or absence of disease. Health involves health of the body, health of the mind and the emotions, and health of the social context in which one lives. While this definition has clear value in broadening our understanding of health, it has limited value from a policy context. It defines a level of health that few can ever hope to achieve. I certainly have relatively few moments when I am in such a complete state of wellbeing. My arm is often bothered by tendonitis; sometimes I have a hard time sleeping because of stressful issues at work. I often wish I could find more time to spend with friends. In addition, it is a rare student in my class who can state that he or she is in a state of complete health. The potential danger in setting what for many may be an unrealistic goal is that it puts us in the position of always falling short, no matter how hard we try.

Beyond setting an expectation that few can hope to attain, this definition gives us little guidance on how to measure health. It seems to create a dichotomy: either we are healthy, or we are not. We have no way of stating, for example, that we are "79 percent healthy." Based on this definition alone, we have no way of following our health over time to determine whether it is improving or declining. Similarly, we have few mechanisms to compare one individual with another.

This is not to say that the WHO definition is without merit. On the contrary, by creating an awareness of the many aspects of health, it gives us an opportunity to explore the three axes of health the definition includes: physical health, mental health, and social well-being. I explore each of these aspects of individual health in sequence, and then ask whether there might be a way to combine them into a composite measure of health that can be used in a policy context.

Physical Health: The Medical Model

Sociologist Andrew Twaddle (1979, pp. 145–46) provided a definition of health that the U.S. medical profession relied on for much of the twentieth century. He stated that "health" must be understood first as a bio-physical state" and that **"illness"** is any state that has been diagnosed as such by a competent professional." Twaddle identified two fundamental dimensions of health according to the medical model:

1. an absence of symptoms—sensations noticed by the patient and interpreted as abnormal
2. an absence of signs—objective characteristics noted by a health professional, of which a patient may often be unaware

Note that this approach to defining health tells us what the concept of health *is not*. A person with abnormal signs or symptoms is not healthy. It does not tell us what health *is*. In the practice of medicine, this might be referred to as a **rule-out definition.** One looks for the presence of abnormal signs or symptoms, and when one determines that there are none, it is possible to rule out ill health. If one does not have ill health, then one is by definition healthy, at least from the medical perspective.

There are potential problems, though, with using this approach in isolation. What if the patient and the doctor disagree? Whose definition of "health" then takes precedence? Say, for example, a person is bothered by a headache (an abnormal symptom) and goes to a doctor for advice. Knowing that headaches can be either benign, with no specific treatment indicated, or serious, with aggressive therapy indicated, the doctor will look for abnormal signs on tests such as a physical examination or a CAT scan. Having looked and found no abnormal signs of illness, the doctor might reassure the person that he is healthy (that is, the doctor has "ruled out" ill health). However, he may still feel the headache and may both feel unhealthy and expect to be treated as unhealthy.

What are we to make of a condition that has no abnormal symptoms? An important example of this is high blood pressure; persons with hypertension develop symptoms only after a number of years. Should we consider a person with somewhat elevated blood pressure to be unhealthy, based on our knowledge that his blood pressure will *eventually* lead to further problems? What might be the consequences of labeling such as person as "unhealthy," even if he feels fine?

Another potential problem with the medical approach to health are the problems that have been identified in the reliability of what would otherwise seem to be objective evidence of abnormal signs of illness. On tests such as EKGs, CAT scans, and certain laboratory tests, different individuals reviewing the tests might interpret the same test as either normal or abnormal. There have even been studies in which the same reviewer has been given the same set of tests to interpret on two occasions, separated by a period of time, with some of the interpretations differing—even though it was the same test. This phenomenon is thought to contribute to the marked variation in the rates at which certain procedures, such as prostate or heart surgery, are done on similar populations of patients. Wennberg and colleagues documented these "area variations" in a number of contexts, variations that seem to involve doctors in different parts of the country interpreting differently what should be considered a "normal finding" and what constitutes an "abnormal finding" (Wennberg et al. 1982; Wennberg 1993).

Health as Functioning at a Normal Level: The Sociocultural Model

Sociologist Talcott Parsons looked at health as reflecting the extent to which an individual is able to maintain a normal level of functioning within his or her social context. He noted that "health may be defined as the state of optimum *capacity* of an individual for the performance of roles and tasks for which he has been socialized" (1972, p. 122). Parsons does state that *"all* processes of behavior on whatever level are mediated through physiologic mechanisms." However, his approach to health focuses more on what a person is able to do with his or her body than on the physiological state of that person's body. Also, rather than comparing a person's level of functioning to some lofty ideal state, as the WHO definition does, it looks at the person in the context of his or her own social circumstances. From this perspective, a person with a medical condition that consistently has abnormal signs or symptoms who is nonetheless able to perform customary roles and tasks should be considered healthy. Thus, from this perspective, health is not the absence of something (signs and symptoms), but rather the presence of something—the ability to function normally.

While there are some attractive aspects of adopting this perspective on health, it too has some potential drawbacks when used in isolation to define health. The same level of physical functioning for two individuals may imply different states of health, depending on the social roles and tasks they face.

Thus, a concert violinist with arthritis in her fingers may be seen as unhealthy and deserving of intervention because of the extent to which the arthritis impairs her ability to perform. A house cleaner with the same degree of arthritis in her fingers may warrant little attention, as it is possible to go on cleaning houses despite the discomfort of the arthritis. Given the degree to which inequalities continue to exist in educational opportunities, with inequalities in educational attainment leading to strikingly different socially defined roles and tasks, adopting the sociocultural model of health in isolation may perpetuate inequalities according to race, ethnicity, or gender.

As we will see when we take another look at the health of the 94-year-old described above as patient 6, the ability to perform common tasks is especially important in evaluating the health of elderly people and of those with physical disabilities. There are five common tasks that most of us take for granted; being unable to perform them directly affects the quality of a person's daily life. These tasks are commonly referred to as **activities of daily living** (ADLs). They are:

1. feeding one's self
2. bathing one's self
3. dressing one's self
4. being able to use the toilet without assistance
5. being able to transfer one's self without assistance (for example, from a bed into a chair)

It should be apparent that a person who is unable to perform any of the ADLs without assistance is in a state of relatively poor health from this perspective. A simple summation of the number of ADLs a person requires assistance with is commonly used as a measure of health and disability. Often this measure is used to determine a person's eligibility for extra benefits, such as home health care.

Health as a General Feeling of Well-Being: The Psychological Model

The first two models of health rely on an assessment of an individual's health by an independent evaluator. The perceptions and attitudes of the individual in question affect the health assessment, but do not determine it. A third model of health relies on the individual himself or herself to provide an assessment of his or her own health. For example, it is possible to ask an individual a question such as, "On a scale of

1 to 10, how would you rate your overall feeling of well-being today?"

A number of scales have been developed to measure a person's health based on that person's own perceptions. These measures are often time specific; a person may give one answer in the face of an immediate stressor and another answer a short time later after that stressor has been removed. Think, for example, of patient 2 above, the Stanford student during final exams. While this student may report a rather low sense of well-being in the midst of final exams, the same student may report a substantially improved well-being after finals are over and he has had a chance to spend time with family and friends at home.

Another Look at Our Six Patients

Having considered three ways to define health (medical, sociocultural, psychological), we can now take another look at our hypothetical six patients to reconsider who is the healthiest and who is the least healthy.

The CEO of a large company who has between six and 10 alcoholic drinks every 24 hours. From the medical perspective, a perceptive physician would determine that this person is quite unhealthy. While the individual may have few symptoms to complain of at this time, the physician knows that chronic alcoholism will, in all likelihood, lead to serious diseases and has the potential to impair significantly social role functioning. This is why many physicians ask probing questions about alcohol consumption as part of routine health screening, and many validated screening instruments have been developed to look for signs of possible alcohol abuse.

From a sociocultural perspective, this person is doing quite well. So long as he can effectively maintain his role as CEO, the alcohol abuse may not impair his health. Once again, however, this person is at high risk of a substantial decline in health if the alcohol abuse begins to impair his functioning at work. In addition, we know little about this person's personal or family situation. If the alcohol abuse were associated with impaired social relations outside of work, then we would have to consider this person to have serious health impairment.

It is difficult to evaluate this person from a psychological perspective. It may well be that the drinking is masking an underlying psychological problem that the person may initially fail to acknowledge.

Were the person to stop drinking, that psychological impairment may become more apparent. It is difficult to predict how this person would rate his own health from this perspective.

In summary, the health of the alcoholic CEO is currently impaired in terms of the medical model, and either impaired or significantly threatened from the standpoint of the other models. We should regard this person as generally unhealthy.

A student at Stanford University in the middle of studying for final exams. This person may report a very high level of stress from the psychological perspective. Stanford students often are short on sleep and experience high levels of anxiety during finals. However, finals only last a week, after which students get at least a week of rest with the opportunity for travel and relaxing with family and friends. For most students, the stress is short-term. From a sociocultural perspective this person is doing quite well. Simply being at Stanford suggests that the student is highly functional in a social context. Most Stanford students will have friends and social networks as well that add to their level of overall social functioning. Similarly, most young adults have little in the way of medical abnormalities that show up as abnormal symptoms or signs. So, even though this person might report experiencing high stress and anxiety right now, we have little to worry about regarding the student's overall health.

A teenager born weighing two pounds who is now exhibiting problems with coordination and cognition. We have little to go on to evaluate the health of this person. Certainly from a strictly medical perspective this person has signs of potentially significant health impairment. The physical and cognitive difficulties many former premature infants face as teenagers often require extra help and support. They may be less able to participate fully in academic, athletic, and social activities. One might expect such a child to feel discouraged or depressed about the life she faces. Later in this chapter I return to this issue by looking at research that has actually followed former premature infants into adolescence, and has asked these types of questions of the children, their teachers, and their parents.

A paraplegic person who bikes to work each morning as an engineer at a major high-tech company. This person has evidence of a health impairment on only one level—the use of his legs. He appears to have compensated for this impairment quite effectively through the use of a mechanical assist devise—the hand-crank bike. I would expect him to have excellent upper-body strength (from all that cranking) and superb cardio-vascular fitness (from biking to work every day rather than driving a car). From a sociocultural perspective this person seems to be doing superbly. Engineers at high-tech companies are generally highly educated, tend to face interesting and challenging work, and enjoy generous incomes. There is no reason to think that this person's family life has been impaired by paralysis. Unless he finds the paralysis itself so discouraging that it affects his own perceptions of his quality of life, one would expect this person to report fairly high perceptions of his own health. An isolated physical impairment does not necessarily make someone unhealthy, and in the face of other signs of positive health takes on less significance in this regard.

A teenager who is 25 pounds overweight and is sad and discouraged because she has few friends. Here is someone we should worry about. This person is showing significant health impairment on all fronts. The obesity itself will very likely be associated with other serious medical problems, either now or in the near future (diabetes and high blood pressure, for example). With few friends this person is showing evidence of poor social role functioning. The sadness and discouragement reported by this teenager is a clear statement of her own perception of poor emotional health. Any health professional who encounters this person would be quite concerned, and would want to evaluate possible interventions on a number of levels.

A 94-year-old who has lived in the same house for 20 years and who has the beginnings of kidney failure and is in the early stages of Alzheimer disease. At first, most of my students place this person squarely in the "unhealthy" category, many at the bottom of the list. In response, I ask the students to consider if their own grandparent were in this situation, how that grandparent would respond to the question, "How are you doing?" This person represents an actual patient I took care of until she eventually died of her worsening kidney failure. There was treatment that would have kept her alive longer, but she refused it. She said she was happy being who she was, and she wanted to die happy. And she did. For her, the impaired memory and physical weakness from her kidneys was of little importance. What *was* important was that at 94 she still lived in the house she had lived in for decades and that she needed no help with her ADLs. She cooked for herself, she dressed herself, and she bathed herself. Her many neighbors and friends helped her with shopping, visited her regularly, and

took her to church every week. From this person's own perspective, life didn't get any better. I knew she had signs of poor memory and an abnormal kidney test, but I believe I enjoyed our visits together almost as much as she did.

So who is the healthiest? For me, the 94-year-old and the bike-to-work engineer are at the top of the list. Who is the least healthy? From my perspective, it has to be either the CEO or the overweight and depressed teenager. For the Stanford student I'll need to wait until after finals to be sure. The former premie who now has substantial impairments may yet surprise us.

Health as a Multidimensional Concept

It seems apparent that each model of health we have considered tells us something about a person's state of health, but tells us little about a person's *overall* state of health. Rather than being one-dimensional, health has multiple dimensions, three of which we have considered so far. Wolinsky (1988) suggests that we think of health as a three-dimensional concept.

Wolinsky suggests that we dichotomize each dimension into "well" and "ill." Overall health is measured by the ratio of "well" dimensions to "ill" dimensions. Someone who is well on the psychological and social dimensions but ill on the medical dimension should be seen as more healthy than someone who is well along the medical dimension but ill along the social and psychological dimensions. The approach suggested by Wolinsky gives equal weight to each of the three dimensions, and does not allow for gradations along the three axes.

What if each dimension is continuous, rather than dichotomous, as suggested by Wolinsky? (That is, what if the measurement on each of the three dimensions can assume any of a wide range of values, rather than simply "well" or "ill"?) From this perspective overall health could be any of a large number of points within the three-dimensional space. If it were possible to measure health reliably at any point along the medical, social, and psychological dimensions, and then combine these measurements into a measurement of overall health, such a tool would be very useful both as a policy tool and in following the health of an individual over time.

John Ware and colleagues developed just such an instrument: the 36-Item Short-Form Health Survey, often referred to simply as the **SF-36** (Ware and

Sherbourne 1992). Developed for use in the Medical Outcomes Study, Ware used the SF-36 to compare the health outcomes over time of patients enrolled in alternative health care delivery systems. The SF-36 uses an approach similar to that proposed by Wolinsky, but treats each dimension of health as continuous rather than dichotomous. It uses 36 individual questions, each asking about a specific aspect of health such as the ability to climb stairs, walk several blocks, or engage in vigorous activities. It also asks about limits on activities as the result of emotional problems.

Using statistical modeling, the SF-36 uses various combinations of these 36 questions to create eight separate scales, each measuring a different dimension of health. It then combines four of these dimensional measures to create an overall measure of physical health, and the other four to create an overall measure of mental health.

The four subscales used to measure overall physical health include:

1. Physical Functioning
2. Role Limitations Due to Physical Problems
3. Bodily Pain
4. General Health Perceptions

The four subscales used to measure overall mental health include:

1. Vitality
2. Social Functioning
3. Role Limitations Due to Emotional Problems
4. General Mental Health

Researchers have translated the SF-36 into other languages and found it to be equally reliable. Changes in an individual's SF-36 score over time have been found to be associated with the cost of providing health care services, with those patients with worse health as measured by the SF-36 requiring more health care.

An excellent example of how the SF-36 can be used in research on health status is a study published by Sjogren and Thulin (2004). The authors wanted to know more about the ways in which heart surgery affected the health status of individuals who were 80 years old or older, concerned that surgery of this magnitude might worsen overall health status rather than improve it. It compared findings on the eight different health status scales incorporated into the SF-36 for patients who underwent surgery, comparing them to age-matched patients without heart disease. They found that those patients who had surgery reported lower physical functioning but less bodily pain than the comparison group. Otherwise the two groups were not significantly different on any of the other six scales.

Using instruments such as the SF-36 allows us to assess health along medical, social, and psychological dimensions. Wilson and Cleary (1995) offer us a way of understanding how these different aspects of health are associated with each other. They suggest that the three dimensions of health are linked causally, with changes in physical health triggering subsequent changes in role functioning and ultimately in emotional health, and that each dimension is influenced by characteristics unique to the individual patient as well as characteristics of the environment in which that person lives. In addition, they suggest that the three aspects of health are not the final outcomes we should focus our attention on, but rather are each intermediate factors that affect in various ways the ultimate thing we should be measuring: quality of life.

In their model, biological and physical abnormalities are the fundamental causes of poor health. These abnormalities in turn lead to symptoms that are characteristic of disease. The person's perception of poor physical health leads to a reduction in functional status. Under this model it is the reduction of functional status in response to perceived illness that leads to a feeling of poor general health. It is the person's perception of a reduction in general health status that then reduces the quality of life he or she enjoys.

For each of these causal links, characteristics unique to the individual and characteristics of the environment in which the individual lives and works can have either buffering or enhancing effects on the chain of causality—from biologic abnormalities to a reduced quality of life. For example, someone with strong social and psychological supports may respond to a given set of symptoms with a smaller reduction in functional status than another person with similar symptoms but a weaker support system. Conversely, someone who tends to amplify the symptoms she or he perceives, or who has little motivation to be healthy, may experience a substantially reduced functional status in response to those symptoms. Similarly, individual motivation and preferences coupled with the nature of one's social and emotional support system will directly affect the quality of life one experiences.

Thus, **quality of life** is powerfully affected by symptoms of illness and functional limitations. However, the presence of these problems does not necessarily mean that a person will experience a reduced quality of life. A case in point is that of premature infants weighing less than 1,000 grams (referred to as extremely low birth weight [ELBW]).

In the 1970s and 1980s, medical science was in the transition from being nearly helpless to being very successful in the treatment of ELBW infants. ELBW babies born in that time frame often survived, but often with substantial levels of physical and cognitive disability. Saigal and colleagues (1996) reported on a study of 141 ELBW babies born between 1977 and 1982 who had survived and were then teenagers, comparing them on a number of scales to a comparison group of teenagers, matched on age, sex, and social class, who were born at full term weighing at least 2,500 grams (normal birth weight [NBW]).

The authors first compared the two groups of teenagers on six scales of disability: cognition, sensation, mobility, self-care, emotion, and pain. For each of the six scales, the ELBW teenagers reported a higher frequency of problems than the NBW group. All these differences were statistically significant ($p \leq$ 05) except for emotion and pain. Using objective measures of disability, the ELBW teenagers had both lower physiological health (cognition and sensation) and lower functional health (mobility and self-care) than the NBW group. From the model proposed by Wilson and Cleary, can we assume that the ELBW teenagers will also report a lower quality of life? Saigal and colleagues addressed this question by assessing each subject's perception of her or his own quality of life, using a standardized assessment tool that measured quality of life on a scale from 0 to 1. What they found was essentially no difference in the distribution of the quality of life score between the two groups.

There is a danger in assuming that an individual who has objective evidence of physiologic abnormalities that are associated with measurable physical impairment will necessarily experience a lower quality of life than someone without those impairments. Nor can we assume that these physiologic and functional impairments will necessarily constrain other important activities of those affected with them. Saigal and colleagues (2006) followed these same teenagers into early adulthood, comparing the ELBW and NBW subjects on educational attainment, employment or educational status, independent living, getting married, and having children. They found few differences, concluding that "a significant majority of former ELBW infants have overcome their earlier difficulties to become functional young adults" (p. 667).

Imagine if, instead of comparing ELBW infants with NBW infants, we were instead comparing 94-year-olds living in their own home with 44-year-olds. On objective scales of dimensions such as cognition, sensation, mobility, self-care, emotion, and pain, the 94-year-olds would likely register worse health than the 44-year-olds, much the same as the comparisons of the ELBW and NBW children above. If we asked the same subjects to rate their quality of life—based on my experience with the 94-year-old woman used as an example at the beginning of this chapter—I might expect something similar to the quality-of-life comparisons of the ELBW and NBW children. Despite their physical frailty and cognitive impairment, when asked about how they feel they are doing these 94-year-olds may well suggest, "I'm doing just fine, thanks."

THE DANGER OF APPROACHING HEALTH AS A MORAL IMPERATIVE

I have described health as a multidimensional concept that is directly affected by individual and environmental circumstances. Should we expect everyone to be healthy? Should we expect those with behavior patterns that are unhealthy to overcome them and to attain the level of health characterized by the absence of abnormal signs and symptoms? There is a hidden danger if we do—especially if we do so in the role of health professionals.

Faith Fitzgerald published a seminal essay in 1994, warning us to avoid what she called the "tyranny of health in which those who are unwell are assumed to have misbehaved" (p. 197). It is easy for a physician or other health professional to look at a person and recognize right away that his or her own behavior (e.g., smoking, lack of exercise, obesity) is impairing the attainment of full health. Should we then blame the person for that behavior and for the resulting ill health? Fitzgerald suggests that as health professionals, or even as friends or family members, it can be problematic, and perhaps harmful to an individual, to approach behaviors associated with poor health as an issue of individual moral worth.

What harm can this do? Much harm. If health (physical, mental, and social) is normal and the failure to be healthy is someone's fault, then when a person becomes ill he or she may have done something wrong. If we root out that wrong-ness, or better yet, prevent it, we can restore that person to normal health and can benefit society. In effect, we have said that people owe it to society to stop misbehaving, and we use illness as evidence of misbehavior. (Fitzgerald, 1994, p. 197)

It is easy to think of behaviors that fall into this category. They include:

- obesity
- smoking
- lack of exercise
- high cholesterol
- poor diet
- alcohol abuse
- drug abuse

Each is known to be associated over time with adverse health outcomes. Each is a behavior over which an individual seemingly has control. Each is also a behavior that differs markedly in terms of the social group to which one belongs. Those who have higher levels of educational attainment, on average, will consistently smoke less than those with lower educational attainment. Often these behaviors will have additional cultural associations, with those from differing racial or ethnic groups yet similar levels of educational attainment having consistently differing patterns of health-related behaviors. Is it the individual that determines behavior based on individual will and choice, or is it a characteristic of human behavior to follow patterns established by the social group? These are issues we will commonly confront, as health professionals, as co-workers, and as friends or family.

What I wish to suggest is that, with regard to health-related behaviors, we separate the issues of blame versus responsibility. A person who develops lung cancer after several decades of smoking certainly bears responsibility for the behavior that contributed to the development of the cancer. Yet it is possible to approach that responsibility in a context devoid of moral judgment—that is, without assigning blame. Blame implies weakness; responsibility acknowledges the causal relationships involved. It is often difficult to look at someone we care for, or someone we are caring for as health professionals, who is engaging in what appears to us to be self-

destructive behavior, without attributing some form of moral weakness to that person. Again in the words of Fitzgerald (1994, p. 197), "we must beware of developing a zealotry about health, in which we take ourselves too seriously and believe that we know enough to dictate human behavior, penalize people for disagreeing with us, and even deny people charity, empathy, and understanding because they act in a way of which we disapprove."

MEASURING THE HEALTH OF A COMMUNITY OR A SOCIETY

Until now I have been discussing how to understand the health of an individual. The available measurements we have identified—symptoms, signs, SF-36 score, and the like—all pertain to a specific individual. What if we want to compare the health of different communities or of different societies? We will need measures that apply to groups of people rather than individuals. Two general categories of health indicator are commonly used to define and compare health at this level: rates of illness and rates of death. Table 7.1 compares the rates of several illnesses and selected rates of death for four states from four different regions of the country: California, Iowa, Mississippi, and New York.

Rate of Illness

Table 7.1 compares the prevalence rates of four common illnesses for the four states. The rates reflect the percentage of adults within the state who were found to have the specified condition. Using these four illnesses, it is fairly straightforward to identify the state with the lowest level of health. Mississippi has substantially higher rates of hypertension (high blood pressure), diabetes, and obesity than any of the other states. However, Mississippi has the lowest rate of asthma, a condition often made worse by the air pollution that is common to large, metropolitan areas. While having the highest rate of asthma, New York has the lowest rate of obesity and the second lowest rate of diabetes—a condition often associated with obesity. California does well with hypertension, while Iowa does well with diabetes.

From these data it should be clear that rates of illness can provide a very interesting look at certain states. The disease or diseases one selects as the measure of comparative health will have a great deal to

Table 7.1   Comparative Health Indexes for Four States

Condition	California	Iowa	Mississippi	New York
Asthma	6.4	6.4	6.1	7.9
Diabetes	7.5	6.0	10.2	7.3
Hypertension	21.3	23.4	34.4	22.7
Obesity	22.5	23.3	27	20.8
Years of potential life lost	6,636	6,341	10,971	6,990
Breast cancer deaths	25.7	24	30.6	27.9
Heart disease death rate	193	232	195	243
Infant mortality	5.4	6.4	10.6	6.4
Median family income	$68,310	$61,951	$49,893	$67,564

Sources: Data from the U.S. Centers for Disease Control and Prevention.
Asthma: Prevalence of current asthma among adults, 2002.
Diabetes: Prevalence of diagnosed diabetes per 100 adult population, by age and state, United States, 2004.
Hypertension: Percentage of adults who reported ever having been told by a health professional that they have high blood pressure, 1997.
Obesity: Percentage of persons age $\geq$ 20 years with body mass index $\geq$ 30.0 kg/m^2, 2001.
Years of potential life lost: Before age 75, age adjusted per 100,000 population, 2000.
Breast cancer deaths: Age adjusted, per 100,000 female population, 2000.
Heart disease death rate: Age-adjusted per 100,000 population, 2000.
Infant mortality: Per 1,000 live births. 2000.
Data for median family income from the U.S. Census Bureau for a family of four, 2004.

do with how a state will fare. Certain diseases will reflect the degree of urbanization within a state. Other diseases, such as obesity, diabetes, and hypertension, will tend to clump together.

Rates of Death

Table 7.1 shows the years of potential life lost due to deaths that occur before the age of 75. This is an aggregate measure that incorporates a wide range of conditions that affect people at various ages. The table also shows the rate of death from three specific causes: breast cancer, heart disease, and infant deaths. Each of the measures is the rate per 100,000 population, and is adjusted for the differing age distribution within the states studied.

The federal government reported that a baby born in the United States in 2003 could expect to live, on average, 77.5 years. Using 75 years as a guideline, the government looks at all the deaths that occur before the age of 75, and calculates how many more years each person who died would have lived had that individual lived to be 75. This number is referred to as the "years of potential life lost." Looking at this number in Mississippi, we see by far the largest gap of any of the four states. Those living in Mississippi lose 57 percent more years of life from premature death than those in New York, 66 percent

more than those in California, and 73 percent more than those in Iowa. Mississippi is the highest of all 50 states in this measure of premature death; Iowa is 47th out of the 50 states.

Mississippi also has the highest rate of infant mortality of all 50 states, while California and Iowa rank in the lowest 10 states in this measure. It is understandable that the state with the highest rate of infant mortality has the most years of potential life lost. An infant who dies in the first year of life has lost 74 years compared to an average expectancy of 75 years.

While Mississippi has one of the highest rates of breast cancer deaths in the country, it is not the highest. In 2000 Delaware had 32.7 deaths per 100,000 adult women, while New Jersey had 31.5 deaths. Iowa had one of the lowest rates of breast cancer deaths in the country, while California and New York were in the midrange of the distribution.

When we look at the rate of death from heart disease, we find New York to have the highest. At 243 deaths per 100,000 population, New York had the highest rate of death from heart disease of all 50 states. Mississippi's rate was third highest among the states. Iowa at 195 deaths and California at 193 deaths were again in the midrange of the distribution among the states.

As with disease rates, rates of death give a fairly consistent picture of the health of a state relative to other states. However, the relative health ranking may change depending on the specific measure one uses.

One should also note the final statistic given in Table 7.1: the median income in that state for a family of four. Mississippi has by far the lowest level of family income of any of the four states studied. In 2004 the median income for a family of four in Mississippi was fourth from the lowest of all 50 states. Only Arkansas, New Mexico, and Oklahoma had lower family income. There is a strong association between economic well-being and health status.

Look at not only the level of income in differing states and differing countries but also at the level of economic inequality—the distance between the best-off residents and the worst-off—among differing states and countries. In addition to being toward the bottom of the distribution in family income, Mississippi has one of the higher levels of economic inequality among its residents. Both the absolute income and income relative to others are associated with health status.

COMPARING HEALTH STATUS GLOBALLY

When comparing health among countries globally, we can use a series of standard indicators gathered and reported by agencies such as the World Health Organization (WHO). Principal among these are

- Male life expectancy at birth—the number of years, on average, a male baby born in the year for which the data are reported can expect to live
- Female life expectancy at birth—the number of years, on average, a female baby born in the year for which the data are reported can expect to live
- Infant mortality rate—of a thousand babies born alive, the number who will die before their first birthday
- Maternal mortality rate—of a thousand women giving birth, the number who will die as the result of complications during the birthing process

It is more difficult to use rates of illness to compare the health of differing countries. While this can be done, different illnesses are unique to certain geographic or climatic areas. In addition, the types of illness found in countries of varying levels of economic development are often quite different. Accordingly, it is more common to use the types of mortality statistics cited above to compare countries.

Using data from the WHO, Table 7.2 shows these indexes for 15 countries from around the globe, drawn from each of the five largest continents. In addition, it presents the per capita share of the gross national income for the countries listed.

There are wide disparities in each of the indicators listed. Infant mortality ranges from 2 per 1,000 births in Singapore to 129 per 1,000 in the Democratic Republic of the Congo. Life expectancy goes from a low of 47 years for women and 42 years for men (again, in the Democratic Republic of the Congo) to 83 years for women and 78 years for men in Canada.

Health status and socioeconomic status are inextricably linked. As socioeconomic status rises over time, health status improves. Using both illness rates and mortality rates, the same is true in comparing health among different states in the United States. To examine this relationship in a global context, I have taken the data from Table 7.2, which lists the countries alphabetically, and instead sorted the countries by per capita income. Table 7.3 shows the 15 countries by income from lowest to highest.

Not surprisingly, of the 15 countries listed, the Democratic Republic of the Congo has the lowest per capita income ($680), while the United States has the highest ($39,710). As we follow the columns showing mortality rates, we see that as we go up the income ladder, infant and maternal mortality declines and life expectancy increases nearly in lockstep. With a few notable exceptions, as the average income within a country goes up, the health of the country improves. Brazil and Colombia are both in South America, have similar levels of per capita income, and have similar levels of life expectancy for men. Despite its higher level of income, Brazil has rates of infant mortality and maternal mortality that are nearly twice those of Colombia, with a corresponding reduction in female life expectancy. (In general, as maternal mortality increases, there will be a corresponding decline in female life expectancy.) We also note that despite relatively low rates of infant and maternal mortality, the Russian Federation has relatively low life expectancy for both men and women when compared to countries with similar levels of per capita income. These discrepancies suggest the need for more focused research on the reasons these countries deviate from the general pattern linking per capita income with these health indexes.

Finally, we see that, despite being the country with the highest per capita income of all those listed, the United States ranks fifth of the five higher-income countries listed for each health indicators.

In comparing health statistics among countries with strikingly different levels of development, there is one caveat. These comparative statistics are valid only to the extent that they are gathered in the same

way, using standardized methods of measurement. Countries may differ in either their ability or their willingness to gather accurate statistics. For example, Liu and colleagues (1992) looked at the way different countries gather and report infant mortality data. In order for the death of an infant to be seen as

Table 7.2   Health Indexes for Fifteen Countries, 2004.

Country	Male Life Expectancy at Birth (years)	Female Life Expectancy at Birth (years)	Infant Mortality Rate	Maternal Mortality Rate	Per Capita Income ($US)
Argentina	71	78	16	70	12,460
Bangladesh	62	63	56	380	1,980
Brazil	67	74	32	260	8,020
Canada	78	83	5	5	30,660
Colombia	68	77	16	130	6,820
Democratic Republic of the Congo	42	47	129	990	680
Greece	77	82	4	10	22,000
Haiti	53	56	74	680	1,680
India	61	63	43	540	3,100
Mexico	72	77	23	83	9,590
Nigeria	45	46	103	800	930
Norway	77	82	3	10	38,550
Russian Federation	59	72	13	65	9,620
Singapore	77	82	2	15	26,590
United States	75	80	6	14	39,710

Source: World Health Statistics 2006 documents and tables, www.who.int/whosis/whostat2006/en/index.html.

Table 7.3   Health Indexes for Fifteen Countries, by per Capita Income, 2004

Country	Male Life Expectancy at Birth (years)	Female Life Expectancy at Birth (years)	Infant Mortality Rate	Maternal Mortality Rate	Per Capita Income ($US)
Democratic Republic of the Congo	42	47	129	990	680
Nigeria	45	46	103	800	930
Haiti	53	56	74	680	1,680
Bangladesh	62	63	56	380	1,980
India	61	63	43	540	3,100
Colombia	68	77	18	130	6,820
Brazil	67	74	32	260	8,020
Mexico	72	77	23	83	9,590
Russian Federation	59	72	13	65	9,620
Argentina	71	78	16	70	12,460
Greece	77	82	4	10	22,000
Singapore	77	82	2	15	26,590
Canada	78	83	5	5	30,660
Norway	77	82	3	10	38,550
United States	75	80	6	14	39,710

Source: World Health Statistics 2006 documents and tables, www.who.int/whosis/whostat2006/en/lndex.html.

contributing to the infant mortality rate, the infant must be born alive. In Western countries this means with a spontaneous heartbeat and other signs of vital organ functioning. However, in a country that has no resources to provide intensive medical care to premature infants the infant has to survive the first 24 hours of life before being counted as a "live birth." In some countries it has become a matter of policy to count as "live births" only those infants who do survive 24 hours following birth. Similarly, if an infant dies close to her or his first birthday, in some countries the health care system may not be aware of the death, and as a result the death may not be counted as an infant death. For these and other similar reasons, comparisons of mortality data among countries globally may have some inherent inaccuracies.

Another measurement instrument that is commonly used in assessing health in a global context is the disability-adjusted life year (DALY). DALY provides a means of estimating the magnitude of the burden created by a disease or condition. DALY builds on the concept of potential years of life lost, by adding to it an estimation of the level of disability attributed to the disease for those who develop the disease but do not die from it. Using a methodology described by the WHO (2006), living one year with a disease that reduces one's level of functioning by 50 percent would mean the loss of 0.50 DALY. Thus, dying 5 years prematurely would create the loss of the same number of DALYs as living with a disease for 10 years with the loss of 50 percent of one's functional ability. Living 10 years with a 50 percent disability and then dying 5 years prematurely would mean the loss of 10 DALYs (5 DALYs for the effect of the disability when alive, and an additional 5 DALYs for the premature death).

Table 7.4 provides an example of the manner in which DALYs are used in the policy context, showing the global burden (measured in millions of DALYs) of four major diseases: diarrhea, worm infection, tuberculosis, and ischemic heart disease. From the table it can be seen that diarrheal illness inflicts by far the largest health burden globally, affecting primarily young children. While ischemic heart disease places a substantial burden on those over 60 years old, its global impact is less than half that of diarrheal illness.

One should not confuse the DALY with another measure, the QALY (quality-adjusted life year). The QALY is commonly used in developed countries as part of cost-effectiveness analysis. Rather than estimating premature death and disability, the QALY is typically used to evaluate the effectiveness of a specific treatment in prolonging the lives of those with specific diseases. It first estimates the number of years a person's life is extended by the treatment, then estimates the health-related quality of life (HRQL) experienced by that person during those additional years. Living an additional year with a 50 percent HRQL constitutes 0.50 QALY; living an additional year with no impairment in HRQL constitutes 1.0 QALY (Miller et al. 2006).

Table 7.4 Global Impact of Four Major Diseases, by Gender and Age Group.

	0–4	5–14	15–44	45–59	60+	Total
Diarrhea						
Male	42.1	4.6	2.8	0.4	0.2	50.2
Female	40.7	4.8	2.8	0.4	0.3	48.9
Worm infection						
Male	0.2	10.6	1.6	0.5	0.1	13.1
Female	0.1	9.2	0.9	0.5	0.1	10.9
Tuberculosis						
Male	1.2	3.1	13.4	6.2	2.6	26.5
Female	1.3	3.8	10.9	2.8	1.2	20.0
Ischemic heart disease						
Male	0.1	0.1	3.6	8.1	13.1	25.0
Female	—[a]	—[a]	1.2	3.2	13.0	17.5

Age (years)

Source: World Bank (1993).
Note: Impact is measured in millions of DALYs.
[a]Less than 0.5 million.

Stress Management

The Nature of Stress

INTRODUCTION

Garfield, the famous cartoon cat says, "In a perfect world, you could breathe under water" as he sticks his head in a fish bowl with a huge smile on his face as a terrified fish is looking on. He goes through additional scenarios that would create a perfect world for him and make his life easier. Unfortunately, we don't live in a perfect world and we don't always have control over what happens to us. In fact,

As we grow up, we learn that even the one person that wasn't supposed to ever let you down probably will. You will have your heart broken probably more than once and it's harder every time. You'll fight with your best friend. You'll cry because time is passing too fast, and you'll eventually lose someone you love. So take too many pictures, laugh too much, and love like you've never been hurt because every sixty seconds you spend upset is a minute of happiness you'll never get back.—author unknown

The fact of the matter is that literally *every day* from the day that you're born until the day that you die, you'll most likely experience some form of stress to some extent. The types of stressors you experience may vary throughout your life-much of your stress as a college student may pertain to school-work (i.e., meeting deadlines, getting good grades), whereas much of your stress as an elderly individual might be dealing with the loss of your spouse or with health problems. Regardless of the type of stressors that you come across, you will encounter a variety of them to varying degrees throughout your entire life.

Not only will the *type* of stressors you encounter vary throughout your life, but the *number* of stressors and the *intensity* of those stressors will vary as well. You might go through a "when it rains, it pours" period when several things go wrong all at about the same time. A friend of mine lost her grandmother (her first experience with death of a loved one), found out that her father had cancer, and went through a major breakup with her boyfriend all within one week. Or instead of experiencing several different major stressors, you might experience only one extremely stressful event or situation, such as being diagnosed with a major illness. Or you might experience many different minor stressors in a relatively short period of time, such as getting a speeding ticket, getting into an argument with your boss, or doing poorly on an exam.

Regardless of the type, amount, or intensity of stressors, life can be stressful! It doesn't matter if you're rich or poor, famous or unknown, intelligent or unintelligent, old or young. *Everyone* will deal with bumps in the road of life. Some might have more bumps and/or steeper bumps than others, but one thing is for sure—you can count on those bumps being there. In other words, everyone will deal with stress throughout his or her life. Some bumps in the road will be self-induced, or stress that you created yourself, and others will be bumps that were just there, or stress that is completely out of your control. Regardless, you will most likely encounter stressors to varying extents all throughout your lifetime.

Yet, how many of us have received some type of training or education as to how to deal effectively with stressors and the accompanying stressful emotions? We're taught how to read and write, but what about how to deal with rejection and devastation? We're taught how to ride a bike, but what about how to deal with despair and depression? We're taught how to drive a car, but what about how to deal with anger and frustration? Unfortunately, many people have not been taught how to deal effectively with

stress. In order to learn how to effectively deal with stress, it's important to gain a basic understanding of stress. In this chapter, we'll discuss the nature of stress in terms of its definitions, its types, and its relationship to health and wellness.

DEFINITIONS OF STRESS

The primary objective for this chapter is to gain a strong understanding of the nature of stress. In order to gain a greater understanding of stress, it's obviously necessary to define it. However, it should be noted that *stress* is not really a useful term for scientists because it's a highly subjective concept. What constitutes stress for one person may not be stressful for another. It's been said that *stress* is one of those words that everyone knows the meaning of but no one can define. In other words, when you initially hear the word *stress*, several thoughts or feelings probably come to mind fairly quickly and easily. We all know how it feels to be stressed, and we all can easily identify our stressors (e.g., finances, meeting deadlines, getting into arguments, traffic). But it might be more difficult and take a little longer to come up with an actual definition of it. Take a look at these definitions.

Stress Affects Body and Mind

- *Stress is any event or situation that brings us out of homeostasis.* **Homeostasis** refers to maintaining internal equilibrium. So basically, homeostasis is when your body is functioning normally and all is well physically. **Internal equilibrium** usually refers to our physiological state. However, the concept of equilibrium also applies to our psychological state. Emotional homeostasis, then, is when your emotional health and well-being are normal and all is well emotionally. So according to this definition, stress consists of (1) a stressor (i.e., event or situation) that threatens to bring us out of physical and emotional equilibrium and (2) the actual state or condition of being out of physical and/or emotional equilibrium.
- *Stress is any outside force or event that has an effect on our body or mind.* This definition implies that stress consists of a stressor and both physiological and psychological reactions.
- *Stress is the nonspecific response of the body to any demand for change.* This definition implies that the body is altered as a result of encountering a situa-

Table 8.1   How Do You Define Stress?

- Stress means many things: peer pressure, relationships, schoolwork, and future events. It is that overwhelming feeling of anxiety that is created and triggered by those events.—Caitie Haynes
- Stress means being faced with a situation that I have no control over and that will eventually hurt me if I do not gain control soon.—Jazmin Beltran
- Stress means when you don't get what you want and when you want it.—Hanh T. Huynh
- Stress is the body's way of rising or reacting to a challenge or situation it is not comfortable with.—Gabe Dalgoff
- That feeling where nothing anyone says or does can make you feel better.—Justin Wang
- Something that takes you out of your normal feeling, whether it is good or bad.—Ali Showkatian
- What causes ones life to seem like an ongoing roller coaster.—Carolyn Rubendall
- Anything that brings you out of your normal routine.—Anonymous
- Anything and everything that makes me question why things are the way they are.—Anonymous
- Something that dampens your day.—Anonymous
- The thing that pushes you to get things done.—Samuel Torrez
- A reactionary mental impulse followed by lack of concentration, fear, conflicting thoughts, restlessness, obsessive/compulsive behavior, anxiety or excitement.—Maryam Dehghan
- The feeling of being overwhelmed, unmotivated, depressed, anxious, worried.—Vu H. Nguyen
- When reality and theory don't meet.—Sabrina Huda
- The motivation to get out of bed in the morning and get things done in life.—Jennifer F. Amagrande
- Anything that causes you to be in anything but a normal relaxed state of mind.—Colt Synder

tion that causes a change or that brings us out of equilibrium.

- **Stress** *is the rate of wear and tear on the body.* This definition implies that stress negatively affects our physiology.
- **Stress** *is physical, mental, or emotional strain or tension.* This definition implies that stress affects our body and mind—our physical health and our emotional health.
- **Stress** *is an organism's total response to environmental demands or pressures.* This definition implies that there are external strains that cause us to react, and that stressors affect us physically and emotionally.

Stress Can Be Good

- **Stress** *is the spice of life.* This definition has a positive connotation and implies that stress can actually be healthy.

Thoughts and Perceptions Play a Role

- **Stress** *is a condition or feeling that occurs when a person perceives that demands exceed the personal and social resources the individual is able to mobilize.* This definition implies that perception plays a significant role in whether we feel stressed.
- **Stress** *is that confusion created when one's mind overrides the body's desire to choke the living #@!*? out of some #@!*? who desperately needs it.* Many of us can definitely relate to this definition, which implies that stressors can stem from our interactions and relationships with others and that our thoughts play a role and/or are influenced by our perceived stress levels.

COMPONENTS OF STRESS

Whenever I ask my students what comes to mind when they hear the word *stress*, many of them usually identify a stressor—schoolwork, a difficult professor, problems with their girlfriend/boyfriend or husband/wife, an obnoxious boss, pressures from friends or family members. However, based on the definitions above, it's clear that stress involves (1) a stressor or some sort of demand, pressure, situation, or event; (2) our perception of that stressor; (3) an emotional reaction(s); and (4) a physiological reaction(s). So the term *stress* involves much more than simply a stressor and refers to a chain reaction involving multiple components, affecting us both psychologically and physically.

TYPES OF STRESS

In addition to defining stress, it's important to understand the nature of stress in terms of its types. There are two general types of stress: eustress and distress.

Eustress

Eustress pertains to the definition of *the spice of life* and is actually considered to be good stress or healthy stress. How is it that stress could actually be good for you? Stressors that elicit positive emotions (excitement, happiness, pleasure, enthusiasm, motivation, invigoration, etc.) are considered to be positive stress or *eustress*. Remember, stress results whenever we're out of homeostasis. Stress that motivates, energizes, or excites technically brings us out of homeostasis, but it's good, healthy stress. Getting married, starting a family, going to college, or interviewing for a job may be examples of eustress. Eustress may also occur when you do something different, break a routine, make a new friend, travel to a new place, or generate some excitement for yourself. Riding a roller coaster (unless you're terrified of roller coasters) or doing something challenging or adventurous may be examples of eustress. It brings you out of emotional and physical homeostasis but in a good way.

Distress

Distress considered bad stress or unhealthy stress and pertains to the definition of *the rate of wear and tear*

Table 8.2 Students' Distressors

- Nearly every moment of every day for the six years I spent in foster care from age 12 to 18. I was transferred to seven different foster homes in six years and had my first son at 16.—Shannon Spilker-Vidal
- College.—Anonymous
- Being laid off and having to apply for unemployment.—Hamzah Jacques
- Being close to graduating from college.—Austin Varner
- When I started college, I got involved in a sports accident that incapacitated me. I was in pain, my GPA tanked, and I missed two full quarters.—Anonymous
- Failing a class for the second time.—Justin Wang
- When my grandma passed away.—Daniel Kim
- When one of my best friends suddenly died from brain cancer.—Ervin Lozano
- My father's substance abuse, which caused me to try to be the surrogate father and spouse while still trying to be a sister and daughter.—Jennifer Rodriguez
- When my uncle got diagnosed with cancer.—Carolyn Rubendall
- When my grandfather was sick with lung cancer.—Kari Nicholas
- When my dad lost his job.—Victoria Timpe
- Being unemployed and not being able to support myself.—Blanca M. Espinoza
- The time that my computer got attacked by a major virus.—Anonymous
- Getting close to graduating—I'm not sure what my future has in store. I hate this type of uncertainty. —Anonymous
- The murder of one of my closest friends and co-worker.—Elene Williams
- Being in a very unhealthy relationship.—Jennifer Estell
- Not being able to be alongside my mother when my grandfather passed away.—Rosemary Garcia
- When I got laid off and fell behind on credit card payments and got numerous threatening calls by creditors every day.—Anonymous
- Choosing where to go to college after graduating from high school.—Samuel Torrez
- Going to school while working full time.—Vu H. Nguyen
- The death of a close friend.—Nicole
- My lack of time management.—Marielle Croudo
- When I was in high school, I was taking too many advanced placement courses, actively participating in student government, working, and had a boyfriend.—Sabrina Huda
- The death of my niece.—Channyn Marasco
- At work because it doesn't matter if I'm absolutely perfect 99% of the time because I'm repeatedly only acknowledged for my mistakes.—Brittany Terrazas
- Senior year of high school when my best friend passed away.—Jennifer F. Amagrande
- The death of my 24-year-old cousin in a car accident who was my best friend.—Colt Synder
- When my dad was diagnosed with a stomach ulcer and needed to go to the hospital immediately to have surgery.—Christina Ta

on the body. You feel bad as a result of encountering a distressful situation and might even experience physical problems as a result of the stressor (e.g., stomachache, acne, hives). It's stress that wears you down and causes you to feel any of the stressful emotions (e.g., frustration, anxiety, anger, burned out, overwhelmed). Examples of distress are having to give a presentation when you hate public speaking, taking 100 million units while working 100 million hours, or being in an abusive relationship. It brings you out of emotional and physical homeostasis in a negative way. When people think of stress, it's usually distress to which they're referring, not eustress.

EUSTRESS VERSUS DISTRESS

Role of Perception

It's important to note that the very same stressors that cause eustress in one person could cause distress in another. Whether the stressor is eustress-ful or distressful depends entirely upon an individual's perception. For example, divorce is a stressor but depending on one's perception, this could be a good thing (eustressful) or a bad thing (distressful). For one person, divorce could feel like the end of the world. Her life is over. For another person, hallelujah—her life is just beginning. We have a family friend who committed suicide after his wife divorced him. But I have another friend who, after her divorce, got into great shape and started tons of hobbies such as sky-diving. She felt that her life began after her divorce. Very different perceptions, yet it's the same stressor. In other words, the same situation produced very different reactions based on the individual's perception. A former student of mine received a "D" and was ecstatic because he passed the class while another student who was enrolled in the same class received a "B+" and was extremely upset and agitated that she didn't receive an "A." Perception is a key factor in determining whether something is eustressful or distressful.

Table 8.3 Healthy Stressors

- Going through Army Basic Training (also known as Boot Camp).—Hamzah Jacques
- Being part of a senior project team that was demanding and stressful but gave me the opportunity to experience how a company is managed and to add something nice to my resume.—Anonymous
- Practicing until I was the number one player on my high school varsity tennis team.—Daniel Kim
- Raising my GPA from 2.83 to 3.0 in 2 quarters so that I could get an internship.—Ali Showkatian
- When I tried out for my high school freshman basketball team.—Ervin Lozano
- My husband's service in the military.—Jennifer Rodriguez
- Midterms.—Kari Nicholas
- Approaching my college graduation.—Victoria Timpe
- Going to college.—Blanca M. Espinoza
- The time when I climbed the 400+ steps of Moro Rock in Sequoia National Park.—Anonymous
- Opening up my own business.—Anonymous
- The day I entered the Los Angeles County Sheriff Academy.—Elene Williams
- Competing in horse shows.—Anonymous
- Graduating and getting my graduation arrangements (photos, announcements, etc) together.—Jennifer Estell
- Having to do well this last quarter in order to graduate.—Rosemary Garcia
- When I left my 9-to-5 job I had been at for eight years in order to pursue my dream career as a fashion photographer.—Anonymous
- Studying to get a perfect score in the math section of the GRE.—Samuel Torrez
- Traveling abroad and meeting people with different socioeconomic or cultural backgrounds.—Maryam Dehghan
- The pressure of graduating from college.—Vu H. Nguyen
- Planning my wedding.—Nicole
- "Crunch time" right before the quarter is over.—Marielle Croudo
- My company had recently merged with another. As a result, we had to learn a whole new list of products, services, procedures, and processing system.—Sabrina Huda
- Buying a house for the first time.—Channyn Marasco
- Going to college.—Jennifer F. Amagrande
- Running in the L. A. Marathon.—Justin Wang

Table 8.4   Examples of Eustress ⇔ Distress

- Being in an abusive relationship (distress) and then deciding to get a divorce and start a new life (eustress).
- Having the perfect job (eustress) and then unexpectedly getting laid off (distress).
- Falling in love (eustress) and then finding that the relationship is turning sour (distress).
- Playing on a sports team for recreational purposes (eustress) and then finding that the time commitment and intensity of practices is too much (distress).
- Putting in a lot of time and effort into studying for a class (distress) and then receiving a good grade at the end of the semester (eustress).
- Riding a fun and exciting roller coaster (eustress) but then finding that it's pushed you past your tolerance, causing you to vomit (distress).

Eustress ⇔ Distress

It's possible for stressors that once caused eustress to eventually cause distress. So, a stressor can switch from being eustressful to being distressful and vice versa. You might learn how to deal with a particular stressor more effectively and thus begin to view the stressor as more of a challenge than a problem. So the stressor that used to be distressful can become eustressful. Hating your job, for example, can be very distressful. But your job might turn into a eustressor because it motivated you to find a better job. Or the stressor that used to be eustressful is now weighing you down and has become distressful. The excitement and butterflies that often accompany the beginning of a relationship are considered to be eustress. But if things turn sour and the relationship becomes abusive, distress results.

Physiology

It's interesting that the physiological responses to distress and eustress are basically the same but the brain processes the experiences differently. If you won the lottery, that would be eustressful for most people, but you would experience the same huge increase in your heart rate and blood pressure after hearing that you won than if you found out that a friend or loved one was killed, which would most likely be distressful. The physiological reactions of encountering eustress are the same as that of distress. Yet, one produces positive emotions and the other results in negative emotions. So although the *physiological* reactions are the same, the *psychological* reactions can be very different. Also, despite the physiological reactions being the same in both types of stress, health consequences are associated only with distress.

Yerkes-Dodson Principle

One of my favorite quotes is "The only difference between a diamond and a lump of coal is that the diamond had a little more pressure put on it." I believe that life is about learning, growing, progressing, and developing. How can we transform from a lump of coal to a priceless diamond if we don't ever experience the pressure that allows us to learn and grow and develop and progress? As illustrated by the concept of eustress, not all stress is undesirable or unhealthy. It's only when our internal defense system begins to break down because of stress-inducing perceptions and ineffective coping methods that stress becomes undesirable or unhealthy. Stress, specifically chronic distress, is unhealthy—no doubt about it. But is too little stress unhealthy? Is there really such a thing as not having enough stress?

In order to increase physical strength, it's necessary to stress the muscles. Lifting weights can stress muscles and cause microscopic tears. It's the building back up from these tears that results in increased physical strength. But if the muscle is stressed too much or you lift too much weight and too often, your muscles can be torn down too much and your body doesn't have a chance to build the muscles back. And if you don't give your muscles a day off and have enough recovery time between workouts, your muscles don't have time to rebuild themselves before you tear them again. So, too, it is with stress. Experiencing and dealing with stressors can cause "microscopic tears" in our emotional health and stamina. But learning to build ourselves back up from stressful experiences results in increased emotional strength. However, if you're dealing with too much stress and are hit with numerous different stressors all at once without enough of a break between those stressors, you might not have a chance to "recover" or deal with the stress effectively. And

Table 8.5   Examples of Acute and Chronic Stress

Acute	Chronic
Seeing the flashing lights of a police car in your rearview mirror	Having a heavy course load while working full time
Giving a presentation	Being in a bad relationship
Watching a scary movie	Having a job you don't like
Hearing a loud, unexpected noise in the middle of the night	Living in poverty
Facing a phobia or fear such as visiting a dentist or going on a bridge	Being in debt
First hearing the news about an unexpected death of a family member or friend	Living with the loss of a family member or friend
Having your computer crash after working on a project for several hours and losing everything	Living with a chronic, debilitating illness or disease
Riding a roller coaster	Living with depression

what was eustress may turn into distress and negatively affect your emotional health.

On the other hand, if you don't sufficiently stress the muscle or you don't lift enough weight, you won't develop your physical strength. A muscle that is never stressed will quickly atrophy or deteriorate. The muscle must be stressed enough to cause microscopic tears so that the body can rebuild the muscle, which, again, results in increased physical strength. So too it is with stress. The challenges and trials that we face serve as the weights we lift in order to strengthen our spirit or character. If we're never faced with emotional stress, we'll never have the opportunity to strengthen our coping capabilities and develop the capacity to effectively handle stress. So the next time you encounter a stressful situation, think of it as your opportunity to "work out" and increase your emotional strength.

Similar to the concept of eustress, the **Yerkes-Dodson Principle** also known as the *Good Stress–Bad Stress Curve*, basically states that too little stress as well as too much stress is unhealthy. In other words, there's an optimal amount of stress that's correlated with an optimal level of both health and overall performance. Studies have shown that athletes perform better when they feel some degree of stress, or when they're "psyched up," prior to a competition. Their performance is below par when they're not psyched up enough or when they're psyched up too much. It's thought that the same is true for non-athletes. In other words, we perform our daily tasks better when we have some stress in our lives. Have you noticed that you're not as productive when you have too much time on your hands? On the flip side, have you noticed that you're not as productive when you have

too much to do because you feel paralyzed and/or overwhelmed? So you don't do anything because you don't know where to start? In addition to our productivity or performance in general, our health is affected when we have too little stress just as it is by having too much stress. In fact, it's thought that some of the same health problems associated with having too much stress can also occur when we don't have enough stress or stimuli in our lives.

So there's an optimal amount of stress that correlates with an optimal level of performance and health. But what is that optimal amount? We're all different in terms of our ability to handle stress. Do you know people who can't handle a lot of stress? They *stress out* at the drop of a dime. On the flip side, can you think of people you know who never seem to stress about anything? What's optimal stress for one person may be too much or too little for another. Learning to find and maintain that optimal level of stress for yourself throughout your life is critical!

TYPES OF DISTRESS

So eustress is "good" or healthy stress and distress is "bad" or unhealthy stress. Not all distress is the same. In other words, not all distress is "bad" or unhealthy to the same extent. There are two types of distress: acute and chronic. **Acute distress** is stress that is intense but doesn't last long. Examples of acute distress would be the dreaded lights of a police car flashing in your rearview mirror while you're driving, giving a presentation, watching a scary moving or hearing an unexpected, loud noise outside your window in the middle of the night. **Chronic stress** that is not as intense but it lingers for prolonged periods of time. Examples of chronic distress would be having a heavy course load for a particular quarter while working full time, being in a bad relationship, living with chronic pain, or having a bad job.

ACUTE VERSUS CHRONIC

The Rabbit and the Fox

The following analogy illustrates the difference between chronic and acute distress: Imagine being a rabbit that has just been spotted by a fox whose eyes say *breakfast*. Yes, the rabbit will experience stress, but that is the only hope the rabbit has. With a surge of fight-or-flight hormones suddenly coursing through its veins, the rabbit takes off—the fox, in a similar physiological state, in hot pursuit. This is acute stress. In that rush of energy, the rabbit's fate is decided. If the rabbit escapes, it probably has a good rest, and then the episode is closed. It won't dream about foxes for a week or go see a psychiatrist for tranquilizers, or join a "Fox Haters Anonymous" group. It just goes on being a rabbit. Anyway, if the rabbit dwells on yesterday's fox, it is going to miss today's fox, and then it may not be nearly so lucky again. Now, imagine some artificial laboratory, in which the rabbit is on a treadmill, just a whisker away from the fox on another treadmill, all arranged so that the fox can't actually reach the rabbit and the rabbit can never get away either. The result: chronic stress!

Most Common and Most Dangerous

Which is the most common type of stress and which is the most detrimental to our health: chronic or acute distress? Unfortunately, the most dangerous type is also the most common type and that is ... chronic distress. Even though acute distress is technically more intense—it causes a greater increase in heart rate and blood pressure—chronic distress lasts longer and tends to be more detrimental to health. Humankind has spent most of its long history living with episodes of acute stress, but modern life seems much closer to chronic stress. It's just one long traffic jam. The *traffic jam syndrome* can apply to school, marriages, bills, and so on. Chronic distress, even if

you believe that you've gotten used to it, can have long-term consequences on your body and your mind.

Types of Stressors

Just as there are different types of stress, so too are there different types of stressors. A **stressor** is defined as *a stimulus with the potential for eliciting a stress response*, can be categorize into four general types:

- A **physiological stressor** pertains to one's level of physical comfort, or lack thereof, and usually stems from illness, injury, or environmental factors such as the weather or noise. Examples include being too hot or too cold or dealing with pain resulting from major surgery. Having grown up in Southern California, I was not accustomed to cold weather (cold weather to me is anything below 60 degrees). Until I moved to the Midwest where I completed my doctoral studies, I never knew it was possible to be so cold that it hurt. I remember wanting to cry because I was so cold one morning walking to class but was afraid that my tears would freeze! I had left my apartment with my hair slightly damp after showering and I couldn't believe when a few strands of my hair actually broke off because they were frozen. Living in cold weather, to me, was definitely an example of physiological stress.

- A **sociological stressor** stems from relationships or interactions with others and can be very stressful. Examples include getting into arguments with friends or family members or dealing with the death of a loved one. Divorce or termination of a relationship is thought to be one of the greatest stressors. In fact, an individual who survived a concentration campus during World War II admitted that feeling rejected from a boy, in a way, was worse than the inhumane experiences she endured in the concentration camp! Not only can it be very stressful when things are not right with friends and family members, it can also be stressful when things are not right with acquaintances or even strangers. It's stressful to feel offended with the rude cashier at the grocery store or to feel frustrated or angry with the abrasive customer service representative on the phone.

- A **psychological stressor** stems from within yourself and pertains to your subconscious perception of yourself or your feelings of self-worth, or lack thereof. Psychological stressors basically have to do with your relationship with yourself and/or your level of self-esteem. Examples of psychological stressors include feeling depressed because you believe that you're not able to handle daily pressures or you feel inadequate to handle a particular situation. You might also feel down because you think that a particular individual dislikes you and you value his or her opinion.

- A **philosophical stressor** comes from not living in congruence with your philosophy or your values and beliefs. Examples of philosophical stressors include guilt resulting from being lazy when you have a strong work ethic or running late when you can't stand people who are always late. Other examples are feeling bad about receiving a

poor grade when you're used to getting only good grades and you have a negative image of those who receive poor grades or living with the knowledge that you cheated on an important exam when you usually have a strong level of integrity.

Which type of stressor is the most stressful or detrimental to our health? It all depends on your perception. Just as your perception determines whether something is eustressful or distressful, your perception also determines which type of stressor is most stressful to you. If you've lived with chronic pain for a long period of time, you might feel that physiological stressors are the most stressful. If you've experienced a horrible divorce that resulted in suicidal thoughts, you may feel that sociological stressors are the most stressful. If you were considered a "nerd" or "geek" while growing up and were constantly made fun of that resulted in your feeling inadequate, psychological stressors may be the most stressful to you. Again, it all depends on your perception, which is largely based on your past experiences.

Stress and Health

Now that we've defined stress and its types, let's discuss how stress affects our health. It's impossible to talk about stress and stress management without addressing the concepts of *health* and *well-being* because these concepts are so closely tied to our perceived stress levels. What is the first thing that comes to your mind when you hear the word *health*? Most people immediately think of physical aspects such as diet or nutrition, exercise, or freedom from disease or illness. Our physical health is definitely important, but the physical aspect is only one of seven components of our health. Health is extremely comprehensive and holistic and includes much more than our physical status. It is defined in terms of each of its dimensions.

DIMENSIONS OF HEALTH

Physical Health

What does it mean to be physically healthy? Do you have to be able to run a marathon in order to be considered physically healthy? **Physical health** is not necessarily measured by whether you can run a

---

Table 8.6 Examples of Types of Stressors

Physiological
- Being too hot or too cold
- Living with chronic pain
- Recovering from a car accident
- Recuperating from major surgery
- Having the flu
- Feeling nauseous or dizzy

Sociological
- Getting into arguments with friends or family members
- Going through a divorce or break-up
- Having to tolerate a roommate's idiosyncrasies
- Feeling offended by the rude cashier at the grocery store
- Feeling frustrated with a strict professor

Psychological
- Feeling depressed
- Living with a poor self-image
- Feeling inadequate to handle daily pressures
- Feeling that everyone dislikes you

Philosophical
- Feeling bad about receiving a poor grade when you're used to getting only good grades
- Feeling guilty about being lazy when you usually have a strong work ethic and are critical of others who are lazy
- Feeling guilty about cheating on an exam when you've never cheated before and you don't believe in cheating
- Feeling frustrated because you're running late and you hate to be late

marathon, but rather it's defined as your ability to adequately perform normal activities of daily living. These activities might include simply being able to get out of bed in the morning, get dressed, walk up a flight of stairs, carry a bag of groceries, and so forth. Our percentage of body fat, weight, blood pressure, cholesterol level, white blood cell count, and other parameters may be indicators of our physical health and may affect our ability to perform those daily activities. Think of someone you consider to be extremely healthy physically. How would you describe this person? Does he or she exercise on a regular and consistent basis? Eat healthy foods the majority of the time? Is he or she at an ideal weight? On the flip side, think of someone who is incredibly unhealthy physically. How would you describe this person? Does he or she smoke? Does he/she constantly have physical health problems?

How is physical health related to stress? Physiological stressors, one of the four types of stressors, can be very distressful. If you have experienced extreme illness or pain for an extended period of time, you probably can relate to feeling stressed when your physical health is not up to par.

Social Health

What does it mean to be socially healthy? Is our social health measured by how many friends we have? Does it mean the more friends you have, the more socially healthy you are? **Social health** is not necessarily measured by the number of friends you have, but rather by how well you relate to other people. Social health has to do with your ability to have satisfying relationships as well as the overall quality of your interaction with others. Think of someone whom you consider to be socially healthy. How would you describe this person? Does he or she get along with just about anyone? Is he or she well liked by others?

Now think of someone you consider socially inept or socially unhealthy. How would you describe this person? Why do you consider him or her to be lacking in social skills or social health? Does this person have a difficult time communicating effectively with other people?

How is social health related to stress? A large percentage of my students have indicated over the years that sociological stressors are the most common type of stressor for them. It can be stressful when things are not right with your relationships or when a relationship has been terminated.

Emotional Health

What does it mean to be emotionally healthy? Is our emotional health measured by how happy we are? Do we always have to be in a good mood to be considered emotionally healthy? **Emotional health,** sometimes called *mental health,* does not necessarily refer to our level of happiness; rather, it has to do with our ability to feel and express the full range of emotions in an appropriate and controlled manner. Emotionally healthy people feel everything from extreme happiness to extreme sadness, but they don't allow their emotions to rule their lives. Their behavior is not necessarily controlled or determined by their feelings and emotions all the time. Think of someone whom you consider to be emotionally healthy. How would you describe this person? In contrast, what about someone whom you consider to be emotionally unhealthy? Why would you consider this person to be emotionally unhealthy? How is emotional health related to stress? Remember that there's physical and emotional homeostasis. Being unable to control your anger, for example, pertains to your emotional health and brings you out of emotional homeostasis (actually because of the strong mind/body connection, it brings you out of physical homeostasis as well). Your emotional health and feelings of stress are closely tied.

Intellectual Health

What does it mean to be intellectually healthy? Do we have to know a lot of facts to be intellectually healthy? Does our GPA or IQ reflect our intellectual health? **Intellectual health** does not necessarily have to do with our GPA or IQ; rather, it refers to our ability to have an open mind and learn new things. Think of someone you consider intellectually healthy. How would you describe this person? Is he or she open minded and like a sponge when it comes to learning new things? Does he or she seek out learning opportunities and love to learn? On the other hand, how would you describe someone who is intellectually unhealthy? Is this person closed minded or unwilling to learn new things? Being asked to "step outside the box" and learn new things might cause stress in some people. So, our intellectual health can be related to feelings of stress.

Spiritual Health

What does it mean to be spiritually healthy? Is our spiritual health measured by how often we go to church? Spiritual health is not necessarily measured by church attendance nor does it necessarily have anything to do with religion. Someone could be extremely spiritual and not necessarily religious or extremely religious and not very spiritual. **Spiritual health** refers to having a strong sense of meaning, purpose, and direction in life. Think of someone you consider extremely spiritual. How would you describe this person? Does he or she have a strong sense of self and where he or she is going in life? Now think of someone you consider spiritually unhealthy. How would you describe this person? Does he or she lack purpose, meaning, or direction in life? How is spiritual health connected to stress? Our spiritual health, or lack thereof, can definitely perpetuate stress-inducing or stress-resistant perceptions.

Environmental Health

The preceding five components of health have to do with things that are going on *inside* a person to a large extent. **Environmental health** refers to *external* factors or factors that occur outside the person that may affect what is going on inside. Environmental health is the one dimension over which we probably have the least amount of control. Environmental health usually has to do with factors affecting our physical health. Quality of air and water are some examples of factors affecting environmental health. But environmental health could also refer to external factors that affect not just the physical domain. Growing up in an abusive home could affect emotional health and could be considered a factor of environmental health. How is environmental health tied to stress? Our individual environments may contribute tremendously to our feelings of stress. For example, living in an extremely rough neighborhood in which you literally have to dodge bullets or run away from muggers would definitely be stressful!

Occupational Health

Occupational health has to do with all of the preceding factors, including environmental health, but as they relate to your place of employment. Because such a significant portion of our lives is spent at our jobs and because the quality of the preceding dimensions of health at work might be very different from that at home, many health promotion professionals agree that occupational health should be an added dimension to our health. Think of how many hours by the end of your life you will have spent at work, whether it be at McDonalds while you're a high school or college student or at a large corporation after you graduate from college. That's a pretty big chunk of your life. One or more of the dimensions of health might be drastically different at home than at work. For example, coal miners' environmental health is undesirable at work (breathing in all the carcinogens in the mines), but if they live in a rural valley free of smog, that aspect of their home environment is positive. Also, emotional health could be completely different at work compared to that at home. You might have a boss who treats you terribly, but you have a wonderful spouse who treats you in a completely opposite manner. Our occupational health, then, is closely tied to our stress levels as well.

Holistic Health

Physical health is the easiest of the dimensions to measure, which is perhaps why we tend to give so much more attention to it compared to the other dimensions. A "physical health" doctor is one of the most, if not *the* most, respected professionals in society. Yet, an "emotional health" doctor carries the negative stigma of "shrink." However, would you consider someone to be healthy if he or she exercised everyday but had absolutely no friends because no one can stand to be around him or her? What if this person ate the most perfect diet—lots of fruits and vegetables, never ate any sweets, etc.—but was unable to relate at all to other people and had absolutely no relationships with others? Would you consider someone to be healthy if he or she was in the best physical shape but had major problems with depression and was suicidal? What if someone had a great body fat percentage but constantly lost his or her temper at the drop of a hat? Would you consider someone to be healthy if he or she was able to run a marathon but was incredibly closed minded to the point of being extremely irrational and had major obsessive-compulsive tendencies? What if this person was at an ideal weight but refused to learn new things? Would you consider someone to be healthy if he or she never got sick but had absolutely no sense of purpose in life, no direction whatsoever? Health is **holistic** and comprehensive and includes so much more than only physical health!

Interrelatedness of Dimensions

The dimensions of health are extremely interrelated—when one dimension is affected, one or more of the others may be affected as well.

In addition to understanding that health is holistic and comprehensive, it's important to understand that the dimensions of health are interrelated: When one dimension is affected, one or more of the others may be affected as well. For example, smoking affects not only your physical health, but also perhaps your social health if you have friends that don't like being around you when you smoke. It might also affect your emotional health if you feel like you need a cigarette in order to relax. Just as your behaviors can affect multiple dimensions of your health, so too can stressors. Getting into a major argument with a good friend, for example, affects your emotional health (you feel frustrated and angry), your physical health (you might get a stomachache or headache), and your social health (you no longer hang out with your friend).

Interrelatedness of Stress and Health

The quality of each dimension of your health may perpetuate and/or exacerbate a stressful life or contribute to homeostasis and a relatively peaceful life. The point is that your stress levels and your health go hand in hand. You might experience stress when any of the dimensions of your health are lacking and/or your dimensions of health are affected by stress. There is usually an inverse correlation with these two concepts: When one is high, the other is low. When all components of your health are in check, your perceived stress levels may be low. When your stress level is high, usually one or more of your health components are out of balance. This is not to say that just because all the dimensions of your health are good, you won't experience any stress. You might be dealing with lots of stressors and yet you're in good health. Or you might be in poor health but you don't feel stressed. However, the better your health, usually the better you're able to deal with your stressors. So when attempting to manage your stress, don't forget to take care of your health!

REFERENCES

Allen, R. *Human Stress: Its Nature and Control*. Minneapolis, MN: Burgess Press, 1983.

Cannon, W. *The Wisdom of the Body*. New York: W. W. Norton, 1932.

Holmes, T. H., and R. Rahe. "The Social Readjustment Rating Scale." *Journal of Psychosomatic Research* 11 (1967): 213–18.

Pelletier, K. *Mind as Healer, Mind as Slayer*. New York: Dell, 1977.

Selye, H. *Stress without Distress*. Philadelphia, PA: Lippincott, 1974.

CHAPTER 9

Public Health

The Public Health System: The Government's Role

Learning Objectives

- Define the concept of public health and give examples of public health activities.
- Explain the role of government in public health.
- List two or more national (federal) public health agencies.
- Explain the role of boards of public health and licensing/regulatory boards.
- Describe at least one major government initiative to protect the public's health.
- Identify the key reporting obligations that health professionals are mandated to uphold.

Key Terms

Assessment

Assurance

Block grants

Case

Centers for Disease Control (CDC)

Centers for Medicare and Medicaid Services (CMS)

Communicable disease

Curative medical care

Drug resistant

Epidemiology

Food and Drug Administration (FDA)

Foundation

Health

Health Resources and Services Administration (HRSA)

Monitoring

Policy development

Prevention efforts

Public Health

Quarantine

Severe Acute Respiratory Syndrome (SARS)

Substance Abuse and Mental Health Services Administration (SAMHSA)

Surveillance

SEVERE ACUTE RESPIRATORY SYNDROME: A PUBLIC HEALTH SUCCESS STORY

Severe acute respiratory syndrome (SARS) is a respiratory illness that was recognized as a global threat in March 2003. The SARS virus can cause fever, headache, body aches, diarrhea, and respiratory problems that are related to low levels of oxygen in the blood. Many people with SARS develop pneumonia. It can also cause death. SARS appears to spread when infected persons cough or sneeze and spread small droplets of saliva and mucus that can land on the mucous membranes of a nearby person

continued.

Austin, Anne; Wetle, Vikki, *The United States Health Care System: Combining Business, Health, and Delivery,* 2nd Edition, © 2012. Reprinted by permission of Pearson Education, Inc., Upper Saddle River, NJ.

or on a surface/object touched by someone who later touches one of their mucous membranes. According to the World Health Organization (WHO), from November 2002 through July 2003, a total of 8,098 people worldwide became ill with SARS (many of them in China). Of this number, 774 died. In the United States, only eight persons were diagnosed with SARS and no one died.

How did the United States avoid a SARS epidemic? The Centers for Disease Control and Prevention (CDC) used strong surveillance techniques and monitoring to keep track of how many people were getting infected and their location. During the 2003 epidemic, the CDC worked with the Council of State and Territorial Epidemiologists to develop surveillance criteria and identify persons with SARS in the United States. Strong communication with state and local health departments helped supply local medical providers with information regarding the symptoms of SARS so that they could identify patients with the disease and report the information to the CDC. Then the agency could take appropriate action to protect the public's health. Epidemiologists investigated how the disease was spread so that prevention recommendations could be created. The science of public health helped prevent a SARS epidemic in the United States.

Source: cdc.gov/ncidod/sars

INTRODUCTION

As individuals, our health is important to us. Yet even though we take care of ourselves, we don't live alone or in isolation. Society is made up of millions of individuals. What affects one member of a community can often affect another member. The health of the nation is the responsibility of the public health system in the United States.

In this chapter, you'll learn about the public health system in the United States: what it is and who's responsible. The history and basic activities of public health are discussed, and the role of government in public health described. Finally, you'll learn about the challenges facing public health in the 21st century. The public health system is not a single system. It is made up of many different agencies coming together to improve the health and lives of Americans. This is a brief overview, highlighting some of the major components of the system.

WHAT IS PUBLIC HEALTH?

To define *public health*, we must first define **health.** The World Health Organization (WHO) defines health as "a state of complete physical, mental and social well-being and not merely the absence of disease or infirmity" (http://www.who.int/en/). According to this definition, being healthy is more than just not being sick. It is a state of well-being in our bodies, our minds, and our lives. Keeping this definition in mind, what happens when we place the word *public* in front of the word *health?* Public in this sense implies the government has primary responsibility for the social good of health, just as it does in public education. **Public health,** therefore, involves the well-being of all of us as we live together in neighborhoods, communities, states, and countries. It is anything and everything that relates to helping us collectively experience "a state of complete physical, mental and social well-being." It touches nearly every aspect of our lives. The large-scale goals of public health are to protect, promote, and restore health and to reduce the premature death and discomfort caused by disease. In short, the goal of public health is to protect the community from the hazards of group life.

Unlike **curative medical care,** which focuses on making us feel better when we are already ill, public health focuses on **prevention efforts** to keep us from getting sick in the first place. Because it focuses on prevention, public health has the power to impact the policies and laws that help us have a healthier society. It helps promote well-being on a societal level and often global level, and it makes the world a better place for all of us.

Public health can be seen in our everyday lives in things as simple as the crosswalk lines on a street that allow us to cross a roadway without getting hit by a car or the laws requiring construction workers to wear hard hats so that they are not injured by falling construction debris. It is also recognizable in state and nationwide campaigns to reduce smoking, heart disease, and cancer. Public health is actualized by activities such as nurses providing free immunizations to low-income children and police officers enforcing laws around seat belt and helmet use.

Most important, public health is the way a society reaches out to protect the health of its most vulnerable members. Using a system of **block grants** and specific public health initiatives, public health programs nationwide provide medical care for the elderly, substance abuse recovery programs, nutritional help for low-income women and infants, free dental care for children, medical care for the homeless, and so much more.

Public health is a wonderful idea, but does it really matter? Shouldn't it be enough for each of us just to take care of ourselves? Although our individual efforts to stay healthy do, in one sense, help us create a healthy community, some things require collective, organized efforts. For example, laws are needed to govern sanitation, waste disposal, food safety, and water purity. The quality of these services can affect an entire community. In the absence of public health efforts, it is easier for disease to spread and make more people ill.

Widespread illness affects not only people but also communities and economies. Think for a moment about the devastating effect of HIV infection in sub-Saharan Africa today. Of the 33 million AIDS cases (each case represents one person) world-wide, 22 million of them are in this one region (www. unaids.org). Young adults in the prime of life are dying. Not only are families devastated and children orphaned, but large sections of the population are not working because of premature death and illness. When people can't work, food is not grown, resulting in starvation, which leads to further problems, and the situation only worsens. Although some health programs are operating in Africa, they are clearly overwhelmed by the demands on their limited resources. The lack of a strong public health system can be the downfall of a society. Public health does more than keep us healthy; it makes civilization possible.

THE HISTORY OF PUBLIC HEALTH

Public health is not a completely new concept in human society. Humans have tried to promote community health in a variety of ways at different points in history. One of the earliest ways was through sanitation efforts. The ancient city of Mojenjo Daro in northern India, built over 4,000 years ago, had paved streets covering sewers that drained waste from bathrooms in residential homes. The classical era of the Greek and Roman civilizations also saw the creation of bathhouses to promote cleanliness and the building of drainage canals (Fairbanks and Wiese, 1998). Early versions of **quarantine** were instituted in the Middle Ages (and earlier) when persons infected with leprosy were placed in leper colonies outside of town limits in an effort to keep the disease from spreading.

In the United States, public health efforts gained strength as the nation grew toward independence in the 1700s. Several key events helped shape public health. Some of the first efforts of organized action to protect community health were the creation of boards of health. These early boards of health were often created in response to an epidemic (Turnock, 1997). For example, in 1793, a terrible epidemic of yellow fever broke out in Philadelphia, then the nation's capital. The epidemic was so devastating that it prompted not only the transfer of the national capital to Washington but also the establishment of Philadelphia's first board of health that same year.

The National Institutes of Health (NIH) traces its roots to 1887 when a one-room laboratory was created within the Marine Hospital Service (MHS), predecessor agency to the U.S. Public Health Service (PHS). The MHS had been established in 1798 to provide for the medical care of merchant seamen. One clerk in the Treasury Department collected 20 cents per month from the wages of each seaman to cover costs at a series of contract hospitals. In the 1880s, Congress had charged the MRS with examining passengers on arriving ships for clinical signs of infectious diseases, especially for the dreaded diseases such as cholera and yellow fever, in order to prevent epidemics. During the 1870s and 1880s, moreover, scientists in Europe presented compelling evidence that microscopic organisms were the causes of several infectious diseases. In 1884, for example, Koch described a comma-shaped bacterium as the cause of cholera. Officials of the MRS followed these developments with great interest. In 1887, they authorized Joseph J. Kinyoun, a young MHS physician trained in the new bacteriological methods, to set up a one-room laboratory in the Marine Hospital at Stapleton, Staten Island, New York. Kinyoun called this facility a "laboratory of hygiene" in imitation of German facilities and to indicate that the laboratory's purpose was to serve the public's health. Within a few months, Kinyoun had identified the cholera bacillus in suspicious cases and used his Zeiss microscope to demonstrate it to his colleagues as confirmation of their clinical diagnoses. "As the symptoms . . . were by no means well defined," he wrote, "the examinations were confirmatory evidence of the value of bacteria cultivation as a means of positive diagnosis" (history.nih.gov/exhibits/history).

One of the key events to shape public health in America was the signing of the Act for the Relief of Sick and Disabled Seamen by President John Adams in 1798 (see Table 9.1). The act provided for a tax of 20 cents a month on the salary of sailors. The funds were used to build and staff hospitals to care for sailors. Over time, this system of hospitals and the person appointed to oversee it became the government body on which we rely today to protect our nation's health: the U.S. Public Health Service, headed by the surgeon general (Fairbanks and Wiese, 1998).

In 1850, Lemuel Shattuck published the *Report of the Sanitary Commission of Massachusetts*. It outlined the existing and future public health needs for that state and became America's blueprint for the development of public health systems. Shattuck's report called for the establishment of state and local health departments to engage in sanitary inspections, **communicable disease** control, food sanitation, vital statistics, and services for infants and children. Although it took several decides for his ideas to catch on, Massachusetts established the first state health department in 1869. By 1900, there were 40 such state health departments (CDC 1999a). The public health system was expanded considerably in the period just after the great influenza epidemic in 1918

(Berry, 2004). Today, every state has a health department and a public health laboratory.

KEY PUBLIC HEALTH FUNCTIONS

In 1988, the Institute of Medicine released a report called *The Future of Public Health* that outlined these three key functions of public health: assessment of the health of the community, policy development, and assurance of the public health. **Assessment** means determining the health needs of the community by surveying disease incidence and prevalence, identifying needs, analyzing why health outcomes are not met, collecting and interpreting data, monitoring health trends research, and evaluating outcomes.

Policy development is the collective decision about what actions are most appropriate for the health of the state or nation. **Assurance** is making sure that the necessary actions are actually taken. To carry out these three functions, information is needed. Public health officials engage in three key activities to satisfy this need: epidemiology, surveillance, and monitoring. These activities provide them with the information they need to assess and assure a community's health and to make policy decisions.

Epidemiology is the study of the history of a disease and its distribution throughout a society. It permits understanding and rational decision-making

---

Career Profile: Epidemiologist

Epidemiologists are sometimes called "disease detectives." Like any good detective, their primary duty is to carry out investigations, in this case of a disease. They study where a disease outbreak occurred, who it affected, and how and when. They examine the relationships among various factors such as lifestyle, environment, person-to-person contact, and geography. They collect information from people using surveys and interview. They also look at existing health information such as local disease statistics or insurance claims information.

Epidemiologists can work in health departments, laboratories, hospitals, and government agencies, such as the CDC. Because disease outbreaks can occur anywhere at any time, some epidemiologists travel the nation, or even the world, for their investigations. Other epidemiologists investigate disease outbreaks closer to home. When not investigating a disease, epidemiologists work at their computers cataloging all the information they have collected.

The conclusions reached by epidemiologists and the data they collect are important in several ways. First, in determining how a disease is spread, epidemiologists can make recommendations about how to avoid further infections. Second, their conclusions can help boards of health and health departments develop policies to protect the community's health. Without the work of epidemiologists, our understanding of diseases and how they pass from person to person would be severely limited. Thanks to epidemiologists, our path to health gets clearer, and a little bit easier, all the time.

Table 9.1 Abbreviated Historical Development—National Institutes of Health

1798	President John Adams signed "an Act for the relief of sick and disabled Seamen," which led to the establishment of the Marine Hospital Service.
1803	The first permanent Marine Hospital authorized to be built in Boston, Massachusetts.
1836	Library of the Office of Surgeon General of the Army established.
1870	President Grant signed a law establishing a "Bureau of the U.S. Marine Hospital Service," Treasury Department, which created central control over the hospitals, and a Supervising Surgeon (later Surgeon General).
1887	Laboratory of Hygiene established at Marine Hospital, Staten Island, New York, for research in cholera and other infectious diseases.
1891	Rocky Mountain Spotted Fever Laboratory established in Hamilton, Montana, as field station of Public Health Service.
1922	Congress authorized National Cancer Institute (NCI) and the awarding of research grants. Rocky Mountain Laboratory became part of NIH.
1938	National Institute of Health moved to land donated by Mr. and Mrs. Luke I. Wilson at Bethesda, Maryland. Cornerstone for Shannon Building laid.
1949	Mental Hygiene Program of Public Health Service transferred to NIH and expanded to become National Institute of Mental Health.
1950	"Omnibus Medical Research Act" authorized the establishment of the National Institute of Neurological Diseases and Blindness and the National Institute of Arthritis and Metabolic Diseases, and the latter absorbed the Experimental Biology and Medicine Institute.
1957	The Center for Aging Research established.
1961	The Center for Research in Child Health established in Division of General Medical Sciences.
1964	Division of Computer Research and Technology established.
1966	Division of Environmental Health Sciences created.
1970	National Institute on Aging created.
1990	National Center for Research Resources was created by consolidating the Division of Research Services and the Division of Research Resources.
1991	National Center for Medical Rehabilitation Research established within the National Institute of Child Health and Human Development.
1992	National Institute on Alcohol Abuse and Alcoholism, National Institute on Drug Abuse, and National Institute of Mental Health were transferred to NIH from the Alcohol, Drug Abuse, and Mental Health Administration.
1993	National Center for Nursing Research was re-titled as the National Institute of Nursing Research.
1994	The Dietary Supplement Health and Education Act of 1993 mandated establishment of an Office of Dietary Supplements within NIH to conduct and coordinate NIH research relating to dietary supplements and the extent to which their use reduces the risk of certain diseases.
2000 to present	The international Human Genome Project public consortium—funded by NIH, DOE, and others—assembled a working draft of the sequence of the human genome.
2003	The International Human Genome Sequencing Consortium led in the United States by NHGRI and the Department of Energy, completed the Human Genome Project
	The complete genetic blueprint of Bacillus anthracis—the microbe that gained notoriety during the 2001 anthrax mail attacks—has been completed by NIAID-funded researchers.
	President George W. Bush visits NIH on Feb. 3 to unveil Project BioShield, a $6 billion, 10-year effort to protect the public from various weapons of bioterrorism.
2004	NIH opens the Mark O. Hatfield Clinical Research Center, a 240-bed successor to the NIH Clinical Center, which opened in 1953
2008	Through legislation enacted by Congress, NICHD was renamed the Eunice Kennedy Shriver National Institute of Child Health and Human Development at the institute's 45th anniversary celebration. In the early 1960s, Shriver persuaded her brother, President John F. Kennedy, to include the proposal for an NIH institute focusing on child health and human development in his first health message to Congress. NICHD was then established in 1963.

Source: http://www.nih.gov/about/almanac/historical/chronology_of_events.htm

Table 9.2   Key Terms in Public Health Measurement

Incidence	Number of new cases of a disease or event such as a motor vehicle accident in a specific population
Morbidity	Number of cases of a specific disease in a specific period of time per unit of population, usually expressed as a number per 1,000
Mortality	Number of people who have died from a given disease or event
Rates	These rates are collected and analyzed from death certificates. **Morbidity and Mortality Weekly Report** is published by the CDC and reports illness and death rates for a variety of diseases.
Prevalence	Total number of infected/affected people (cases) over a given period of time
Relative risk	How an individual's risk may change relevant to a specific factor (e.g., a smoker has a higher relative risk of getting lung cancer than a person who does not smoke)
Risk	Likelihood that someone will become infected/affected

regarding actions that need to be taken. Epidemiologists investigate where a disease outbreak occurred, who it affected, and how and when. Popularized recently as "disease detectives," epidemiologists help determine not only where a disease came from but also how to protect people from it. For example, in 1993 in the state of Washington, 477 people became ill from *Escherichia coli*, a deadly bacterium that causes severe intestinal problems and sometimes death. Epidemiologists kept track of who had the disease. They investigated what activities the infected persons had engaged in up to the time when they got sick. Their research led them to a local fast-food restaurant that had been undercooking ground beef. Thanks to epidemiologists, the cause of the problem was discovered and further illness prevented. To learn more about the career of epidemiology, see the Career Profile Box.

The term *surveillance* is used to describe the actions of police as they watch a suspect and take note of what takes place. Similarly, in public health, **surveillance** refers to the continuous search for and documentation of disease. If public health departments were not always on the lookout for new diseases or outbreaks of disease, diseases could run rampant. Surveillance keeps track of all kinds of things, from sexually transmitted infections, to episodes of violence, to the number of cases of the flu.

Monitoring refers to the use of surveillance data to determine changes in the number of infected persons so that the appropriate action can be taken when the infection rate gets too high. Monitoring helps answer questions about whether or not there is more or less of a particular disease present now than in the past.

Several basic measurements can help us understand the information uncovered through surveillance and monitoring activities. Often you hear these terms used in the news or in reports about a current health concern. These measurements are used to create a picture of how a disease is affecting society. Table 9.2 lists some key public health terms.

Where do the data for surveillance and monitoring come from? State health departments are required by law to report on cases of specific diseases or conditions. Some of this data, such as the number of persons infected with a particular disease, are collected for statistical purposes and to alert health authorities to a possible epidemic. Other conditions, such as child abuse, are reported because it allows someone to intervene in the situation and ideally prevent any further abuse from occurring. Whenever health or social service providers come across one of these conditions or diseases, they are required to report the information to the state. This information can be reported confidentially. For example, although the number of people infected with HIV is reported to the state, their names are not. As of 2009, 72 diseases had to be reported at the national level, including HIV, cholera, rabies, sexually transmitted infections, tuberculosis, hepatitis, and anthrax exposure (see Table 9.3).

ROLE OF GOVERNMENT IN PUBLIC HEALTH

The government plays a key role in assuring the public's health. Government in action can be seen at the local (county, neighborhood), state, and federal levels. Prior to the Great Depression (1929–41), U.S. citizens did not think the federal government should intervene in people's health. Health is not a power granted to the federal government in the Constitution. Therefore, individuals, with some help from the state government, took care of their health themselves. But the situation was so desperate during the

Table 9.3 Infectious Diseases Designated as Notifiable at the National Level During 2007

Acquired immunodeficiency syndrome (AIDS)	Meningococcal disease
Anthrax	Mumps
Domestic arboviral diseases	Novel influenza A virus infections
California serogroup virus disease	Pertussis
Eastern equine encephalitis virus disease	Plague
Powassan virus disease	Poliomyelitis, paralytic
St. Louis encephalitis virus disease	Poliovirus infection, nonparalytic
West Nile virus disease	Psittacosis
Western equine encephalitis virus disease	Q fever
Botulism (foodborne, infant, other)	Rabies (animal, human)
Brucellosis	Rocky Mountain spotted fever
Chancroid	Rubella (congenital syndrome)
Chlamydia trachomatis, genital infection	Salmonellosis
Cholera	Severe acute respiratory syndrome-associated coronavirus
Coccidioidomycosis	
Cryptosporidiosis	Shiga toxin-producing Escherichia coli (STEC)
Cyclosporiasis	Shigellosis
Diphtheria	Smallpox
Ehrlichiosis (human granulocytic, human monocytic, human with other or unspecified agent)	Streptococcal disease, invasive, group A
	Streptococcal toxic-shock syndrome
Giardiasis	Streptococcus pneumoniae, invasive disease (drug resistant—all ages, nondrug resistant—age < 5years)
Gonorrhea	
Haemophilus influenzae, invasive disease	Syphilis (congenital)
Hansen disease (leprosy)	Tetanus
Hantavirus pulmonary syndrome	Toxic-shock syndrome (other than streptococcal)
Hemolytic uremic syndrome, postdiarrheal	Trichinellosis
Hepatitis A, acute	Tuberculosis
Hepatitis B (acute, chronic, virus—perinatal infection)	Tularemia
Hepatitis C (acute, virus infection—past or present)	Typhoid fever
Human immunodeficiency virus (HIV) infection (adults age > 13 years, pediatric age < 13 years)	Vancomycin-intermediate Staphylococcus aureus infaction (VISA)
Influenza-associated pediatric mortality	Vancomycin-resistant Staphylococcus aureus infection (VRSA)
Legionellosis	
Listeriosis	Varicella infection (morbidity)
Lyme disease	Varicella (mortality)
Malaria	Vibriosis (non-cholera Vibrio infections)
Measles	Yellow fever

Source: www.cdc.gov/mmwr/preview/mmwrhtml/mm5653a1.htm (latest available data).

Great Depression that the federal government was expected to take action (Turnock, 1997).

Since then, the federal government's role in health has expanded. Two sections of the Constitution have been interpreted as allowing the federal government to intervene in the nation's health. The first is the ability to tax people to provide for the "general welfare." This allows for the collection of money to be used in support of health programs. In fact, today the government's main role in public health is financial support of public health programs.

Second, the federal government has the ability to regulate commerce. Only the government can en-force policies that limit the personal and property rights of individuals or businesses. This power allows for the regulation of restaurants, sewage and water companies, product and drug safety, and other businesses that sell products to consumers.

Federal Government

Public health at the federal level is represented by numerous agencies, each dedicated to a specific aspect of the public's health. The Department of Health and Human Services (DHHS) is the U.S.

government's principal department protecting the health of the nation. *As of 2004, DHHS included over 300 programs and several key agencies* (Berry, 2004). Here is a list of some of these key agencies:

- The **Food and Drug Administration** (FDA) assures the safety of foods, cosmetics, and medications.
- The **Centers for Disease Control** (CDC) works with state health departments and other community organizations to monitor disease, help prevent outbreaks, maintain national health statistics, and operate disease prevention and health promotion programs.
- The **Health Resources and Services Administration** (HRSA) provides access to health care services for low-income and uninsured people or for people who live in areas where health care is not easily available. HRSA-funded health care centers provide medical care for more than 13 million people in over 3,600 health centers across the nation.
- The **Centers for Medicare and Medicaid Services** (CMS) provides health care insurance through third-party carriers for about one in every four Americans. Medicare provides insurance for more than 41 million elderly and persons with disabilities. Medicaid additionally covers 44 million low-income persons, including 19 million children. State children's health insurance programs administered by CMS cover an additional 4.2 million children.
- The **Substance Abuse and Mental Health Services Administration** (SAMHSA) works to improve the availability and quality of substance abuse prevention, addiction treatment, and mental health services. Funding from SAMSHA helps more than 650,000 Americans with serious substance abuse problems or mental health problems.

As mentioned earlier in the chapter, public health is the way a society cares for its most vulnerable citizens. The government's financial involvement is clearly crucial to this effort. Without this support, literally millions of individuals would be without adequate medical care. Our ability to control disease would be severely hampered. A government's investment in public health is a symbol of how much it supports and cares for its citizens.

State Government

At the state level, there are two kinds of public health bodies: boards of health and state health departments. Boards of health are the policymaking bodies for a state's Department of Health. Twenty-four states have boards of health that oversee financing and policy development (Fairbanks and Wiese, 1998). States that do not have boards of health have other mechanisms to make policy. They have the power to adopt and amend rules and regulations and to make recommendations. State health departments are charged with promoting the public's health and implementing public health laws. States regulate things like newborn screening. Forty-eight states and the District of Columbia have regulations requiring PKU and other genetic disorders screening. Many have provisions for treating these defects with special formulas and other necessary interventions through the Health Departments (http://www.hrsa.gov).

Additional responsibilities of state departments of health include:

- Carrying out national and state mandates designed to protect health
- Managing environmental education and personal health services
- Collecting, analyzing, and disseminating information on threats to the community's health
- Responding to statewide health crises such as hepatitis and flu outbreaks
- Setting policies and standards for health care and medical professionals
- Conducting inspections of restaurants and factories
- Conducting the planning and evaluation of health programs

There are two models of a state health department. In most states, the health department is a freestanding agency that reports directly to the state governor. In other states, the health department is part of a larger institution, such as the state's Department of Health and Human Services. The Affordable Health Care Act of 2010 will impact the scope and responsibility of state health departments (http://www.healthcare.gov/).

In addition, licensing and regulatory boards help protect the public's health by assuring that health care professionals and others, such as food handlers, are held to basic standards of care, cleanliness, and safety. For example, state health inspectors evaluate whether or not laboratories are using proper techniques, if restaurants have adequate food safety efforts, or if a factory has strong enough pollution control measures. As you read about health professionals, licensing boards assure consumers that their health or service professionals have been tested and trained on specific knowledge. Not only are health professionals licensed, but in many states so are service personnel such as food handlers and cosmeticians.

Local Health Departments

Local health departments can serve an individual county, city, or region. They are responsible for the delivery of services mandated by the state or by local statute. They can be independent or part of a state department of health.

In 1999, the National Association of County and City Health Officials surveyed 1,100 local public health agencies nationwide in an effort to better understand their activities. They determined that the most common programs and services included adult and child immunizations, communicable disease control, community assessment, community education, environmental health services, epidemiology and surveillance, food safety, restaurant inspections, and tuberculosis testing. These local agencies rarely provided direct medical care. Because state government has so many administrative, legal, and inspection responsibilities, it is important to have local health systems that can provide more direct service to community members.

OTHER PUBLIC HEALTH PARTNERS

Public health is not solely in the hands of the government. Organizations like the Red Cross, March of Dimes, and the American Cancer Society play an important role. In addition, smaller local social service organizations are able to work directly with the community members whose health they want to protect. These may be not-for-profit organizations or community-based organizations. They provide services in their local communities for specific populations and for one or two targeted health problems. For example, an organization could choose to

help inner-city homeless youth or young women with substance abuse problems. **Foundations** are a particular kind of not-for-profit organization. They raise funds to support a cause of their choice and then distribute the funding to other community-based organizations in support of their work.

The importance of these nongovernmental partners cannot be underestimated. In particular, community-based organizations often go directly to the person needing services. Sometimes this means visiting people in their homes or finding them in parks or on the street. Thus many people who might not make it to the health department receive the help they need. By specializing in a specific health issue, these organizations can also provide expert advice to their patrons. Nongovernmental efforts help complete and strengthen the public health system.

PAST SUCCESSES AND FUTURE CHALLENGES

According to the CDC, the life expectancy of persons living in the United States has increased by 30 years since 1900; 25 years of this gain are attributable to successful public health interventions. Although the successes of public health are many, the CDC selected key program areas as having the most impact on lowering death rates and decreasing illness and disability in the United States (CDC 1999b). These 10 great achievements are related to the following areas:

1. Vaccination: The development of vaccines and vaccination campaigns has led to decreased incidences of many illnesses such as diphtheria. Also, vaccinations have eradicated diseases such as smallpox and, in the Western Hemisphere, polio.
2. Safer workplaces: New safety standards in industries such as mining, construction, manufacturing, and transportation have led to a 40 percent reduction in the rate of job-related injuries.
3. Healthier mothers and babies: Improvements in hygiene, nutrition, and availability of antibiotics, greater access to health care, and technological advances have helped reduce infant and maternal mortality.
4. Control of infectious diseases: Improved sanitation and clean water have helped control many diseases such as cholera and typhoid. Also, new

---

Medical Reserve Corps

The Medical Reserve Corps (MRC) was founded after President Bush's 2002 State of the Union Address, in which he asked all Americans to volunteer in support of their country. It is a partner program with Citizen Corps, a national network of volunteers dedicated to ensuring hometown security. The U.S. Surgeon General assigns MRC units specific areas to target that strengthen the public health infrastructure of their communities each year. These reflect the priorities for the health of individuals, and the nation as a whole. The goal, in addition to providing well-trained volunteers in an emergency, is to improve health literacy, and in support of this, she wants us to work toward increasing disease prevention, eliminating health disparities, and improving public health preparedness. Units are community-based and function as a way to locally organize and utilize volunteers who want to donate their time and expertise to prepare for and respond to emergencies and promote healthy living throughout the year. MRC volunteers supplement existing emergency and public health resources.

MRC volunteers include medical and public health professionals such as physicians, dentist, pharmacists, dentists, veterinarians, and epidemiologists. Many community members—interpreters, chaplains, office workers, legal advisors, and others—fill key support positions.

MRC volunteers can also choose to support communities in need nationwide. When the southeast was battered by hurricanes in 2004, MRC volunteers in the affected areas and beyond helped communities by filling in at local hospitals, assisting their neighbors at local shelters, and providing first aid to those injured by the storms. During this 2-month period, more than 30 MRC units worked as part of the relief efforts, including those whose volunteers were called in from across the country to assist the American Red Cross (ARC) and the Federal Emergency Management Agency (FEMA).

During the 2005 hurricane season, MRC members provided support for ARC health services, mental health, and shelter operations. MRC members also supported the HHS response and recovery efforts by staffing special needs shelters, community health centers, and health clinics and by assisting health assessment teams in the Gulf Coast region. More than 1,500 MRC members were willing to deploy outside their local jurisdiction on optional missions to the disaster-affected areas with their state agencies, the ARC, and HHS. Of these, almost 200 volunteers from 25 MRC units were activated by HHS, and more than 400 volunteers from more than 80 local units were activated to support ARC disaster operations in Gulf Coast areas. During the 2009 flu pandemic, volunteers set up vaccination stations in schools, public meeting places, and fire stations.

MRC volunteers attend training sessions and must be certified in Incident Command Strategy to facilitate the integration of the volunteers with Emergency Response teams to avoid some of the confusion found in early large-scale disasters.

Sources: http://www.medicalreservecorps.gov/; Photo: http://www. medicalreservecorps.gov/image/PhotoGallery/Training/ExerSep09–006.jpg

medications have helped control the spread of diseases like tuberculosis and sexually transmitted infections.

5. Coronary heart disease and stroke prevention programs: Education regarding smoking cessation, blood pressure control, and the importance of early detection has led to a 51 percent decrease in death rates since 1972.

6. Safer and healthier foods: The identification of essential nutrients and food fortification programs (e.g., adding iodine to salt or vitamin D to milk) has nearly eliminated diseases such as rickets and goiter.

7. Family planning: Access to family planning has provided health benefits such as smaller family sizes and longer intervals between the births of children. In addition, the use of barrier contraceptives (condoms) has helped prevent unwanted pregnancies and the transmission of HIV and other sexually transmitted diseases.

8. Motor vehicle safety: Improvements in both car and highway design and successful education programs to change personal behavior (e.g., wearing seat belts, helmets, not drinking and driving) have led to large reductions in vehicle-related deaths.

9. Fluoridation of drinking water: Since 1945, fluoride has been added to drinking water and has helped to reduce tooth decay in children (40% to 70%) and tooth loss in adults (40% to 60%).

10. Recognition of tobacco as a health hazard: Anti-smoking campaigns have helped prevent initiation of tobacco use, promoted quitting, and reduced environmental tobacco smoke. The prevalence of smoking among adults has decreased, and millions of smoking-related deaths have been prevented.

Even with all these successes, there remains much work to be done. What are the new challenges for public health in the next 100 years? Public health must meet several new challenges in the future, such as changing patterns of disease, increasing numbers of chronic conditions, new and emerging infections, injuries, violence, and curable genetic diseases (Turnock, 1997). Diseases once thought under control, like tuberculosis, are making a comeback because of global travel in and out of countries where these diseases are common and in specific populations such as those with compromised immune systems. Antibiotics, one of our most powerful weapons in the fight against disease, are becoming increasingly ineffective as many bacteria become **drug resistant** (i.e., the bacteria are no longer killed by the antibiotic). Global travel allows for the quick spread of disease across borders. The United States faces a range of wholly preventable diseases and conditions that have reached epidemic proportions, such as HIV/AIDS, obesity, and stress-related conditions. In the next 100 years, public health must continue to adapt and expand its capacity to address these new health concerns.

SUMMARY

In this chapter, you read about the history of public health both globally and in the United States. Public health refers to any and all organized and collaborative efforts that are undertaken with the goal of protecting community health. The basic public health activities are assessment of the health of the community, policy development, and assurance of the public health. Health professionals who study disease and monitor key data perform these activities. The government is involved at the federal, state, and local level to carry out these activities. Foundations and other private partners also play a role in assuring the nation's health.

REFERENCES

Berry, J. 2004. *The great influenza: The epic story of the deadliest plague in history.* London: Penguin Books.

Centers for Disease Control and Prevention. 1999a. Achievements in public health, 1900–1999: Changes in the public health system. *Mortality and Morbidity Weekly Report* 48(50): 1141–47.

Centers for Disease Control and Prevention. 1999b. Ten great public health achievements: United States 1900–1999. *Mortality and Morbidity Weekly Report.* 48(12): 21–243.

Centers for Disease Control and Prevention (http://www.cdc.gov).

Fairbanks, J., and W. Wiese. 1998. *The public health primer.* Thousand Oaks, CA: Sage. Health Resources and Services Administration (http://www.hrsa.gov/heritabledisorderscommittee/correspondence/NBStatementStatutesRegs.htm).

HealthCare.gov (http://www.healthcare.gov/).

Medical Reserve Corps, (http://www.medicalreservecorps.gov/).

National Institutes of Health (http://www.nih.gov/about/almanac/historical/chronology_of_events.htm).

National Institutes of Health. *A short history of the National Institutes of Health.* (http://www.history.nih.gov/exhibits/history).

Turnock, B. 1997. *Public health: What it is and how it works.* Gaithersburg, MD: Aspen.

UNAIDS: The Joint United Nations Programme on HIV/AIDS (www.unaids.org).

World Health Organization (http://www.who.int/en/).

FOR ADDITIONAL INFORMATION

Mullan, F. 1989. *Plagues and politics: The story of the United States public health service.* New York: Basic Book.

National Association of County and City Health Officials. 2001. *Local public health agency infrastructure: A chartbook.* Washington, DC: National Association of County and City Health Officials.

Centers for Disease Control and Prevention, Emergency Preparedness and Response (http://www.bt.cdc.gov/).

International Network for the History of Public Health (http://www.liu.se/tema/inhph/).

State and Local Government on the Net (http://www.statelocalgov.net/).

United States Department of Health and Human Services (http://www.hhs.gov). United States General Accounting Office. 2004. *HHS bioterrorism preparedness programs: States reported progress fell short of program goals for 2002.*

10

Culture

Intracultural Communication

Learning Objectives

- Define culture and its impact on health care.
- Describe the difference between individualism and collectivism and its impact on culture.
- Identify the role of cultural contexts in communication.
- Describe the common barriers to communication in relation to culture.
- List steps that can be used when working with people from different cultures.
- Identify problems caused by ethnocentrism and how to cope with them.

Key Terms

Acculturation	Enculturation	Intracultural
Avoidance	Equality	Language
Behavior	Ethnocentrism	Learning
Context	Ethnorelativism	Nonverbal communication
Cross-cultural	Hippocratic Oath	Prejudice
Cultural competency	Indifference	Sensitivity
Cultural empathy	Intercultural	Stereotyping
Cultural sensitivity	Interethnic	Subculture
Culture	International	Translation
Culture shock	Interpretation	Xenophobia
Disparagement	Interracial	

Newton Bennett (1986) describes **ethnorelativism** as relationships that are mediated by empathy, "the ability to temporarily shift one's frame of reference to see the world 'as if' through the eyes of another person." Nunez (2000) stated, "**culture** is the lens through which you give your world meaning." Betancourt (2003) defined culture as "an integrated pattern of learning beliefs and behaviors that can be shared among groups and includes thoughts, styles of communicating, ways of interacting, views of roles and relationships, values, practices, and customs."

In *Intercultural Communication: A Contextual Approach*, Neuliep (2003), explained, "It is predicated in terms of demographic information that by 2025, Caucasians will make up 62% of the population. By 2050, only half of the U.S. population will be Caucasian." To contrast, in 1960, 90% of the population of the United States was of European decent. Between 1990 and 2000, the Hispanic population in the United States increased by 60% (predominately

From *Applied Communication for Health Professionals* by E. Phillips Polack, Virginia P. Richmond, James C. McCroskey. Copyright © 2008 by Kendall Hunt Publishing Company. Reprinted by permission.

in the west and southwest). By 2025, Hispanics will account for 18% of the total population of the United States. This will be true not just in the west and southwest but throughout the country. In the first decade of the 21st century, Hispanics make up about 12.5% of the population; in comparison, the African American population, which is the second largest non-Caucasian group, makes up just over 12%. The African American population is expected to remain relatively stable, increasing by only one percentage point to 13% of the population by the year 2025.

Miscommunication may occur from assigning different meanings for different words to express healthcare problems. For instance, we may consider a certain set of symptoms to be signs that we're coming down with a cold; Hispanics may consider a cold to consist of different symptoms. Davis and Flannery (2001) found that Puerto Rican women trusted health information when the sources were compatible with their cultural beliefs. This was further reinforced by Kakai et al. (2003) when they observed very different patterns among Caucasian, Japanese, and Pacific Islander cancer patients in how they obtained health information and what sources they found to be most reliable. In this study, ethnicity *overrode* any educational background in forming health choices. The only credible source for a Japanese or Pacific Islander, for instance, is a physician of the same or similar ethnicity.

On the subject of **cultural competency,** Michael Katz (personal communication, November 1998) wrote on the U.S. Department of Health and Human Services (the Office of Minority Health) website:

"In sum, because healthcare is a cultural construct arising from beliefs about the nature of disease in the human body, cultural issues are actually central to the delivery of health services, treatment, and preventative interventions. By understanding, valuing, and incorporating the cultural differences of America's diverse population and examining one's own health related values and beliefs, healthcare organizations, practitioners, and others can support a healthcare system that responds appropriately to and directly serves the unique needs of the populations whose cultures may be different from the prevailing culture."

Hofstede (1983), in analyzing IBM employees around the world, introduced the concept of individualism (low context-verbal) and collectivism (high context-nonverbal). In summary (Klopf & McCroskey, 2007), there are societies such as in the United States, notably among those of European descent, that are highly individualistic—the individual trumps the group. We are a verbal or left-brained culture. Among the current minority cultural groups in the United States, there is far less individualism. The Native Americans have many shared (collectivistic) views. Collectivistic cultures are more right-brained (nonverbal) in behavior. The 28.3 million Hispanic Americans are more collectivistic (Klopf & McCroskey, 2007). The Hispanics share a cultural value with a strong identification and attachment to extended families. Another important value is simpatíca. Chong (2002) noted that this is a harmonious physician relationship not only with the patient but also with their family. The Hispanics respect the dignity of others, avoid confrontation, and avoid words or actions that might hurt the feelings of others. Simpatíca can be achieved only by the provider who demonstrates a warm and caring attitude. The provider who is described as simpatíco is considered a dear friend to whom the patient and her family can turn when they need help.

Physical pain is also experienced very differently across cultures. One of the most noted works is that of Zborowski (1952), who compared various ethnic groups in a large New York Hospital. When comparing Italian, Jewish, Irish, and native-born Anglo-Saxon patients, the Jewish and Italian patients responded more emotionally with heightened expressions of pain.

A studied phenomenon is that of childbirth. Weber (1996) looked at childbirth and the value of silence in the Chinese. The Chinese women endured the pain quietly because they feared "loss of face." If they were highly emotional, it would dishonor them and their family. Conversely, Pakistani women believe that the more they scream and display suffering, the more caring their husbands will be during the following weeks (Ahmad, 1994).

Cultural differences can also be found in the way physicians and patients interact. In Western cultures, the power distance between physician and patient has diminished. Contemporary information transfer is based on a patient's right to know information, and this is notably true with delivering "bad news." Conversely, physicians in Japan hide bad news from the patient at any cost. Elwyn, Fetters, Sasaki, and Tsida (2002) researched the reversal of the "patient's right to know bad news" in Japan, finding that physicians, the majority of whom choose not to tell the patient, will paint an optimistic, as opposed to a bleak, picture of the prognosis to the patient and yet report the pessimistic view to the family.

WHAT IS CULTURE?

Bohannan (1992) stated that "culture is an interlinked web of symbols." It consists of intimately related parts of a complex whole learned by humans as members of society. According to Lustig and Koester (1993), culture is "a learned set of shared perceptions about beliefs, values, and norms that affect the behaviors of a relatively large group of people." Devito (1992) further elaborated that this is passed on from one generation to the next. **Enculturation,** or learning our native culture, allows us to learn from others and know what choices are suitable for specific circumstances. Bohannan (1992) stated that culture is thus "a means of standardizing choices of sharing successful results of choices made with others in the past."

Bohannan (1992) also points out that cultures must exist both in people's minds (in the meaning they attach to symbols) and in the environment, either as behavior or as artifact. He finally writes that transforming the culture (meaning) in our minds to the outside world is **behavior,** and transforming the culture from the outside world to our minds is **learning.**

Klopf (1995) noted that culture may be thought of as "a set of rules for constructing, interpreting, and adapting to the world." Cultures are values, and values grow and change very slowly and have many means of protecting themselves. A culture is cumulative and can grow, expand, and adapt to change, albeit slowly. When a group's culture is· passed onto its children through a learning process, it is then called enculturation—this is taught by schools, churches, parents, peers, and senior members of the community as well as the mass media. **Acculturation** is almost always a host culture influencing a newcomer who has *moved into* its environment. Interestingly, cultures are pervasive. They are omnipresent, and we seldom notice our own culture until we are somewhere where it *isn't.*

Many subcultures exist within large cultural groups. In the United States, there are groups like New Englanders, Midwesterners, and Westerners based on geographic residency. There are also cohorts of people living in communities based on ancestry or ethnicity, for example, Asian American, German American, and Hispanic American communities.

THE NATURE OF CULTURE

Context is one of the critical components of the communication process (Klopf & McCroskey, 2007). **Context** focuses on *roles* (job descriptions) and *rules* (governing principles). Thus, as a healthcare practitioner, you are primarily responsible for defining the communication roles and rules required in cross-cultural communication.

When you try to communicate with someone from another culture (with whom you do not share the enculturated [inborn] knowledge of their culture), you will realize how helpless you become because you do not understand or share the other person's point of view.

In America, we are a "mosaic" of diverse cultures. As a healthcare practitioner, you will be required to take on many different sets of rules and roles, depending on the cultural context in which you must function. Considering the vast demographics of the United States and our current cultural mix, *all of us* are likely to find ourselves in an intercultural communication context on any given day.

CULTURAL CONTEXTS

There are six cultural contexts for communication (Klopf & McCroskey, 2007; McCroskey & Richmond, 1996). You must remember the tenet of modern communication theory that "meanings are in people, not words." This includes (1) **intracultural** (within the same culture) communication, (2) **intercultural** (between cultures) communication, (3) **cross-cultural** (between cultures) communication, (4) **international** (governmental) communication, (5) **interethnic** (between ethnic groups) communication, and (6) **interracial** (between racial groups) communication. In any communication context, the largest margin of error comes in *nonverbal* communication. This is particularly true with the use of gestures. When traveling and mixing with other cultures, Americans place great emphasis on learning "words," whereas communication failure will most likely be predicated on nonverbal misunderstandings. One educational tool that the authors find useful as a dictionary to intercultural behavior is Roger

Axtell's (1991) *Gestures: Do's and Taboos of Body Language around the World*. In this book, Axtell identifies more than 70,000 different physical signs and customs globally.

Intracultural communication refers to communication between the same culture or subculture group (Klopf & McCroskey, 2007). This is the most common form of communication for most people, and the proportion of shared words and nonverbal behaviors is quite high. Meanings can develop differently within cultures. Within a given culture, people learn through the educational process and the experience of everyday living what messages are intended to mean. The major differences are predicated on membership in different "groupings" within the same culture. Chugh et al. (1994) noted that cross-cultural communications of health beliefs "within ethnic groups" can be more diverse than those between ethnic groups, for example, more variations within the Hispanic community than between the Hispanic and Asian communities.

Cooper-Patrick et al. (1999) conducted a telephone survey from November 1996 through June 1998 that polled 1816 adults between the ages of 18 and 65 (mean age, 41 years). These were individuals who had recently been treated at a large managed care organization primary care practice in an urban setting. The study, which looked at the participatory decision-making (PDM) styles of the physicians, concluded that African Americans rated their visit with physicians as less participatory than did their Caucasian counterparts. Yet if an African American had visited with an African American physician, he or she rated the physician's participatory decision-making style at a higher level. Increased PDM styles are translated to higher levels of patient satisfaction and ultimate improvement in health outcomes. As part of their conclusions, the researchers summarized that cross-cultural communication with a diverse group of primary care physician providers may result in higher PDM as well as greater patient satisfaction, and that this translated to better health outcomes according to the rules of homophily (Rogers & Bhowmik, 1971).

In *intercultural communication*, the people are members of different cultural groups. Intercultural communication can also refer to communication between members of two subcultures if there is a wide diversity. An example may be a member of the Asian American community communicating with a member of the Hispanic American community.

We need to look at medical communication from an interpersonal perspective. You must obtain information from the patient's perspective, which may be quite different from yours. This will require exploration of patients' health beliefs and views. Some common barriers to this include the following:

1. **Language:** A language barrier might be so insurmountable that a well-trained interpreter may be required. Ngo-Metzger et al. (2003), in studying Chinese and Vietnamese immigrants to the United States, determined that patients would rather use a professional interpreter of the same sex than a family member and that they were frequently frustrated by the Western healthcare providers' lack of information about "traditional Asian medical beliefs and practices."

2. **Nonverbal communication:** Remember that most nonverbal communication is *not* pancultural, notably gestures, touch, proxemics, eye contact, and demonstration of relational behavior. Nilda Chong (2002) has written an excellent book on the Latino patient titled The *Latino Patient: A Cultural Guide for Healthcare Providers*. In the acknowledgments of the book, she identified herself as being the daughter of a Chinese father and a Latina mother and stated that she was raised in the multiculturalism of Panama. She is not only bilingual but also bicultural, and she has listed multiple acronyms for a culturally competent care model for Latino patients.

3. **Cross-cultural communication:** "Cross-cultural" is a synonym for "intercultural," yet it refers to communication behaviors across cultures from different nations.

4. **International communication:** This refers to communication between governmental representatives of different cultures. These gaps can be quite wide, such as the cultural differences between England and Japan, or very narrow, such as between Canada and the United States. Most international communication is complicated by politics, which adds to the challenges of intercultural communication.

5. **Interethnic communication:** This is communication between members of different ethnic groups, for example, all Irish American person communicating with an Italian American person.

6. **Interracial communication:** This is communication between members of different racial

groups. This is exemplified by an African American person communicating with a Korean American person, but it would not pertain to an Irish American communicating with an Italian American.

CULTURAL EMPATHY

Culture empathy (relativism) is the best policy in healthcare. You can still maintain your preference for your own culture (remain ethnocentric) but you must learn to understand how other cultures see things from their vantage points rather than through the evaluative filter of your belief system. This is **cultural sensitivity.** We accept other people *as they are.*

Our intercultural communication can be improved through anyone of 12 ways: (Neuliep, 2003)

1. Recognize your own ethnocentrism; your patients are likely to have values different from yours.
2. Avoid derogating anyone else's culture.
3. Demonstrate respect for the other person and his or her culture.
4. Be empathic.
5. Develop a higher tolerance for ambiguity.
6. Reduce the level of evaluation in your messages.
7. Be exceptionally careful in interaction management. It is the roles and rules of the patient's culture, not yours, that you must learn.
8. Be sensitive to relational/social needs. Is the patient's culture high context (nonverbal, e.g., Japanese or Hispanic) or low context (verbal, e.g., United States and Canada)?
9. Do not assume that nonverbal messages, particularly gestures, are pancultural.
10. Be sensitive to both differences and similarities.
11. Work to build better stereotypes; do not prejudge.
12. Never forget that meanings are in people, not in cultures; diversity remains in any culture the same as it is in ours.

In summary, these 12 suggestions may read like the "12 commandments," but if you follow them you will increase the likelihood that your intercultural communication and experiences with your patients will be much more positive and effective.

It is vital in our diverse nation to provide both culturally and linguistically appropriate services to people who may be of limited English proficiency. As you are sensitive to the needs of the hearing impaired with the federal mandate, that is, that a "signer" be available, so are you also ethically bound to have linguistically appropriate interpreter for your patients (Ngo-Metzger et al., 2003).

The authors would caution that there is a distinction between *interpretation* and *translation*. Although these terms are frequently used interchangeably, they are very different. **Interpretation** is associated with culturally sensitive oral communication, whereas **translation** refers to written text. As you might imagine, including an interpreter requires triangulation of the relationship. A culturally sensitive interpreter is one who is trained in all aspects of ethics, impartiality, accuracy, and completeness. He or she must be able to translate with linguistic accuracy and convey the affective components of the communication without changing the meaning or injecting his or her own bias or opinions.

It is crucial, as with all interpersonal communication, that the triangulated communication be carried out at eye level. Herndon (2004) suggests that the interpreter be seated side by side with the patient and that both parties face the practitioner. Lee (1997) recommends that the practitioner initiate the communication and clearly identify the role of the interpreter. This should prevent the patient from developing a primary relationship with the interpreter. Lee (1997) further advises the following:

1. The practitioner should be aware of age, gender, class, and other ethnic differences between the patient and the interpreter. For example, it would be considered irreverent and disrespectful to use a young female interpreter with an older Asian male, according to the Asiatic bias of patriarchy, which demands deference to the elderly.
2. Prior to the physician-patient encounter, if an interpreter is to be used there should be a preliminary discussion that explains the medical terms and the condition that will be discussed (preconsultation education). This includes emphasizing that you and the interpreter are both part of the interdisciplinary clinical team. The interpreter serves as the "culturally sensitive" broker, ultimately enhancing the clinical interaction.

A valuable website for health information translations is www.healthinfotranslations.org. It offers translations in Arabic, Bosnian, Chinese (simplified and traditional), English, French, Hindi, Japanese, Korean, Marshallese, Portuguese (Brazilian), Russian, Somali, Spanish, Tagalog, Ukrainian, and Vietnamese; it is a collaborative facilitated by the Ohio State University Medical Center, Ohio Health, Mount Carmel, and the Nationwide Children's Central Ohio Hospital Council.

ETHNOCENTRISM

Ethnocentrism is the view that the customs and practices of one's own culture are superior to those of other cultures (McCroskey & Richmond, 1996). Although ethnocentrism tends to make intracultural communication more effective, it generates problems for communication in all other contexts. There are few messages (verbal or nonverbal) that are found to be "pancultural," with the exception of facial expressions, notably the smile. People of all cultures are ethnocentric to various degrees.

Ethnocentrism is a combination of two Greek words: *ethnos,* meaning "nation," and *kentron,* "center" (Klopf, 1998). There are both positive and negative aspects of ethnocentrism. Throughout the ages, ethnocentrism has been valuable. Ethnocentrism helps maintain the integrity of the culture against *external threats.*

Ethnocentrism is a source of cultural identity. In times of trouble, it will promote positive and effective communication among members (intracultural) of the culture.

Xenophobia is ethnocentric behavior to the extent that there is a fear of strangers.

Culture Shock, Stereotypes, and Prejudice (Communication Subsets of Ethnocentrism)

Although ethnocentrism has some positive aspects, there are potential communication problems that can be caused by ethnocentrism. These include culture shock, stereotyping, and prejudice.

Culture Shock

Oberg (1960) first described **culture shock** as something almost everyone experiences when *moving into* a new cultural environment. This is the degree of

trauma that is likely to be experienced and is another meaning for the word "shock" (not a drop in blood pressure, but rather a life *stressor*). Researchers Bellini, Baime, and Shea (2002) found this to be true as they viewed variations in doctors' moods throughout the intern year, including depression, hostility, and fatigue. These stages include (1) *the honeymoon phase,* when you feel like you are a "vacationer" (first 3 months of the internship); (2) *the culture shock phase,* which is very similar to depression (second 3 months); (3) *the adjustment phase,* when you are getting used to things (months 6 through 9); and (4) *the acculturation phase,* when you are becoming less apprehensive that everything is different around you. You take on some of the values of the new culture that you have "moved into" (months 9 through 12), the culture of being a physician. Yet authors Bellini et al. (2002) cautioned that the culture of an internship year with its associated moods of depression, hostility, and fatigue may have long-term effects on empathic behavior in later years. They point out the need for further research from internship and beyond. Many physicians do not survive the culture shock of a specialty internship year, leading to changes in career specialty.

Kathryn Andolsek and Robert C. Cefalo, with support from the Josiah Masey, Jr., Foundation, developed a CD-ROM teaching series with accompanying teacher's guide (Andolsek, 2005). The program is known by the acronym LIFE (learning to address impairment and fatigue and enhance patient safety) and is available free of charge from www. lifecurriculum.info. Topics covered include residency fatigue, management of the disruptive physician, burnout, boundary violations, impairment, stress and depression, and substance abuse; there also is a section on communication and cultural differences.

Stereotyping

Stereotyping (Neuliep, 2003) is a way of trying to make sense out of infinite variations in our environment. It is a generalization. When you stereotype, you tend to make three kinds of errors: *overestimating* the differences, *underestimating* the differences, and seeing what you *expect* to see. When overestimating, you exaggerate the differences. With underestimating, you stereotype people from other cultures as being the same as you. When you see only what you

---

Hippocratic Oath—Classical Version

I swear by Apollo Physician and Asclepius and Hygieia and Panaceia and all the gods and goddesses, making them my witnesses, that I will fulfill according to my ability and judgment this oath and this covenant;

To hold him who has taught me this art as equal to my parents and to live my life in partnership with him, and if he is in need of money to give him a share of mine. Similarly I will not give to a woman an abortive remedy. In purity and holiness I will guard my life and my art.

I will not use the knife, not even on sufferers from stone, but will withdraw in favor of such men as are engaged in this work.

Whatever houses I may visit, I will come for the benefit of the sick, remaining free of all intentional injustice, of all mischief and in particular of sexual relations with both female and male persons, be they free or slaves.

What I may see or hear in the course of the treatment or even outside of the treatment in regard to the life of men, which on no account one *must* spread abroad, I will keep to myself, holding such things shameful to be spoken about.

If I fulfill this oath and do not violate it, may it be granted to me to enjoy life and art, being honored with fame among all men for all time to come; if I transgress it and swear falsely, may the opposite of all this be my lot.

Translation from the Greek by Ludwig Edelstein. From *The Hippocratic Oath: Text, Translation, and Interpretation*, by Ludwig Edelstein. Baltimore: Johns Hopkins Press, 1943.

---

expect to see, you tend to be "blinded" even though the stereotype is not true. Stereotypes are highly resistant to change. You look for ways to reinforce your stereotypes, and you will find those that fit your expectations so the stereotype is easier for you to deal with. When patients go to a clinic, they expect people to wear a white coat, and if they don't, the patients may choose not to talk to them.

Prejudice

Prejudice refers to prejudgment (a priori), and it is based on stereotypes. These are judgments made in advance of the time when they are employed. In short, prejudice means to prejudge a person or the person's behavior based on very limited information about the culture or subculture. For example, "All football players are tough."

COPING WITH ETHNOCENTRISM

McCroskey and Richmond (1996) caution that ethnocentrism can be destructive to communication if one person is highly ethnocentric. Devito (1992) outlined ethnocentrism along a continuum of five steps (from least to most severe): equality, sensitivity, indifference, avoidance, and disparagement.

1. **Equality:** This is the lowest level of ethnocentrism. If both communicators approach the communication situation with this orientation, the probability of effective communication is quite high. Regrettably this is the least common circumstance under which intercultural communication is likely to be undertaken.

2. **Sensitivity:** If the health care provider is sensitive that you are somewhat ethnocentric, you must want to communicate without offending patients from another culture. You must do the hard work necessary to be "on your best behavior."

3. **Indifference:** This happens when you really don't care much about people of other cultures or subcultures and prefer to communicate with your "own." People who are indifferent if forced to communicate with people of other cultures tend to become more ethnocentric.

4. **Avoidance:** When you want little or nothing to do with other cultures and given a communication situation, you avoid the communication. This is probably a wise choice because the communication likely will not be effective.

5. **Disparagement:** This is with a great deal of negative prejudice. The communication will likely involve hostility and is best avoided.

THE OATH

In healthcare, we recognize a cross-cultural document in that we all take the Greek oath of Hippocrates. This is a 2500-year-old statement of ethics that requires equality for humankind.

REFERENCES

Ahmad, S. (1994). *Culturally sensitive care giving for the Pakistani woman.* Lecture presented at the Medical College of Virginia Hospitals, Richmond, VA.

Andolsek, K. M. (2005). Life Curriculum. Retrieved on June, 21, 2007, from http://www.lifecurriculum.info

Axtell, R. E. (1991). *Gestures: Do's and taboos of body language around the world.* Hoboken, NJ: John Wiley and Sons.

Bellini, L. M., Baime, M., & Shea, J. A. (2002). Variation of mood and empathy during internship. *Journal of the American Medical Association, 287,* 3143–3146.

Bennett, N. J. (1986). A developmental approach to training for intercultural sensitivity. *International Journal Intercultural Relations. 10,* 197–213.

Betancourt, J. R. (2003). Cross cultural medical education conceptual approaches and frameworks for evaluation. *Academic Medicine, 78,* 560–565.

Bohannan, P. (1992). *We, the alien: An introduction to cultural anthropology.* Prospect Heights, IL: Waveland Press, Inc.

11

Medicolegal

Should You Be Deposed: What to Expect

Learning Objectives

- Recognize medicolegal terminology.
- Review judicial process
- Describe importance of depositions
- Discuss individual liability and importance of self-protection.

Key Terms

Arbitration	Expert witnesses	Percipient witnesses
Defendants	Individual liability	Plaintiff
Deponent	Judicial process	Subpoena
Depositions	Mediation	

Please note that when reading this chapter, although it uses the example of clinical engineering and biomedical technology, the judicial process is the same no matter what area of healthcare you are entering.

Litigation! This is a word that no one wants to hear—except maybe lawyers. However, being involved in litigation is a possibility that those in the field of clinical engineering and biomedical technology must consider. Unfortunately, few, if any, in the field have received any advice or training on what to do if they become involved in litigation. Most commonly, biomedical equipment technicians and clinical engineers will be called on to act as percipient or, "fact" witnesses if an investigation of a patient injury or death leads to suspicion that a medical device caused or contributed to the event. The question then becomes, what is my role? What should I expect? Who will help me? This chapter will at-tempt to provide answers to these questions and provide some guidance on how to fulfill your role in litigation.

OVERVIEW OF THE JUDICIAL PROCESS

It may first be helpful to have a general overview of the judicial process involved in medical injury litigation. If a patient or relatives or representatives **(plaintiff)** believe that the patient's injury or death was caused by some form of negligence or failure on the part of the healthcare provider, they may contact a plaintiff attorney to seek damages. The attorney will discuss the circumstances with the plaintiff and determine whether there is merit to the proposed case. If so, the attorney will initiate an investigation of the matter.

If this initial investigation supports the case, a complaint will be filed with the court. At this time, the parties against whom the complaint is being filed **(defendants)** will be notified of the filing of the suit and the allegations against them. Both parties will then begin preparing their cases through review of documents, requesting production of records and documents from the opposing side, and retention of experts to provide advice on the case and interviews of individuals who are involved in their position. Note that attorneys are not permitted to interview members of the opposing side to obtain information without the permission of the attorney representing that side. When record and document reviews are completed, information is obtained from involved individuals and experts through depositions.

During depositions, questions are asked to obtain additional information, and designated experts are asked to provide their opinions and the justifications for those opinions. Prior to being deposed, experts will have reviewed depositions of percipient witnesses and any available information that pertains to their role in the matter.

After completion of depositions, each side reviews its position and decisions are made concerning possible settlement of the case. If negotiations for settlement do not succeed, **arbitration** or **mediation** is often used as a means to attempt to reach a settlement. It should be noted that the majority of cases are settled out of court and never go to trial. If such measures fail or are rejected, the case is scheduled for trial.

In the intervening period before trial, both sides will prepare their positions and strategies. They will also make decisions concerning who will be called to testify at trial. If equipment failure is an issue to be considered at trial, it is likely that at least one person responsible for support of the equipment allegedly involved will be asked to testify at trial. Most trials in medical injury cases are conducted before a judge and jury, so testimony will occur in open court under oath. The attorneys for each side will present their positions to the jury and question both percipient and **expert witnesses,** after which final arguments will be made and the jury will be requested to arrive at a verdict in favor of either the plaintiff or defense. Trials may last for only a few days or up to a month or more, depending on the complexity and seriousness of the matter.

All medical support personnel have the potential to be involved in patient incidents. This may occur because the person is an operator of equipment or devices used for treatment or diagnosis, or has set up a device to be used on a patient. For biomedical/clinical engineering personnel, they are usually peripherally involved by maintaining and managing equipment. However, they may be part of a clinical team in helping to set up and operate equipment, particularly in smaller healthcare facilities. Simply being in the same room at the time an injury occurred means that an individual is a source of information on the event.

ROLE OF THE CLINICAL ENGINEERING PROFESSIONAL

There are several scenarios in which clinical engineering personnel may become involved in litigation. The primary ones are having performed or having been responsible for the maintenance and repair or assisting in the setup or use of a medical device deemed to be involved in a patient injury or death. Another possible means of involvement is having performed (or failed to perform) incoming inspections of a device brought into the healthcare facility for purchase evaluation or a patient-owned item that is suspected of malfunctioning. For a person with this kind of responsibility, chances of being involved in litigation as an information source are high. In some case, it may simply be a matter of the plaintiff's attorney casting a wide net to attempt to get information from all possible sources.

As an example, assume that a patient expired during a code and it is alleged that the defibrillator failed to convert the fatal rhythm. Such a case involves questions of whether the patient had an intractable rhythm, there were errors in therapy, the defibrillator was not used properly, or there was a failure of the defibrillator to operate properly. This is a not uncommon, but complex, scenario. Allegations of equipment failure will be made, and aimed at the biomedical service. This will require production of maintenance and repair records, any functional tests or inspections performed in-house after the event occurred, and other records as requested by the defense or plaintiff attorneys. The manager of the service, the technician who last performed maintenance on the device, and the person who checked the device after the event (if any) will be incorporated into the litigation as employees of the biomedical service, whether an in-house department or an outside service contractor. Although these people were not at the actual event, they are considered sources of information, or percipient witness. As such, they can expect to be involved in some phase of the litigation process.

A complaint must be flied with the court within a certain period of time, which will vary between jurisdictions. It is not uncommon for a period of two to three years to pass before the defendant becomes aware of an action being filed. If investigation determines that a device was involved in a patient injury, the plaintiff will include this in the complaint or may amend the complaint after it has been filed. Allegations of device malfunction, failure to properly use the device, failure to properly maintain the device, or improper application of the device are common charges brought against the health care provider. The plaintiff's attorney will make an effort to determine all staff involved in the use and support of the device. Commonly, an expert in medical devices will be hired by the plaintiff attorney to review the case and assist the attorney in understanding what happened. The expert will review medical records, reports related to the incident, and information about the device alleged to be involved. After this review and inspection of the device(s) in question, the expert will formulate opinions concerning how the injury occurred and fault.

As part of the review and preparation process, the opposing counsel will subpoena all records and documents related to the event. Although the actual incident reports and some other communications are *protected* and cannot be obtained by plaintiff counsel, biomedical service documentation is not. Consequently, all manuals, maintenance records, and personnel records are potential targets of the plaintiff. The facility's biomedical service will be required to provide the complete maintenance and repair history of the device in question. This is often the "Achilles' heel," where scheduled maintenance or operational checks were not done or were inadequately documented. Another problem can be the lack of manuals or written procedures, which will bring up questions of how a device can be properly calibrated or given functional specification checks without the manufacturer's procedures and tolerances. Adequacy of staff training to maintain and operate equipment will also need to be documented. The facility's risk manager and defense counsel will generally coordinate the process of obtaining this information in response to a Request for Production from the opposing side. Biomedical personnel will often be asked to assist by researching and copying records, providing manuals, and participating in discussions with risk management and/or legal counsel.

IMPORTANCE OF DEPOSITIONS

After the plaintiff has completed its investigation and initial case preparation, it will then subpoena facility staff for depositions. **Depositions** are the process by which attorneys gather information by questioning witnesses under oath. This process will be explained in more detail later in the chapter. Many cases are settled after depositions have been completed through negotiations between the parties or through mediation. If the matter cannot be settled by this means, it then goes to trial, generally in the form of a jury trial. Many of the people who were deposed will be required to testify at trial, with the questions asked being based on the information gathered during depositions. The entire process from the filing of a complaint to settlement will often take between two to five years.

In the event testimony at trial is required, the attorney representing the defense will spend time briefing the witness on procedures and what is likely to be asked at trial. The witness should ask the attorney about the line of questioning to be expected and any strategies likely to be used by the opposing side. The procedures are similar to the questioning done during a deposition, except that testimony will be made in front of a judge and jury in a courtroom and the proceedings are more formal and structured. During trial, each side will ask questions and attempt to obtain answers designed to sway the jury to their position. However, it is important that the witness not be affected by these techniques and provide forthright and truthful information.

The deposition is often the crucial part of litigation proceedings, and can result in a settlement or the case going to trial. As mentioned previously, anyone with knowledge of the events surrounding the case is subject to being deposed as a **percipient witness.** Such witnesses are expected to provide information concerning the event. Healthcare staff with knowledge of the event or who were involved in a support role related to the event will be asked questions concerning their role, what they observed, their actions, and their education and training as related to the event. Biomedical personnel will be asked about their background and education, qualifications for their position, level of knowledge about the device involved, any investigations or testing they performed, and information that they may have concerning the event. This process is usually done in the conference room of an attorney's office or the healthcare facility. A court reporter takes down the entire proceeding and generates a transcript, which the witness is usually asked to read and make any factual corrections within a period of time after completion of the deposition.

During the deposition, attorneys for all parties involved will usually attend and be allowed to ask questions of the **deponent.** If you are an employee of a healthcare facility or service company, you will be accompanied by the attorney representing your employer. It is this person's responsibility to explain the deposition process to you and act as your advocate during the deposition. This attorney may object to opposing attorneys' questions and either allow the deponent to answer or direct him or her not to answer. It is important that the deponent pause before answering a question for two reasons: 1) to take time to make sure he or she understands the question, and 2) to allow time for objections from the attorney representing the healthcare facility. Although the process is intimidating for most people, the deponent should not hesitate to ask for water, take breaks, and request to confer with their attorney. In general, questions should be answered with yes or no when feasible; don't volunteer information that is not specifically requested. Only factual information should be provided; percipient witnesses are not generally asked or allowed to express opinions.

INDIVIDUAL LIABILITY

The question is often asked: Can I be sued personally? In general, the answer is that an employee will be defended by his or her employer and have the resources of the employer's defense counsel available at no cost, under the concept of corporate liability. This will also generally occur in the event the employee is named individually. The exception is when an employee has been found to have disobeyed instructions or has been grossly negligent, and these actions are considered to have contributed to the event in question. In such cases, the employee will be the subject of allegations from all parties and will be in the position of having to retain counsel and defend him/herself.

For those employed by outside service contractors, the situation is somewhat different than em-

ployees of a healthcare facility. Outside contractors will likely be named as a co-defendant in the suit, and will retain their own counsel. At this juncture, the facility and the contracting company may put up a joint defense and cooperate, or the facility may file a cross-complaint against the contractor, alleging that negligence on the contractor's part led to failure of equipment and the subject injury to the plaintiff. If a joint defense is mounted, the biomedical staff may find themselves acting as cooperative third parties at arm's length to the facility management. If a cross-complaint is filed, they will be in the position of defending their actions against allegations by both the plaintiff and the contracting facility. In both cases, they must be careful to follow the directives of the contracting company's counsel to preserve the position of the contractor in the litigation. This often results in a "good guy—bad guy" situation in which the relations between the contractor and the facility become strained due to the posture taken by the facility's management and counsel. In such cases, staff members must be particularly careful to be objective and not make derogatory statements or statements that could be used as admissions of fault by adverse parties. They must also be prepared to defend against accusations made by the facility as part of its defense strategy. This will require close cooperation with counsel to maintain the balance between the parties to the litigation.

IMPORTANCE OF SELF-PROTECTION

With all of these things going on, who will look after me? The best answer is that biomedical staff members must prepare to defend themselves by ensuring that all work is done properly, on time, and documented. Lack of performance allows the opposing party to use this as a weakness and opens opportunities to attack credibility of the biomedical service. Beyond this, when litigation ensues, there should be several support resources. In a healthcare facility, the risk manager is often the initial interface between the employee, an untoward event, and the legal system. It is important that the risk manager be aware of the assistance that can be provided by the biomedical/clinical engineering service. The service should volunteer to assist with investigation of patient injuries considered to be related to the use of medical devices. This person is responsible for the in-house investigation of adverse events, gathering

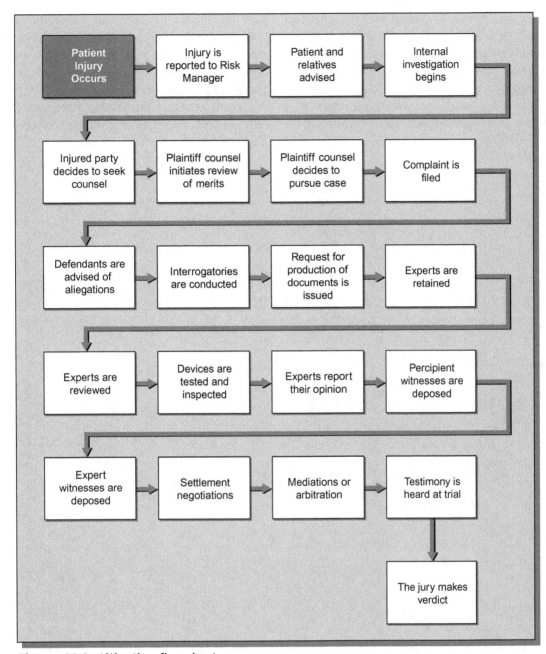

Figure 11.1 Litigation flowchart

information for counsel, and coordinating counsel and employee interactions. The attorney for the employer should interact with employees as necessary, informing them of proceedings and assisting them in participating in the various phases of litigation as needed. Such services should be part of the representation provided by the attorney in pursuing the case.

It is important that a person understand the limits of his or her role if participating in litigation as an employee involved in service and support of medical devices. As already indicated, you are considered a percipient witness, not an expert witness. As such,

you generally will be asked only to provide factual information about what you did and saw. You will not be in the position to offer opinions unless specifically asked to and designated as an expert. Although everyone has opinions, litigation is not the time to express them unless specifically asked to, and your counsel does not object. It is also very important that when being questioned, you do not stray from your area of experience and expertise. For example, you may be asked a technical question about x-ray equipment, and may have general knowledge of it, but you primarily work on patient monitoring equipment. If you answer the question inaccurately or incorrectly, this will be discovered by the opposition through their experts. This will then cast doubt on your knowledge and credibility, and can endanger the strategy of the defense counsel, as well as reflecting poorly on your reputation. It is much better to simply say you don't know than be found to be wrong!

The chances of becoming involved in medical injury litigation are remote for most clinical and biomedical engineering personnel. However, having an understanding of the process and knowing what is necessary to support your position in the matter can mean success or failure, should the time ever come that suit is brought against you or your employer.

CHAPTER **12**

Ethics

Introduction to Medical Law, Ethics, and Bioethics

Learning Objectives

- Define the glossary of terms.
- Describe the similarities and differences between laws and ethics.
- Discus the reasons for studying law, ethics and bioethics.
- Describe how to apply the three decision-making models discussed in the chapter.
- Explain why ethics is not just about the sincerity of one's beliefs, emotions, or religious viewpoints.

Key Terms

Amoral	Honesty	Principle of beneficence
Applied ethics	Humility	Principle of justice
Beneficence	Integrity	Principle of nonmaleficence
Bioethictists	Interpersonal ethics	Privacy/confidentiality
Bioethics	Justice	Quality assurance
Comparable worth	Laws	Respect
Compassion	Litigious	Responsibility
Cost/benefit analysis	Loyalty	Rights-based ethics/natural
Deontological theory	Medical etiquette	rights
Dr. Bernard Lo's Clinical	Medical ethics	Sanctity of life
Model	Medical law	Seven-step decision model
Due process	Medical practice acts	Sexual harassment
Duty-based ethics	Moral virtue	Sympathy
Empathy	Morality	Teleological theory
Ethics	Perseverance	Three-step ethics model
Ethics committee	Plagiarism	Tolerance
Fairness	Precedent	Utilitarianism
Fidelity	Preventive medicine	Virtue-based ethics
Gentleness	Principle of autonomy	Work

Fremgen, Bonnie F., *Medical Law and Ethics*, 3rd Edition, © 2009, pp. 1-24. Reprinted by permission of Pearson Education, Inc., Upper Saddle River, NJ.

THE CASE OF MARGUERITE M. AND THE ANGIOGRAM

Marguerite M., an 89-year-old widow, was admitted into the cardiac intensive care unit in Chicago's Memorial Hospital at 3:00 A.M. on a Sunday morning with a massive heart attack (myocardial infarction). Her internist, Dr. K., who is also a close family friend, has ordered an angiogram to determine the status of Marguerite's infarction (heart attack). Dr. K. has found that the angiogram and resulting treatment need to be done within the first six hours after an infarction in order to be effective, and the procedure is going to be done as soon as the on-call surgical team can set up the angiography room. The radiologist, who lives thirty minutes from the hospital, must also be in the hospital before the procedure can begin. At 4:30 A.M. the team is ready to have Marguerite, who is barely conscious, transferred from the intensive care unit (ICU) to the surgical suite.

Coincidentally, at 4:30 A.M., Sarah W, an unconscious 45-year-old woman, is brought in by ambulance with a massive heart attack. The emergency room (ER) physicians, after conferring with her physician by phone, conclude that she will need a balloon angiography to save her life. When they call the surgical department to have the on-call angiography team brought in, they are told that the room is already set up for Dr. K's patient. They do not have another team or surgical room for Sarah W. A decision is made that Sarah, who needs the balloon angiography in order to survive, will receive the procedure.

Dr. K is called at home and told that his patient, Marguerite, will not be able to have the angiogram. The hospital is going to use the angiography team for Sarah, since she is younger than Marguerite and has a greater chance for recovery. Unfortunately, it took longer than expected to stabilize Sarah before and after the procedure and the six-hour "window" when the procedure could be performed on Marguerite passed. Sarah survived, made a full recovery, and returned to her family. Marguerite expired (died) the following morning.

1. Do you believe that this case presents a legal or an ethical problem or both?

2. What do you believe should be the criteria for a physician to use when having to choose between a solution that will benefit one patient at the expense of another?

3. How can Dr. K. justify this decision when speaking to the family of Marguerite M.?

INTRODUCTION

Medical professionals encounter healthcare dilemmas that are not experienced by the general population. They are faced with individual choices that must, of necessity, always take into consideration the common good of all patients. Medical-ethical decisions have become increasingly complicated with the advancement of medical science and technology. The topics of medical law, ethics, and bioethics, while having very specific definitions, are interrelated. One cannot practice medicine in any setting without an understanding of the legal implications for both the practitioner and the patient. Medical ethics is an **applied ethics,** meaning that it is the practical application of moral standards that concern benefiting the patient. Therefore, the medical practitioner must adhere to certain ethical standards and codes of conduct. **Bioethics,** while closely related to applied ethics, is a field resulting from modern medical advances and research. Many medical practitioners, pa-

tients, and religious organizations believe that advances in bioethics, such as cloning, require close examination, control, and even legal constraints.

One teacher of medical law and ethics clearly stated that our primary goal is to teach students to think independently and become sensitive to the risks and issues that pervade the field. The ultimate goal in teaching this topic is that students will be able to understand complex health care public policy from all sides of an issue, regardless of personal beliefs. We want our students to be able to conduct themselves in a manner that is ethical, legal, and exemplary.

WHY STUDY LAW, ETHICS, AND BIOETHICS?

Without a moral structure for one's actions, people would be free to pursue their own self-interests. In many cases, people would behave in a moral fashion within the constraints and framework of their culture and religious beliefs. However, upon closer examination of living without the constraints and limitations imposed by moral standards and laws, a state of hostility may arise in which only the interests of the strong would prevail. The words *justice* and *injustice* would have little meaning. We all believe we know the difference between right and wrong. We may firmly believe that while some decisions are difficult to make, we would intuitively make the right decision. However, there is ample proof in medical malpractice cases that in times of stress and crisis, people do not always make the correct ethical decisions. Because what is illegal is almost always unethical it is important to have a basic understanding of the law as it applies to the medical world.

We must always remember that our primary duty is to protect our patients from harm. We should also understand that we live in a **litigious** society in which people have become excessively inclined to sue healthcare practitioners. In addition, healthcare agencies, hospitals, nursing homes, and manufacturers of medical products and equipment are all at risk of being sued by patients and their families. In fact, in our society anyone can sue anyone else. Lawsuits take a great toll in terms of stress, time, and money for all parties involved. While being sued does not indicate guilt, nevertheless, it can affect the reputation of a person or an institution even if judged to be innocent in a court of law.

MED TIP

A basic understanding of law and ethics will help to protect you and your employer from being sued.

Another reason for studying ethics and the law is that people often convince themselves that what they are doing is not wrong. For example, **plagiarism,** which is using someone else's words or ideas, may be both unethical and illegal, depending on the circumstances. It's understandable that an author who has worked hard to write a book would not want another author to use his or her written material without permission or giving credit to the original author. In fact, lawsuits have been won when this is proven to be true. In this case, it is both illegal and unethical. But what happens when a student has someone else do his or her work? Or if students lift passages from another book and then claim the words as their own? Is this also illegal and unethical? It may be both. There are computer programs such as MyDropBox.com and TurnItIn that allow students to check their work before they turn their papers in to see if they have provided the proper citation or sourcing for their material. These relatively new anti-plagiarism software programs can also uncover writing that has been copied from other student's work in the class. A student entering the medical field is held to a high standard. Strong ethical values can begin with a matter as simple as turning in honest papers.

Medicine is based on the professional skills of many persons, including physicians, nurses, physician assistants, medical assistants, radiology technicians, pharmacists, and a multitude of other allied health professionals. The healthcare team, composed of these professionals, with the addition of healthcare administrators, often must decide on critical issues relating to patient needs. In some cases, the decisions of these professionals are at odds with one another. For example, when an obstetrician withholds resuscitation attempts on a severely handicapped newborn, such as one born without a brain (anencephalic), he or she may be acting in opposition to the law in many states and the ethics of many people. Does a nurse have an ethical responsibility to override this order if he or she believes it to be wrong? Is there a better way to handle such an ethical dilemma without the patient's suffering in the process? It is generally understood that nurses and other allied healthcare professionals carry out the orders of their employer/physician. However, as illustrated in the above case, in some situations, confusion arises about what is the right thing to do.

It is generally accepted that some behavior, such as killing, is always wrong. But even this issue has been in the news when, as Hurricane Katrina roared through New Orleans in 2005, several critical hospital patients who could not be moved and would certainly die were allegedly given a lethal injection of morphine by a doctor and two nurses. In 2007 a grand jury determined not to indict the physician and cleared her of all accusations.

MED TIP

A study of law, ethics, and bioethics can assist the medical professional in making a sound decision based on reason and logic rather than on emotion or a "gut feeling."

Ethics asks difficult questions, such as "How should we act?" and "How should we live?" The answers to such questions are often subjective and can change according to circumstances, so it is realistic to ask, "Why study ethics?" The short answer is that in spite of the many gray areas of ethics, we are expected to take the right action when confronted with an ethical dilemma. We must consider the consequences of wrongdoing. We must learn how to think about the ethics of an action and then how to translate those thoughts into action. So, even if the "right thing" isn't always clear, we can prepare our minds to think about action and to see how the experiences of others can influence our own actions. The important thing is to be able to think and then take action!

While studying ethics, ask yourself the following questions. Do you know what you would do in each of the following situations? Do you know whether you are exposing yourself to a lawsuit?

- A fellow student says, "Sure, I stole this book from the bookstore, but the tuition is so high that I figured the school owed me at least one book." What do you do?

- An orderly working in a skilled-nursing facility is left alone in the dining room in charge of a group of elderly residents who are finishing their dinner. One of the residents does not want to eat but wishes to go back to his own room, which he cannot find by himself. The orderly has been instructed never to leave patients alone. Since he cannot leave the dining room full of patients, nor can he allow the one elderly resident to find his own room, the orderly locks the dining room. The elderly resident claims he has been falsely imprisoned. Is he correct?

- You are drawing a specimen of blood on Emma Helm, who says that she doesn't like having blood drawn. In fact, she tells you that the sight of blood makes her "queasy." While you are taking her blood specimen, she faints and hits her head against the side of a cabinet. Are you liable for Emma's injury? If you are not liable, do you know who is?

- You are a recently hired registered nurse working in the office of an internist. You have agreed to answer the phone calls in a physician's office while the receptionist is having lunch. A patient calls and says he must have a prescription refill order for blood-pressure medication called in right away to his pharmacy, since he is leaving town in 30 minutes. He says that he has been on the medication for four years and that he is a personal friend of the physician. No one except you is in the office at the time. What do you do?

- Terry O'Rourke, a 25-year-old female patient of Dr. Williams, refuses to take her medication to control diabetes and is not following her dietary plan to control her disease. After repeated attempts to help this patient, Dr. Williams has decided that she can no longer provide care for Terry. The office staff has been advised not to schedule Terry for any more appointments. Is there an ethical or legal concern (or both) regarding this situation? Is there anything else that either Dr. Williams or her staff should do to sever the patient relationship with Terry?

- You drop a sterile packet of gauze on the floor. The inside of the packet is still considered sterile; however, the policy in your office is to resterilize anything that drops on the floor. This is the last sterile packet on the shelf. The chances are very slight that any infection would result from using the gauze within the packet. What do you do?

- The pharmaceutical salesperson has just brought in a supply of nonprescription vitamin samples for the physicians in your practice to dispense to their patients. All the other staff members take samples home for their families' personal use. They tell you to do the same, since the samples will become outdated before the physician can use all of them. It would save you money. What do you do? Is it legal? Is it ethical?

- You feel a slight prick on your sterile glove as you assist Dr. Brown on a minor surgical procedure. Dr. Brown has a quick temper, and he will become angry if you delay the surgical procedure while you change gloves. Will it hurt to wear the gloves during the procedure, since there was just a slight prick and the patient's wound is not infected? Who is at fault if the patient develops a wound infection? Is this a legal and/or ethical issue?

- Demi Daniels calls to as you to change her diagnosis in her medical record from R/O (rule out) bladder infection to "bladder infection" because her insurance will not pay for an R/O diagnosis. In fact, she tested negative for an infection, but the physician placed her on antibiotics anyway. What do you do? Is this legal? Is it ethical?

- A physician from another office steps into your office and asks to see the chart of a neighbor whom he believes may have an infectious disease. He states that the neighbor is a good friend and that she will not mind if he reviews her medical chart. Is it legal for you to give the chart to this physician?

- A well-known baseball Hall of Fame fielder received a liver transplant in 1995. It took only two days for Baylor Medical Center's transplant team to locate an organ donor for this national hero when his own liver was failing due to cirrhosis and hepatitis. The patient was a recovering alcoholic who also had a small cancerous growth that was not believed to be life-threatening. Since there are relatively few liver donor organs available, there were mixed feelings about speeding up the process for a famous person. He subsequently died a few years later from cancer. What are the ethics of giving a scarce liver to a recovering alcoholic? What are your thoughts about the statement "People should not be punished just because they are celebrities"?

■ A physician used his own sperm to artificially inseminate his patients. He told the court that he didn't see anything wrong with this practice because these women came to him wanting to have a child. However, his patients were unaware that he was using his own sperm for the procedure. Some of his office staff became suspicious of the physician's methods but failed to report their suspicions immediately. Many children were conceived as a result of this physician's sperm being implanted into their mothers. Is this a legal, ethical, or bioethical issue? Was the office staff also at fault? What are the issues for this physician's community?

■ A 55-year-old man, Glenn Ross, with pancreatic cancer has been told by his physician that he has only a few months to live. He has received several series of chemotherapy that were of little or no benefit. Mr. Ross, who is now bedridden in a nursing home for the terminally ill, has requested that he receive no further treatment. His son, who lives in another state, demands that his father be hospitalized and placed back on chemotherapy. When the physician explains that there is little hope for the father's recovery, the son threatens to sue the physician for withdrawal of care. What are the ethical issues in this case?

MEDICAL LAW

Laws are rules or actions prescribed by an authority such as the federal government and the court system that have a binding legal force. **Medical law** addresses legal rights and obligations that affect patients and protect individual rights, including those of healthcare employees. For example, practicing medicine without a license, Medicaid fraud, and patient rape are violations of medical laws that are always illegal and immoral or unethical.

It is easy to become confused when studying law and ethics, because, while the two are different, they often overlap. Some illegal actions may be quite ethical—for example, exceeding the speed limit when rushing an injured child to the hospital. Of course, many unethical actions may not be illegal, such as cheating on a test. Law and ethics exist in everyday life and, thus, are difficult to separate. An insurance company denying payment for a life-saving heart transplant on a 70-year-old male is not illegal in most cases, but it may well be unethical.

MED TIP

In general, an illegal act, or one that is against the law, is always unethical. However, an unethical act may not be illegal. For instance, when an employee looks at a neighbor's medical record out of curiosity, it is not necessarily against the law, but it is unethical.

There is a greater reliance on laws and the court system, as our society and medical system have become more complex. In fact, some physicians have been practicing a form of medicine called **"preventive medicine."** This means that they may order unnecessary tests and procedures in order to protect themselves from a lawsuit since they can then say "I did everything that I could to treat the patient." This type of preventive medicine is not only costly but also may put the patient through needless and uncomfortable tests and procedures. In some cases, physicians may even avoid ordering tests or procedures that may carry a risk for the patient since they do not want to take a chance that a lawsuit may result if the patient outcome is poor.

The law provides a yardstick by which to measure our actions, and it punishes us when our actions break the laws. Many of the actions punishable by law are considered morally wrong, such as rape, murder, and theft. The problem with measuring our actions using only the law, and not considering the ethical aspects of an issue, is that the law allows many actions that are morally offensive, such as lying and manipulating people. Laws against actions such as adultery, which most people agree is immoral, exist, but they are rarely enforced. Some situations involving interpersonal relationships between coworkers, such as taking credit for someone else's work, are difficult to address with laws. Other work issues such as lying on job applications, padding expense accounts, and making unreasonable demands on coworkers are usually handled on the job and are typically not regulated by laws.

A further caution about relying on the law for moral decision making is the concern that the requirements of the law often tend to be negative. The standards of morality, on the other hand, are often seen to be positive. The law forbids us to harm, rob, or defame others; but in most states it does not require us to help people. Morality would tell us to give aid to the drowning victim even if the law does not mandate that we do so.

Many people believe that something is wrong, or unethical, only if the law forbids it. Conversely, they reason that if the law says it's all right, then it is also ethical. Unfortunately, these people believe that until the law tells them otherwise, they have no ethical responsibility beyond the law. Finally, laws are often reactive and may lag behind the moral standards of society; slavery is the most obvious example. Sexual harassment and racial discrimination existed as moral problems long before laws were enacted to suppress this behavior.

There are a multitude of laws, including criminal and civil statutes (laws enacted by state and federal legislatures) as well as state medical practice acts that affect healthcare professionals. **Medical practice acts,** established in all 50 states by statute, apply specifically to the way medicine is practiced in a particular state. These acts define the meaning of the "practice of medicine" as well as requirements and methods for licensure. They also define what constitutes unprofessional conduct in that particular state. While the laws vary from state to state, the more common items of unprofessional conduct include the following:

- Practicing medicine without a license.
- Impaired ability to practice medicine due to addiction or mental illness.
- Conviction of a felony.
- Insufficient record keeping.
- Allowing an unlicensed person to practice medicine.
- Physical abuse of patients.
- Prescribing drugs in excessive amounts.

As we study law and ethics as they relate to medicine, we will frequently use court cases to illustrate points. For our purposes it is not necessary to memorize the specifics of a lawsuit, such as the legal cita-

tion, that has been decided in a court of law. But it is important to keep in mind that unless a decided case is overturned in an appeals court, it is considered to have established a **precedent.** This means that the decision of the case acts as a model for any future cases in which the facts are the same.

ETHICS

Ethics is the branch of philosophy related to morals, moral principles, and moral judgments. **Morality** is the quality of being virtuous or practicing the right conduct. A person is said to be **amoral** if he or she is lacking or indifferent to moral standards. However, the terms *ethics* and *morality* are used interchangeably by many people. Ethics, as part of philosophy, uses reason and logic to analyze problems and find solutions. Ethics, in general, is concerned with the actions and practices that are directed at improving the welfare of people in a moral way. Thus, the study of ethics forces us to use reason and logic to answer difficult questions concerning life, death, and everything in between. In modem terms, we use words such as *right, wrong, good,* and *bad* when making ethical judgments. In other cases, people refer to issues or actions that are *just* and *unjust* or *fair* and *unfair.* **Medical ethics** concerns questions specifically related to the practice of medicine. This branch of ethics is based on principles regulating the behavior of healthcare professionals, including practitioners such as physicians, nurses, and allied health professionals. It also applies to patients, relatives, and the community at large.

MED TIP

Medical ethics mandates that the welfare and confidentiality of the individual patient must be the chief concern.

Ethics is meant to take the past into account, but also to look to the future and ask, "What should I do now?" Unfortunately, using moral views based only on those of parents and peers can lead to radical subjectivism that can make ethical discussion of issues such as euthanasia, abortion, or cloning difficult if not impossible. While most healthcare practitioners, other than physicians, will not be required to make life and death decisions about their patients, it is still important for everyone to develop his or her own personal value system. Whenever you are involved in an ethical dilemma, you must analyze actions and their consequences to all concerned parties. Law also does this by directing actions into "legal" and "illegal" human actions. As we study ethics, we will also analyze various actions and their effects.

MED TIP

Remember that ethics always involves formal consideration of the interests of others in deciding how to act or behave.

Basic questions relating to the study of ethics have been the subject of much debate and analysis, particularly among philosophers. Various philosophers have defined ethics under several categories, such as utilitarianism, natural rights or rights-based, duty-based, and virtue-based ethics. A division is often made between *theological* and *deontological* theories in ethics. A **teleological theory** asserts that an action is right or wrong depending on whether it produces good or bad consequences. Utilitarianism is an example of this theory. **Deontological ethical theory** asserts that at least some actions are right or wrong and, thus, we have a duty or obligation to perform them or refrain from performing them, without consideration of the consequences. Duty-based ethics is an example of deontological theory.

Utilitarianism

Utilitarianism is an ethical theory based on the principle of the greatest good for the greatest number. This ethical theory is concerned with the impact of actions, or final outcomes, on the welfare of society as a whole. Additionally, utilitarianism is a consequences-based ethical theory that follows the premise that the ends (consequences) justify the means (methods for achieving the ends). For example, in the case of limited financial resources, money would be spent in a way to benefit the greatest number of people. In this respect, utilitarianism is considered to be an efficient allocation of resources. In a professional context, a **cost/benefit analysis** justifies the means of achieving a goal. In other words, if the benefit (or well-being) of a decision outweighs the cost (financial or otherwise) of achieving a goal, then the means to obtain the goal would be justified. A problem arises when utilitarianism, or cost/benefit analysis, is used for making ethical decisions, since some people will inevitably "fall through the cracks."

The nation's Medicare system, in which all persons over the age of 65 receive healthcare benefits, is one example of utilitarianism. Congress has limited amounts to allocate for medical coverage and uses those funds to cover the elderly and others, such as the disabled, under the Medicare Act. However, not *all* people require the benefit. In the case of Medicare, for example, not all elderly persons need to have medical coverage provided for them, since some are wealthy and can afford their own coverage.

Another example of utilitarianism occurs when there is a limited supply of donor organs. Under a utilitarianism approach, patients with the most immediate need (and who would benefit the most) would receive the organ. Using this approach to organ distribution, terminally ill or elderly persons with a limited lifespan would not be the first to receive a scarce resource such as a new heart.

Rights-Based Ethics

A **natural rights,** or **rights-based,** ethical theory places the primary emphasis on a person's individual rights. This theory, based on justice, states that rights belong to all people purely by virtue of their being human. Under our rights-based democracy, all Americans have the right to freedom of speech. Employees have the right to due process, which entitles them to a fair hearing in the case of dismissal from their jobs. In the previous example of limited donor organs, using a rights-based ethical approach, every patient needing a donor organ would have the same right to receive the available organ.

Duty-Based Ethics

Duty-based ethics focuses on performing one's duty to various people and institutions such as parents, employers, employees, and customers (patients). Americans have a duty to adhere to laws enforced by government authorities. One of the problems encountered with a duty-based approach is that we may hear conflicting opinions about what is our "duty" or responsibility. If our employer asks us to do something that we are sure is wrong or unethical, we have a duty not to perform the action. However, this violates our duty to our employer. Most religions have statements that address one's duty as a member of that faith or religion. However, many people do not accept their faith's beliefs concerning issues such as birth control and working on the Sabbath, but do adhere to other doctrines of their religion.

Virtue-Based Ethics

A **moral virtue** is a character trait that is morally valued. The emphasis of virtue-based ethics is on persons and not necessarily on the decisions or principles that are involved. Most people agree that virtues are just good habits, such as fairness and honesty. Other examples of virtues and good character traits are integrity, trust, respect, empathy, generosity, truthfulness, and the ability to admit mistakes.

Virtue-based ethics, or seeking the "good life," is our legacy from the philosopher Aristotle. According to him, the goal of life, for which we all aim, is happiness. He believed that happiness is founded not solely on what we gain in life, but also on who we are. For example, the joy of being a medical professional cannot be present without having the traits or virtues that make one a good nurse, medical assistant, technologist, or physician.

While each of these four ethical theories can have positive outcomes and are useful in certain circumstances, no one ethical theory or system is perfect. See Table 12.1 for a comparison of the advantages and disadvantages of the four ethical theories.

Ethical standards that relate to the medical profession are set and defined by professional organizations such as the American Medical Association. All professional disciplines, such as nursing, have their own organizations and standards of guiding ethical codes of conduct.

In general, people believe an action is wrong or unethical if it

- Causes emotional or physical harm to someone else.
- Goes against one's deepest beliefs.
- Makes a person feel guilty or uncomfortable about a particular action.
- Breaks the law or traditions of their society.
- Violates the rights of another person.

Table 12.1   Advantages and Disadvantages of Four Ethical Theories

Utilitarianism: The principle of the greatest good for the greatest number. Also called a cost/benefit analysis. A consequence-based theory—or a means to an end.

Advantages: Encourages efficiency and productivity by looking beyond the individual to access the impact of decisions on all who will be affected. It is consistent with profit maximization: getting the most value (benefit) for the least cost.

Disadvantages: Virtually impossible to quantify all important variables. It can result in a biased allocation of resources, especially when some people lack a representation of voice (i.e., the poor, elderly, and handicapped). The rights of some people may be ignored in order to achieve a utilitarian outcome.

Rights-based ethics: Based on the premise that there are moral entitlements by virtue of being human (i.e., the right to healthcare, the right to free speech).

Advantages: Protects the individuals from injury; consistent with rights to freedom and privacy. It is consistent with an accepted standard of social behavior, independent of outcomes.

Disadvantages: Can imply individualistic selfish behavior that, if misinterpreted, may result in anarchy. Can foster personal liberties that may create obstacles to productivity and efficiency.

Duty-based ethics: Based on absolute moral rules. This theory is based on the premise that universal principles should guide all actions. These absolute rules or principles will help us to determine what constitutes our duty toward others.

Advantages: People are not treated as a means to an end with this theory. There is a mandate for respect and impartiality toward people.

Disadvantages: Difficult to identify who should determine what the rules and principles of moral behavior should be. Who determines what our duty is to one another?

Virtue-based ethics: Based on the premise that there is an acquired human quality that tends to enable us to achieve those goods (or rewards) that are the result of virtuous practices.

Advantages: Virtuous behavior includes such attributes as perseverance, courage, integrity, compassion, fidelity, humility, and justice.

Disadvantages: While there are few disadvantages with this ethical theory, there is a concern that persons can be taken advantage of if they become too complacent and trusting.

Principles or Values That Drive Ethical Behavior

Most people have established throughout their lifetime their own set of principles or values that drive their ethical behavior. Benjamin Franklin included in his list of virtues such things as cleanliness, silence, and industry. In today's world, we don't think of these things as virtues; they are assumed by many people to be a part of everyday life.

However, in today's fast-paced healthcare environment, it is important to slow down enough to consider some of the most respected virtues. Some of these virtues include beneficence, fidelity, gentleness, humility, justice, perseverance, responsibility, sanctity of life, tolerance, and work.

- **Beneficence**—The action of helping others and performing actions that would result in benefit to another person. It cautions all those working in the healthcare field to do no harm to anyone. In fact, when we prevent harmful actions from happening to our patients, we are using this virtue to its fullest extent.
- **Fidelity**—Loyalty and faithfulness to others. Fidelity implies that we will perform our duty. We must use caution when practicing fidelity. A strict adherence to a sense of duty or loyalty to an employer does not mean that we must perform actions that are wrong or harmful to our patients.
- **Gentleness**—A mild, tender-hearted approach to other people. Gentleness goes beyond compassion since it can exist in the absence of a person's pain and suffering. A gentle approach to patient care is considered by patients to be one of the most welcome virtues. Both men and women have the ability to demonstrate gentleness.
- **Humility**—Acquiring an unpretentious and humble manner. Humility is considered to be the opposite of vanity. It has been said, "honesty and humility are sisters." This means that to be truly humble, we must be entirely honest with ourselves. Humility requires that we recognize our own limits. Vanity and a sense of self-importance have no place in medicine. When mistakes are made, they must be reported so that corrections can take place. It takes a humble—and honest—person to admit mistakes.
- **Justice**—Fairness in all our actions with other people. It means that we must carefully analyze how to balance our behavior and be fair to all. Justice implies that the same rules will apply to everyone. This means that as healthcare workers we cannot demonstrate favoritism with our patients or our coworkers. The four cardinal virtues are justice, temperance, prudence, and courage. Of these four, only justice is considered to be an absolute good. To emphasize this point, the philosopher Immanuel Kant said, "If legal justice perishes, then it is no longer worthwhile for men to remain alive on this earth."
- **Perseverance**—Persisting with a task or idea even against obstacles. This virtue implies a steady determination to get the job done. For example, it takes perseverance to complete one's education. This is an outstanding virtue for a healthcare worker to have. It implies that one will finish the job even if it is difficult.
- **Responsibility**—A sense of accountability for one's actions. Responsibility implies dependability. A sense of responsibility can become weakened when one is faced with peer pressure. Medical professionals must be able to "answer" or be accountable for their actions. Taking responsibility is a sign of maturity.
- **Sanctity of life**—The sacredness of human life. All human beings must be protected. This means that we may have to become an advocate for people who cannot speak out for themselves, such as children and many elderly.
- **Tolerance**—A respect for those whose opinions, practices, race, religion, and nationality differ from our own. Tolerance requires a fair and objective attitude toward opinions and practices that differ from our own.
- **Work**—An effort applied toward some end goal. Work, if performed well, is clearly a virtue that almost everyone enters into at one time or another. In its broadest sense, work is part of our everyday existence that includes activities such as studying, childrearing, home maintenance, gardening, hobbies, and religious activities. The work we do to earn a living can be performed with pride or can be performed poorly and grudgingly. The most satisfying work involves achieving a goal that we believe is worthwhile and worthy of our talent.

Interpersonal Ethics

The expectation of employees in the workplace is that they will be treated ethically with respect, integrity, honesty, fairness, empathy, sympathy, compassion, and loyalty. Professional healthcare employees are no different in their expectation of receiving such treatment.

MED TIP

Remember to treat each person, whether patient or coworker, the way you wish to be treated.

- **Respect** implies the ability to consider and honor another person's beliefs and opinions. This is a critical quality for a healthcare worker, since patients come from a variety of racial, ethnic, and religious backgrounds. Co-workers' opinions must also be respected, even if contrary to one's own.
- **Integrity** is the unwavering adherence to one's principles. People with integrity are dedicated to maintaining high standards. For example, integrity means that healthcare professionals will wash their hands between each patient contact even when no one is looking. Dependability, such as being on time for work every day, is a key component of integrity.
- **Honesty** is the quality of truthfulness, no matter what the situation. Healthcare professionals must have the ability to admit an error and then take corrective steps. Anyone who carries out orders for a physician has a duty to notify the physician of any error or discrepancy in those orders.
- **Fairness** is treating everyone the same. It implies an unbiased impartiality and a sense of justice. This is a particularly important characteristic for supervisors.
- **Empathy** is the ability to understand the feelings of others without actually experiencing their pain or distress. Acting in this caring way expresses sensitivity to patients' or fellow employees' feelings.
- **Sympathy,** on the other hand, is feeling sorry for or pitying someone else. Most people, including patients, react better to empathetic listeners than to sympathetic ones.
- **Compassion** is the ability to have a gentle, caring attitude toward patients and fellow employees. Any illness, and in particular a terminal illness, can cause fear and loneliness in many patients. A compassionate healthcare professional can help to ease this fear.
- **Loyalty** is a sense of faithfulness or commitment to a person or persons. Employers expect loyalty

from their employees. This loyalty should be granted unless the practice of one's employer is unethical or illegal. For example, it is never appropriate to recommend that a patient seek the services of another physician unless instructed to do so by the employer. By the same token, employees expect loyalty, or fair treatment, from their employer.

MED TIP

Loyalty to one's employer does *not* mean hiding an error that has been committed by that employer or by a physician.

Additionally, there are specific issues that affect the workplace such as privacy, due process, sexual harassment, and comparable worth:

- **Privacy,** or **confidentiality,** is the ability to safeguard another person's confidences or information. Violating patient confidentiality is both a legal and ethical issue that carries penalties. Employees have a right to expect the contents of their personnel records to be held in confidence by their employer. By the same token, it is inappropriate for employees to discuss the personal life of their physician/employer.
- **Due process** is the entitlement of employees of the government and public companies to have certain procedures followed when they believe their rights are in jeopardy. The Fourteenth Amendment of the Constitution acts to prevent the state's deprivation or impairment of "any person's life, liberty, or property without due process of the law." The Fifth Amendment also restricts the federal government from depriving individuals of these rights without due process of the law. In a work environment, this means that employees of the government and public companies accused of an offense are entitled to a fair hearing in their defense. Due process is also a protection guaranteed to healthcare workers as it relates to their state certification, license, or registration to practice. To remove a person's license to practice his or her profession is the same as removing a person's livelihood. Thus, the removal of this documentation is not to be taken lightly. If there are allegations (accusations) made claiming that a healthcare worker, such as a medical technologist, nurse, or a physician, has committed malpractice, then their rights to defend themselves

and due process must be protected. This means that they must receive a notice of the charges, an investigation of the allegations, and a hearing if enough evidence is found. If these allegations are proven to be false, then the individual must not be penalized.

- **Sexual harassment** is defined in the Equal Employment Opportunity Commission guidelines, which are part of Title VII of the Amended Civil Rights Act of 1964:

  > Unwelcome sexual advances, requests for sexual favors, and other verbal or physical conduct of a sexual nature constitute sexual harassment when (1) submission to such conduct is made either explicitly or implicitly a term or condition of an individual's employment; (2) submission to or rejection of such conduct by an individual is used as the basis for employment decisions affecting such individual; or (3) such conduct has the purpose or effect of interfering with an individual's work performance or creating an intimidating, hostile, or offensive working environment.

Both males and females working in the healthcare field have reported sexual harassment.

- **Comparable worth,** also known as pay equity, is a theory that extends equal pay requirements to all persons who are doing equal work. The principle of fairness and justice dictates that work of equal value performed by men and women in the workplace should be rewarded with equal compensation. However, research demonstrates that there is a wage gap, with some estimates as high as 36 percent, due to the undervaluation of work performed by women. This results in injustice; equals are not treated equally. Since pay scales are the same for males and females in many of the healthcare professions, the situation is not as intense as it is in the business world. However, employers and supervisors who are involved in the hiring process must be committed to providing equal pay for equal work.

MED TIP

Any type of gender harassment is seen as one person exerting power over another.

MODELS FOR EXAMINING ETHICAL DILEMMAS

The decision maker must always be objective when making ethical decisions. It is critical to examine all the facts of a given situation by gathering as much information or data as possible. Alternative solutions to the problem must be assessed if they are available. Both sides of every issue should be studied before ethical decisions are made. The following are three decision-making models that can be helpful when resolving ethical issues: the three-step ethics model, the seven-step decision model, and Dr. Bernard La's clinical model.

Three-Step Ethics Model

Kenneth Blanchard and Norman Vincent Peale advise the use of a three-step model when evaluating an ethical dilemma. The three steps are to ask yourself the following questions:

- Is it legal?
- Is it balanced?
- How does it make me feel?

When applying this model, if the situation is clearly illegal, such as inflicting bodily harm on another, then the matter is also clearly unethical, and you do not even have to progress to the second question. However, if the action is not against the law, then you should ask yourself the second question—["Is it balanced?"]—to determine if another person or group of people is negatively affected by the action. In other words, is there now an imbalance so that one person or group suffers or benefits more than another as a result of your action? For example, in the case of a scarce resource such as donor organs, does one group of people have greater access? The final question—["How does it make me feel?"]—refers to how the action will affect you emotionally. Would you be hesitant to explain your actions to a loved one? How would you feel if you saw your name in the paper associated with the action? Can you face yourself in the mirror? If you can answer the first two questions with a strong "Yes" and the final question with a strong "Good," then the action is likely to be ethical.

For example, student cheating is clearly unethical. By using the three-step ethics model, we have an even clearer idea of why it is unethical to look at even one answer on another student's test. We ask the three questions:

1. Is it legal? Yes, as far as we know there is no law against cheating.
2. Is it balanced? No, it is not. This question is where the model really helps us. One group or person (in this case the cheater) does have an advantage over another group or person. In addition, the grades will be skewed for the entire class, since the person who cheated will receive a higher grade than what he or she earned.
3. How does it make me feel? Remember that we have to live with ourselves. The philosopher Thomas Aquinas said, "We become what we do," meaning that if we lie, we become a liar. Or in this case, if we cheat, we become a cheater.

MED TIP

The three-step ethics model is a quick way to check yourself when you are uncomfortable about an ethical decision. Use it often!

The Seven-Step Decision Model

1. Determine the facts by asking the following questions:
   What do we need to know?
   Who is involved in the situation?
   Where does the ethical situation take place?
   When does it occur?
2. Define the precise ethical issue.
3. Identify the major principles, rules, and values. For example, is this a matter of integrity, quality, respect for others, or profit?
4. Specify the alternatives. List the major alternative courses of action, including those that represent some form of compromise. This may be a choice between simply doing or not doing something.
5. Compare values and alternatives. Determine if there is one principle or value, or a combination of principles and values, that is so compelling that the proper alternative is clear.
6. Assess the consequences. Identify short-term, long-term, positive, and negative consequences for the major alternatives. The short-term gain or loss is often overridden when long-term consequences are considered. This step often reveals an unanticipated result of major importance.

7. Make a decision. The consequences are balanced against one's primary principles or values.

The seven-step decision model forces us to closely examine the facts before we make an ethical decision.

Dr. Bernard Lo's Clinical Model

Dr. Lo has developed a clinical model for decision making to ensure that no important considerations relating to patient care are overlooked. He believes this approach can be used to help resolve important patient-care issues, such as when to proceed with life-sustaining interventions (for example, cardiopulmonary resuscitation [CPR] or kidney dialysis).

1. Gather information.
   If the patient is competent, what are his or her preferences for care?
   If the patient lacks decision-making capacity, has he or she provided advance directives for care?
   If the patient lacks decision-making capacity, who should act as surrogate? What are the views of the healthcare team?
   What other issues complicate the case?
2. Clarify the ethical issues.
   What are the pertinent ethical issues?
   Determine the ethical guidelines that people are using.
   What are the reasons for and against the alternative plans of care?
3. Resolving the dilemma.
   Meet with the healthcare team and with the patient or surrogate.
   List the alternatives of care.
   Negotiate a mutually acceptable decision.

Dr. Lo emphasizes that patients should play an active role in decisions. Everything should be done to ensure that the patient has been well informed by providing information in an easy-to-understand way. He requires that the entire healthcare team—including medical students, nurses, social workers, and all others who provide direct care for the patient—be involved in the decisions. These caregivers should voice any moral objections they have to the proposed care. Finally, the patient's best interests must always be protected. This model is more commonly used in a hospital or clinic setting.

WHAT ETHICS IS NOT

Ethics is not just about how you feel, the sincerity of your beliefs, or your emotions; nor is it only about religious viewpoints. Feelings, such as in the statement "I feel that capital punishment is wrong," are not sufficient when making an ethical decision. Others may feel that capital punishment is right in that it helps to deter crime. All people have feelings and beliefs. However, ethics must be grounded in reason and fact. For example, a statement such as "I feel that cheating is wrong" doesn't tell us why you believe it is wrong to cheat. A better statement reflecting ethics would be, "I think cheating is wrong because it gives one student an unfair advantage over another student."

The sincerity with which people hold their beliefs is also not an adequate reason when making an ethical decision. For example, Hitler sincerely believed that he was right in exterminating more than 6 million Jews. His sincerity did not make him right.

Emotional responses to ethical dilemmas are not sufficient either. Emotions may affect why people do certain things, such as the woman who kills her husband in a rage after discovering he had an affair. However, we should not let our emotions dictate how we make ethical decisions. We may have helplessly watched a loved one die a slow death from cancer, but our emotions should not cloud the issue of euthanasia and cause us to kill our ill patients.

Ethics is not just about religious beliefs. Many people associate ideas of right and wrong with their religious beliefs. While there is often an overlap between ethics and what a religion teaches as right and wrong, people can hold very strong ethical and moral beliefs without following any formal religion.

MED TIP

Our determination of what is ethical or moral can have serious consequences in human action.

BIOETHICS

Bioethics, also known as biomedical ethics, is one branch of applied, or practical, ethics. It refers to moral dilemmas and issues prevalent in today's society as a result of advances in medicine and medical research. The term *bio,* meaning life, combined with *ethics* relates to the moral conduct of right and wrong in life and death issues. Ethical problems of the biological sciences, including research on animals, all fall under the domain of bioethics. Some of the bioethical issues discussed in this text include the allocation of scarce resources such as transplant organs, beginning-of-life issues, cloning, harvesting embryos, concerns surrounding death and dying, experimentation and the use of human subjects, who owns the right to body cells, and dilemmas in the treatment of catastrophic disease.

Bioethics uses a form of moral analysis to assist in determining the obligations and responsibilities of unique issues relating to modern healthcare. Today's modern medical care requires that decision-makers carefully examine facts, identify the moral challenges, and then look carefully at all alternatives. There are basically four principles that can serve as guidelines when confronting bioethical dilemmas. These include the principles of autonomy, beneficence, nonmaleficence, and justice.

The **principle of autonomy** means that people have the right to make decisions about their own life. The concept of "informed consent" is included in this principle. It means that patients must be informed and understand what they are told before they can provide consent for the treatment. They must be told what the treatment involves, the risks involved, the chance for success, and the alternatives.

The **principle of beneficence,** or the principle of doing good, means that we must not harm patients while we are trying to help them. This principle recognizes that medical science must do what is best for each individual patient. If there are risks involved, then the principle of autonomy must be invoked so that decisions are made in conjunction with patient's wishes.

The **principle of nonmaleficence** is taken from the Latin maxim *Primum non nocere,* which means "First, do no harm." This is a warning to all members of the healthcare profession. Nonmaleficence completes the principle of beneficence since we are now asking the medical profession to not only do good for the patient, but also to do no harm in the process. In some cases the risks of a treatment may outweigh the benefits. For example, when a surgeon removes a pregnant woman's cancerous uterus to save her life, her unborn child will not live. The principle of nonmaleficence causes the medical profession to stop and think before acting.

Finally, the **principle of justice** warns us that equals must be treated equally. The same treatments must be given to all patients whether they are rich, poor, educated, uneducated, able-bodied, or disabled.

These four bioethical principles are guidelines for physicians and health care professionals to use when patients are unable to provide their personal wishes. For example, there have been cases of "wrongful life" in which a fetus is delivered too soon before development is complete. These infants, if they survive, may have severe disabilities. Physicians may be requested by parents to "do nothing" to re-suscitate or save their undeveloped child. Issues such as these weigh heavily upon the shoulders of all medical professionals. Having a set of guidelines, such as the above four principles, to follow has helped in some of the decision making.

Bioethicists, specialists in the field of bioethics, give thought to ethical concerns that often examine the more abstract dimensions of ethical issues and dilemmas. For example, they might ask, "What are the social implications of surrogate motherhood?" Bioethicists are often authors, teachers, and re-searchers. This branch of ethics poses difficult, if not impossible, questions for the medical practitioner.

THE ROLE OF ETHICS COMMITTEES

Hospitals, as well as other healthcare organizations and agencies, have active ethics committees that ex-amine ethical issues relating to patient care. This type of oversight committee consists of a variety of members from many health-care fields as well as other disciplines, including physicians, nurses, clergy, psychologists, ethicists, lawyers, healthcare administrators, and family and community mem-bers. The ethics committee can serve in an advisory capacity to patients, families, and staff for case re-view of difficult ethical issues, especially when there is a lack of agreement as to what is in the patient's best interests. They also develop and review health policies and guidelines regarding ethical issues such as organ transplantation. After examining the facts surrounding the ethical issue, the committee often determines a recommendation based on predeter-mined criteria. These criteria might include the severity of the patient's medical condition, the age of the patient, and the chance for ultimate recovery.

The ethics committee may examine issues such as when hospitalization or treatment needs to be discontinued for a patient. For example, a hospital ethics committee will assist in determining the best

action to take for a terminally ill patient who is on a respirator. In some cases, the committee may be asked to examine if a patient received the appropri-ate care.

Ethics committees have tremendous power in today's healthcare environment. Patients are holding their doctors and hospitals to a high standard of care. While it is necessary for the committee meet-ings to be confidential in order to protect the pa-tient's privacy, nevertheless, there should be a strong set of policies that govern how the meetings are con-ducted. In some cases members of an ethics commit-tee will never see or talk to the patient whose life and care they are discussing. Mistakes can be made when a group of people makes a judgment without review-ing all the facts.

MED TIP

It has been suggested that ethics committees make an effort to have disabled people represented on their committee either as a member or as a resource person to represent the viewpoint of the handicapped patient. In some cases decisions are made based on committee members own prejudice against living with a disability.

QUALITY ASSURANCE PROGRAMS

In addition to ethics committees, most hospitals and healthcare agencies have a quality assurance (QA) program. These programs were established in the early 1960s as a response to the increasing demand from the public for accountability in quality medical care. **Quality assurance** (QA) is gathering and eval-uating information about the services provided, as well as the results achieved, and comparing this in-formation with an accepted standard.

Quality assessment measures consist of formal, systematic evaluations of overall patient care. After the results of the evaluations are compared to standard results, then any deficiencies are noted and recom-mendations for improvements are made. The types of issues that are reviewed by a QA committee are

- Patient complaints relating to confidentiality.
- Errors in dispensing medications.
- Errors in labeling of laboratory specimens.

- Adverse reactions to treatments and/or medications.
- Inability to obtain venous blood on the first attempt.
- Safety and monitoring practices for radiology and laboratory.
- Infection control.

MEDICAL ETIQUETTE

There are certain rules of **medical etiquette,** or standards of professional behavior, that physicians practice in the relationship or conduct with other physicians. These are general points of behavior and are not generally considered to be medical ethics issues. For instance, physicians expect that their telephone calls to fellow physicians will be taken promptly and that they will be seen immediately when visiting a physician's office. This courtesy is extended to physicians because they are often consulting about patients with other physicians. However, ethical issues are present when one physician overlooks or "covers up" the medical deficiencies of another physician.

MED TIP

The outdated medical courtesy of physicians providing free medical care to their colleagues is not advisable. If their colleagues were to need further treatment, their insurance coverage may be in jeopardy because of the initial "free" care.

REFERENCES

Blanchard, K., and N. Peale. 1988. *The power of ethical management.* New York: William Morrow.

Boatright, J. 2005. *Ethics and the conduct of business.* New York: William Morrow.

Brincat, C., and V. Wike. 2000. *Morality and the professional life.* Upper Saddle River, NJ: Prentice Hall.

Comte-Sponville, A. 200 1. *A small treatise on the great virtues.* New York: Henry Holt.

Espejo, R. ed. 2003. *Biomedical ethics.* New York: Greenhaven Press.

Levine, C. 2004. *Taking sides.* New York: McGraw Hill.

Lo, B. 1995. *Resolving ethical dilemmas: A guide for clinicians,* New York: Lippincott, Williams, & Wilkins.

Mappes, T., and D. DeGrazia. 2001. *Biomedical ethics.* New York: McGraw Hill.

Munson, R., 2002. *Raising the dead.* New York: Oxford University Press.

Nossiter, A. 2007. "Grand jury won't indict doctor in hurricane deaths." *The New York Times* (July 25, p. A10).

Pilon, M. 2006. "Anti-plagiarism programs look over student's work." *USA Today* (May 23, p. 100).

Skipp, C., and A. Campo-Flores. 2006. "What the doctor did." *Newsweek* (July 31, p. 49).

Healthcare Economics

Financing

INTRODUCTION

Health care is like no other sector of the economy. In his seminal 1963 article, "Uncertainty and the Welfare Economics of Medical Care," Kenneth Arrow identified these differences as uncertainty, asymmetries of information, and non marketability of risks inherent in medicine and medical practice. Even after a millennium of observation and study, our knowledge about the human body, disease, and medicine is very much incomplete. In addition, whereas the physician nearly always has more medical knowledge, patients generally know more about their own history so that there is usually a serious information asymmetry between patient and provider. Furthermore, patient behavior is guided by perception of risk. For example, **moral hazard** is the change in an individual's behavior that results from having insurance coverage, which modifies the costs of misfortune. Social scientists predict that people make less effort to avoid misfortune when they are insured. If an accident costs a person $2,000 but insurance pays $1,500, the insured person has less incentive to avoid the accident than if the insurance paid only $500.

Financing health care is a tension among the ethics and values we place on human life, the asymmetries of information, and uncertainty about care wrapped in nonmarketable risks. The implication is that the health care market would collapse if entirely governed by market forces, even though the health care sector exists within a general market economy. That is, at some level, health care competes for resources (e.g., workers, supporting goods and services) against the production of food, the construction of homes, the creation of movies, and the seemingly infinite number of other goods and services that a nation of 300 million people and associated businesses consume. At some level, providing resources for an additional surgeon to perform cardiac surgeries means that fewer houses can be constructed or that the quality or quantity of food produced will be diminished. Within the health care sector itself, tradeoffs are also made: Money spent on an MRI machine is money not spent on additional doctors, money spent on research is money not spent on providing care, and money spent researching one disease is money not spent on another. Thus, financing health care in the United States is a complex matter of workarounds, redundancies, and contradictions. Furthermore, because the United States lacks a single national health care payment system, just how the money is paid to the providers of health care has become very complicated (Igelhart, 1999a).

This chapter describes the basics of health care financing and the system that handles its functions: how much money is spent on health care in the United States, where the money comes from, what the money is spent on, and how the money is paid to providers.

HOW MUCH IS SPENT

Thus far, the United States has increased the rate of health care spending every year, at least since 1960. In both absolute and relative terms, national health expenditures have grown considerably over the years. Between 1980 and 2005, national health care

payments sextupled in current dollars. In 1980 health care expenditures accounted for only 9.1% of the Gross Domestic Product GDP, in contrast to 16.0% of the GDP in 2005. During the 1980s, the annual rate of increase in health care expenditures was constantly in the double-digit range, even when inflation and the GDP growth rates were not. Why this happened is a matter of much controversy.

Starting in the 1990s, with the advent of managed care and its downward pressure on both physician and hospital usage, a brake was put on health care cost increases, at least for the time being: the rates of increase from 1970 through 1990 had been over 10% per year. By 1993, the rate of increase had fallen to 8.5%, and from 1997 through 1998 it was about 6%. In 1999, the rate of increase began an upward trend, going from 6.2% to 9.1% in 2002. In 2003 there was another period of decline, with the rate of increase going from 8.1 % in 2003 to 6.9% in 2005.

In 2003, health care spending accounted for 15% of the GDP. That figure is about 36% higher than the percentage of the GDP spent by the country with the next highest spending rate—Germany (U.S. Census Bureau, 2005, Table 1323). Germany has a comprehensive national health insurance program. In fact, it is the oldest such program in the world. National health expenditures accounted for 16% of the GDP in 2004 and 2005.[1] Only when housing, household operation, and residential investment (not a common grouping) are combined into a supercategory (i.e., "Shelter") is there any larger spending category (Bureau of Economic Analysis, 2006). In 2004, 13.5 million people were employed in health care—13.1 million were wage and salary workers and about 411,000 were self-employed (Bureau of Labor Statistics, 2006).

In 1980, health care expenditures totaled about $254 billion, an increase of 13% over the previous year. About 85% of total expenditures went for personal health care. The balance was paid for research facilities construction, program administration, private health insurance administration, and public

---

[1]This category does not include public health, government administrative costs for Medicare, and health-related construction and other infrastructure investments such as hospital construction and renovation. Also, like all elements of the GDP, unpaid work is not counted. This is particularly significant in health care because most medical symptoms are self-diagnosed and treated (Dean, 1981). Additionally, it is very common for people to receive care from family and loved ones in the course of mild illness. When people stay home from work because of illness, the GDP is reduced. On the other hand, if those same people were taken care of by a paid caregiver, the GDP would increase.

health services. In 1990, just 10 years later, health care payments totaled about $714 billion, an increase of 11% over the previous year, and about 2.8 times higher than total expenditures in 1980. Again, personal health care accounted for 85% of spending. In 2005, health care payments totaled about $1.99 trillion, an increase of about 7% over the previous year, and about 2.8 times higher than the total in 1990. Changing little since 1980, about 84% of total expenditures went for personal health care. As in previous years, the balance was paid for research, facilities construction, program administration, private health insurance administration and profits, and public health services.

Regardless of whether health care cost inflation will outstrip the general inflation rate by a lot or a little, using fairly conservative estimates, Heffler and colleagues came to some rather startling conclusions. They projected expenditures of close to $2.2 trillion, 16.1% of the GDP, in 2007, and more than $2.8 trillion, 17% of the GDP, in 2011 (Heffler et al., 2002).

A considerable part of the constant upward trend in health care spending in the United States has been caused by factors other than simple utilization, such as the ever-intensifying use of expensive technology-based diagnostic and procedural interventions, especially at the beginning and the end of life (Franks, Clancy, & Nutting, 1992; Meier & Morrison, 2002). Thus, it remains to be seen how long the increase in expenditure rate will remain at a relatively modest level (although still above the general rate of inflation), or whether it will return to its previously astronomical (double-digit) levels, as in the 1970s and 1980s.

WHERE THE MONEY COMES FROM, WITHIN THE SYSTEM

In the United States, health care is paid by some combination of the patient, the provider, and a third-party payer. Money paid directly be a patient for health care costs is referred to as **"out-of-pocket." Charity care** and **forgiven debts** are the terms providers use when they have borne the cost of providing care. Anyone responsible for payment of a health care cost other than the patient (or the patient's family) or the provider is a **third-party payer.** Third-party payers include the patient's or their relative's employer, private insurance or managed-care organization (MCO) engaged by the patient or another party, charity organizations, and federal, state, and local governments. In many cases, several of these parties—patient,

provider, and third-party payers—come together to pay a single bill. To use a typical example, a child might visit a pediatrician who would then receive a small "copay" from the mother ("out-of-pocket") during the visit. Then the pediatrician's office would bill a private insurance firm (perhaps an MCO contracted by the father's employer), which would pay some or the remainder of the bill. Very complicated relationships can enjoin three or more payers.

In the United States, payers are generally categorized as private or public. Within the **private sector,** private health insurance companies and out-of-pocket expenditures are primary. Within the public sector, federal, state, and local governments all provide funding for health care. The public sector may act as a provider of services or as a third-party payer. For example, some health care programs paid for directly by government: the federal Department of Veterans Affairs health care system, the states' mental hospitals, and public general hospitals operated by local governments. These are all supported mainly by tax revenues. On the other hand, the Medicare program acts as a third-party payer in that it does not provide services, but only the money to pay for health services supplied by hospitals, physicians, and others.

Traditionally, for many patients, health care has been provided under a direct, private (usually unwritten) contract between themselves and the provider of care. But that care is usually paid for by a third-party payer as defined previously. This system has been further complicated by the development of **managed care.** Patient care is still paid for by a third party, but the patient now has a written contract with the MCO, not the physician, describing in detail what care he or she will be entitled to under what circumstances, delivered by whom, in return for the payment made to the MCO, usually by the patient's employer. This written contract with the payer replaces the old unwritten contract with the provider. Among other things, this change in contract type has had a major impact on just who is ultimately in charge of patient care decisions.

Private Health Insurance[2]

The current and historical financial involvement of the private health insurers will be briefly examined

[2]A comprehensive overview of private health insurance is Gary Claxton's "How Private Insurance Works: A Primer," available from the Kaiser Family Foundation's Web site, www.kff.org.

here. The salient feature of private insurance in the United States is that most people obtain it through their employer (or spouse's or parent's employer). One can almost say that employers (and employees, through their contributions to health insurance premiums) are the true payers in this case and that private insurance companies are the administrators of payments. Outside of employer-sponsored plans, private health insurance can be difficult to obtain because of the inherent problems of moral hazard and asymmetries of information discussed earlier. In the state of New York, for example, insurance purchased outside of employer (or other group) sponsored plans can cost as much as $3,000 per month for a family even though the benefits are not more generous than a typical employer plan, which would cost far less to the same family.

About 69% of Americans have some type of private health insurance coverage (U.S. Census Bureau, 2005, Table 142). This is a decrease from 73% in 1990. Generally speaking, insurance companies are either for-profit or nonprofit. Blue Cross/Blue Shield (BC/BS) has been a major private health insurer since 1929. According to the Blue Cross Blue Shield Association (BCBS, 2007):

> Over the past 75 years, we've grown from our humble beginnings assuring hospital care to Texas teachers and providing physician care to lumber and mine workers in the Pacific Northwest. Now we're the largest health benefits provider in America, serving more than 98 million people in all regions of the country.

Originally, BC/BS was entirely nonprofit, although a move to convert to for-profit status began for some BC/BS companies in the mid-1990s (Cunningham & Sherlock, 2002). The commercial insurance companies such as Metropolitan Life and Aetna, either independently or in partnership with an MCO, have always operated on a for-profit basis only. Some of their surplus of income over expenditures is paid to the owners of the company as profit.

The private sector—through health insurance companies, out-of-pocket payments, and other sources—paid about 55% of health care expenditures in 2005, down from about 60% in 1990. Private health insurance companies alone paid about 35% of national health care expenditures in 2005, of which about 86% was for personal health care services in-

cluding hospitalization, physician services, and prescription. The remaining 14% was for administrative costs. In 2000, private health insurance companies paid slightly less of national health care expenditures (34%), of which 88% was for personal health care services and 12% for administrative costs.

Out-of-Pocket Expenditures

Out-of-pocket expenditures include direct payments to providers for noninsured services, extra payments to providers of insurance-covered or managed care-covered services that bill at an amount higher than the insurance/managed care company pays for that service, and deductibles and coinsurance on health insurance/managed care benefits.

A **deductible** is a flat amount, for example, $200 per individual or $500 per family, that a health care beneficiary must pay out-of-pocket before the insurance company will begin paying for any health services received during some time period (usually a calendar year). **Coinsurance** is a share, for example, 20%, of the payment for each service covered by insurance for which the beneficiary is responsible.

Under managed care, beneficiaries receiving health services from a provider of their choice within the plan or out-of pocket entirely will usually pay for some or all of the excess charges out-of-pocket. Today however, there are an increasing number of **"luxury" MCO plans,** available at an extra cost above that normally borne by the beneficiary's employer. They provide for unfettered patient choice of physician, without prior authorization and without additional payment beyond the usual deductible or coinsurance. Obviously, only higher paid employees can take advantage of such plans.

Out-of-pocket expenditures accounted for about 14.8% of national health care expenditures in 2005. This was about the same as in 2000. Reflecting the different levels of third-party coverage for different health services, out-of-pocket payments accounted for about 3% of hospital expenditures, about 10% of physicians' fees, and over 25% of the costs of prescription drugs in 2005.

Government Spending

Government spending has accounted for an increasing proportion of the health care dollar since 1960.

At that time, 5 years before Congress enacted the Medicare and Medicaid programs, government's share was about 25% of the total. By 1970, it was 37.6%. It reached 41.9% in 1980. In 1993, the government's share of health care expenditures reached about 44% and has stayed above that level ever since (45.4% in 2005). In 2005, government entities covered close to 57% of hospital care and almost 66% of nursing home and home health care costs.

Medicare.[3] The first national social insurance program to finance medical care in the United States was established by Congress in 1965 as part of President Lyndon Johnson's "Great Society" program. Called **Medicare,** it is authorized by Title XVIII of the Social Security Act (Hoffman et al., 2001; Igelhart, 1999c; Moon, 2001). Originally, it provided payment for some health services for persons 65 years of age and older who were eligible for Social Security or Railroad Retirement benefits, whether they took them or not. In 1973, its coverage was broadened to include those permanently disabled workers and their dependents who were eligible for old age, survivors', and disability insurance under Social Security, as well as persons with end-stage renal diseases.

Medicare has four parts: hospital insurance **(Part A),** which also covers skilled nursing facility care on a very limited basis, as well as hospice and home health care; supplementary medical insurance **(Part B),** which covers physician and certain other health professional services, hospital outpatient care, and certain other services; Medicare+Choice **(Part C),** which permits Medicare beneficiaries to enroll in MCOs; and the Medicare Prescription Drug Coverage **(Part D),** which was designed to lower the costs of prescription medication for Medicare beneficiaries. Medicare Part A is funded primarily from Social Security taxes, whereas about two thirds of Part B is funded from general revenues, with the balance coming from enrollee premium payments. Medicare prescription drug coverage is funded through premiums.

Medicare is operated by the Centers for Medicare and Medicaid Services (CMS, formerly called the Health Care Financing Administration) of the U.S. Department of Health and Human Services. Its administrative costs are remarkably low compared to those of

the private health insurance sector, ranging from 1% to 2% (Hoffman, Klees, & Curtis, 2000, p. 11).

Medicare Pan D, which was part of the **Medicare Prescription Drug Improvement and Modernization Act** (MMA) of 2003, began on January 1, 2006. Part D provides eligible patients with prescription drug benefits, designed to reduce the cost of medications. Coverage is provided through private entities, both stand-alone prescription drug plans (PDPs) and the more comprehensive Medicare Advantage (MA) plans. The financial risk of the program is shared by both private entities and the government.

Enrollment into Medicare Part D is voluntary for those who did not previously receive drug coverage through Medicaid. The population subset that is eligible for both Medicaid and Medicare is known as **"dual eligibles."** Before 2006, their drug coverage was provided by the Medicaid program. In the beginning, beneficiaries had the option to choose which plan best suited their needs. Later, they were automatically enrolled in what the government decided was the appropriate plan.

For those not covered under dual-eligible status, there is a monthly premium, estimated to be $35 in 2006. This premium is in addition to the annual premium for Medicare Part B (about $420). Under the plan's current structure, there is a $250 deductible to be paid by the individual. After the deductible is paid, Medicare pays 75% of prescription drug costs, up to $2,250 in total drug costs. Between $2,250 and $5,100, Medicare Part D provides no coverage. This gap in coverage is known as the **"donut hole."** After the gap, Medicare pays 95% of drug costs. In every category, the individual is expected to pay the remaining portion of costs, either out-of-pocket or through additional private insurance coverage. The deductibles, premiums, and limits will increase annually (Burns, Glaun, & Lipschutz, 2005).

Most Medicare beneficiaries use providers of their choice. Physicians are paid on a fee-for-service basis, according to a fee schedule constructed on the so-called resource-based relative value system (RBRVS). In the mid-1980s, it replaced the old inflation-stimulating "usual and customary fee" system. Because the "usual and customary fees" were set by the physicians themselves, the inflation factor was built in.

Unfortunately, as payments to physicians began to decline in the early 2000s as a result of the federal Balanced Budget Amendment (BBA) of 1998, an increasing number of physicians refused to accept Medicare fees as payment in full. In this instance, the

[3]An ongoing series of reports on and guides to the Medicare system is available from Medpac, the Medicare Payment Advisory Commission to the U.S. Congress, at www.medpac.gov.

physician sees only those Medicare patients who agree to accept responsibility for the total charges and then submit the bill to the Medicare program to obtain whatever reimbursement they can.

Hospitals are reimbursed on an **episode-of-care-basis,** the amount of payment for each case determined by a formula based on a fiscal construct called the **Diagnosis-Related Group** (DRG), one form of the prospective payment system (PPS). Managed care was introduced into the Medicare program in the mid-1990s (Himmelstein & Woolhandler, 2001, chapter 5; Zarabozo, Taylor, & Hicks, 1996). However, MCOs claimed that Medicare reimbursement levels were too low (Moon, 2001), and they dumped almost 1 million beneficiaries on January 1, 2001, as a result.

In 2005, total Medicare expenditures were $331.4 billion for personal health care expenditures (CMS, 2007a, Table 5), covering some of the health care costs for about 42 million enrollees, up from $146.2 billion for almost 37 million beneficiaries in 1993. In 1998, although about 75% of Medicare enrollees incurred some expenses, about 50% of the total paid for care went to only 6% of beneficiaries who received care (Hoffman et al., 2001, pp. 32, 93). Medicare financed 32% of all spending for hospital care and 22% of physician services costs (Hoffman et al., 2001, Tables 2 and 3). As noted by Meier and Morrison (2002), "In 2002, 50 percent of deaths of Medicare beneficiaries occurred in hospitals, often after stays in intensive care units, visits to multiple physicians in the months before death, and enormous expenditures for treatments intended to prolong life" (p. 1087).

Looking toward the mid-21st century, the Medicare program is seriously in need of rescue and reform (Igelhart, 1999c; Moon, 2001). The **"baby boomers"**—those people born in the immediate post-World War II era—will become eligible for Medicare starting in 2010, whereas the number of working people available to finance the system through the payroll tax that presently supports it will, in relative terms, continue to decline.

Though not yet widely recognized, any permanent rescue of Medicare will require some kind of national health care system that covers everyone. Medicare covers that part of the population that requires the most medical services (i.e., the elderly). But it is financed narrowly by the limited payroll tax. It is hard to see how it will be possible for the program to avoid bankruptcy with the expanding elderly population and the shrinking financing base

that is projected in this century. However, as the fight over the Clinton health plan in 1993–1994 showed a national financing system covering all Americans equally and the regulatory controls that would come with it are something that many private stakeholders in the U.S. health care system continue to fight hard to avoid.

Medicaid. Along with Medicare, Congress created the Medicaid program in 1965, authorized by Title XIX of the Social Security Act (Hoffman et al., 2001; Igelhart, 1999b; Rosenbaum, 2002). **Medicaid** is a needs-based program that provides coverage for some health services for some of the poor on a "means-tested" basis. Therefore, to receive Medicaid coverage, unlike Medicare coverage, a person must apply for it. Also, in contrast to Medicare, the Medicaid program then applies a series of income-level determinations to each applicant, thus "testing their means." Only those persons whose incomes and other assets fall below a certain level as specified by law or regulation (varying from state to state) are declared eligible for coverage.

Medicaid is supported by federal and state tax levy funds and is administered by the states. Each state program is distinct and unique. Therefore, benefits and coverage vary widely from state to state. Like Medicare, Medicaid generally reimburses providers on a fee-for-service/episode-of-care basis, although in the mid-1990s managed care was introduced into the Medicaid program, as it was to Medicare.

Title XIX, as amended, requires a state to provide a set of 14 services in order to be eligible to receive federal funds for its program, with a very complicated set of requirements governing just who may be considered eligible for Medicaid and who may not. The 1996 Welfare Reform Act has had a major impact on Medicaid because of its elimination of the Aid to Families with Dependent Children (AFDC) program, since the time of the New Deal the principal welfare program in the United States. As of this writing, the overall nature of that impact remains far from certain.

A combination of low income eligibility requirements and low fees paid to providers (many of whom have therefore chosen not to participate) has led to very limited coverage in many states. A few of the wealthier states now provide Medicaid coverage for the **medically indigent.** These are persons in an income range deemed not to be low enough to qualify them for income, but low enough to make paying for health services a heavy burden.

Some states (e.g., New York) allow elderly persons with assets to divest themselves of those assets by passing them on to their children over a period of time. They can thus artificially **"spend down"** (by this divestiture to family members) to the stipulated Medicaid-eligible income and assets levels without actually spending the money to pay for care. Of course, this means that the taxpayers of the state pick up the costs of care of a person otherwise ineligible for Medicaid.

It is interesting to note that in 2003, whereas 49% of Medicaid beneficiaries were children and 26% were nonelderly, nondisabled adults (most of them the mothers of the covered children), about 70% of all Medicaid expenditures were for the benefit of the aged (28%) and the disabled (42%) (Kaiser Family Foundation, 2006). Eligible elderly accounted for 11% of Medicaid beneficiaries, and eligible disabled accounted for 14%. In 2003, Medicaid covered over 17% of all personal health care spending, with 55 million people receiving some kind of Medicaid coverage.

State Children's Health Insurance Program. Created with the Clinton Administration's Balanced Budget Act (BBA) of 1997, the **State Children's Health Insurance Program** (SCHIP) provides health coverage for uninsured children who are not eligible for Medicaid. It is jointly financed by the federal and state governments and administered by the states. Within broad federal guidelines, each state determines the design of its program, eligibility groups, benefit packages, payment levels for coverage, and administrative and operating procedures. SCHIP provides a capped amount of funds to states on a matching basis for federal fiscal years (FY) 1998 through 2007. Federal payments to states are based on state expenditures under approved plans.

Other Government Programs. Among other major government health programs are, at the federal level, those offered through the Department of Defense, the Department of Veterans Affairs, and the National Institutes of Health (the federal government's major biomedical research arm); at the state level, the state public health and mental hospital services; and, at the local level, the local public general hospitals and local public health services.

These government programs are paid for primarily with broad-based tax levy funds. Together, they consume a relatively small proportion of the national health care budget. For example, in 1999, national expenditures on public health services ac-

counted for about 2.8% of the total. By way of comparison, payments for program administration and the net cost of private insurance (administration and profit) together were about 2.5 times higher than expenditures for public health services.

WHERE THE MONEY GOES

National health expenditures (NHE) are calculated by the Centers for Medicare and Medicaid Services (CMS), Office of the Actuary, National Health Statistics Group (CMS, 2007a). NHE comprise the following two major categories: (1) Health Services and Supplies; and (2) Investments, a category made up of Research and Structures and Equipment. Most expenditures fall within Health Services and Supplies, and most of these are for personal health care (hospital care; physician and other professional services including dentistry; nursing home and home health care; and medical products including prescription drugs and durable medical equipment). Complementary and alternative medicine (CAM) is included under Other Professional and Personal Health Care services, and vitamins, supplements, and minerals are included under Other Medical Products. The other two categories within Health Services and Supplies are: (1) Government Administration and Net Cost of Private Health Insurance; and (2) Government Public Health Activities. NHE do not include a much broader definition of health care that might include expenditures for dieting and weight loss, health and fitness clubs, sporting goods and related recreation, and healthy foods.

How does the United States spend its health care dollar? In 2005, 93.6% of NHE were for Health Services and Supplies; investment accounted for the balance of 6.4%. Of the Health Services and Supplies, 89.3% were for Personal Health Care; 7.2% for Government Administration and Net Cost of Private Health Insurance; and 2.8% for Government Public Health Activities. Of the major groups within Personal Health Care, hospital care accounted for 30.7% of the NHE, physician and clinical services for 21.2%, nursing home and home health care accounted for 8.5%; prescription drugs accounted for 10.1%; and durable medical equipment for 1.2%.

How are NHE allocated by health condition and characteristics of patients? Through its Medical Expenditure Panel Survey (MEPS) program, the Agency for Healthcare Research and Quality (AHRQ) maintains the most complete source of data on the cost and use of health care and health insurance coverage.[4] Through large-scale surveys of families and individuals, their medical providers (doctors, hospitals, pharmacies, etc.), and employers across the United States, MEPS collects data on the specific health services that Americans use, how frequently they use them, the cost of these services, and how they are paid for, as well as data on the cost, scope, and breadth of health insurance held by and available to U.S. workers (Agency for Healthcare Research and Quality [AHRQ], 2006).

Ranked by expenditure, in 2003 the top 12 diseases or conditions accounted for 55.7% of MEPS-captured spending (Center for Financing, Access, and Cost Trends, 2005). It should be emphasized that different (e.g., broader or narrower) categorizations of disease may produce different rankings.

Older people use more health care than younger people, on average. For men, the expenditures jump suddenly between the ages of 18 and 21 and then fall until after age 40. Expenditures for women jump after age 21 but then plateau until age 50, when they begin to rapidly rise along with those of men.

Health care spending is disproportionately distributed in the population. In 2002, half the population accounted for only 3% of total health care spending. Five percent of people accounted for 49% of spending and 1% accounted for 22% of expenditures (Stanton & Rutherford, 2006). Or, to put it another way, for every $100 spent by someone in the bottom half, someone in the top 1% spent more than $35,000.

Roughly a quarter of this small group remained in the top 1% of health care expenditures in 2003,

and clearly, 75% did not.[5] But of the people who were in the top half of expenditures in 2002, most remained in the top half the following year. Mirroring this, most of the people who were in the bottom half of expenditures in 2002 remained in the bottom half the following year. The implication is that there is both a strong chronic and episodic utilization of health care. High or low use in one year is a strong predictor of similar use in the next. However, even over short periods of time, a sizable segment of the population moves between percentiles.

Although numerous studies advise of the relatively significant resources spent during the last year of life—and even more during the last 6 months—Ezekiel J. Emanuel and Linda L. Emanuel (1994) argue:

> Cost savings due to changes in practice at the end of life are not likely to be substantial. The amount that might be saved by reducing the use of aggressive life-sustaining interventions for dying patients is at most 3.3 percent of total national health care expenditures.

They also assert that these savings "would not restrain the rate of growth in health care spending over time. Instead, this amount represents a fraction of the increase due to inflation in health care and less than [the amount] needed to cover the uninsured population. Accepting this, we cannot assume that less aggressive care at the end of life will solve the financial problems of the health care system.

HOW THE MONEY IS PAID: PROVIDERS, PAYERS, AND PAYMENTS

Provider Payment Approaches

In the health care market, professional services from physicians, therapists, dentists, and so forth accounted for 31.3% of NHE in 2005. These providers are considered to drive the utilization of much of the remainder of NHE including hospital care, nursing home and home health care, prescription drugs, and medical equipment, devices, and supplies. Prescription drugs and other medical products are also mar-

---

[4]The expenditures included in the MEPS survey are a subset of those included in the Personal Health Care component of the NHE. Although the sample of U.S. civilian noninstitutionalized population surveyed in the Household Component of MEPS represents 98% of the U.S. population, the nature of the population excluded from the MEPS sample is such that they are likely to have very different health care expenditures. In addition, the NHE includes expenditures on nonpatient services (gift shops, cafeterias, etc.) as well as other expenditures not counted by MEPS (e.g., nonprescription nondurable goods and CAM services). In 1996, the expenditures of MEPS Household Component made up about 60% of the Personal Health Care component of National Health Expenditures, and in 2003. MEPS accounted for $895.5 billion or slightly less than 62% of the estimated $1,446 billion spent on Personal Health Care. The author strongly recommends that anyone planning to use either NHE or MEPS data for analysis or decision making should supplement their understanding of the inclusions, exclusions, and limitations of such data with the article "Reconciling Medical Expenditure Estimates From the MEPS and the NHA," by T. M. Selden and colleagues (Selden et al., 2001).

[5]The MEPS data also indicate that of the people who dropped out of the top percentiles of 2002, only a small percentage can be explained by death, institutionalization, or ineligibility in the following year (Cohen & Yu, 2006).

kets with their own dynamics, but this discussion focuses on how the services of health care providers and institutions (e.g., hospitals, nursing homes) are paid.

In general, there are six payment modes that people and organizations use to buy and sell services. These are cost/cost-plus, hourly or time and materials, fee-for-service, fixed-price, capitation, and value. We will discuss each in relationship to the provision of personal health care services.

Cost/Cost-Plus. **Reimbursement** is how hospitals describe payment received for services they have already provided. Under a **cost payment method,** the organization providing the service tracks all costs associated with each customer and then asks to be paid that amount. This is similar to how an employee might be reimbursed for expenses incurred during a business trip. The employee would offer receipts for plane fare, hotel, food, and other allowable items and then expect to receive exactly that amount in return. An **indemnity plan** is one under which the covered party is reimbursed for all expenses he or she incurs.

An organization is often paid on a **cost-plus basis** (so-called because a contract specifies that the organization will be reimbursed for actual costs plus an additional percentage of those costs). The cost-plus method provides an additional margin out of which the providing organization can generate profit after any nonproject expenses are paid.

In practice, any independent entities have to be paid in a cost-plus manner. Of course, a profit-generating organization will never survive under a pure cost-only reimbursement model, but even non-profits need more than cost reimbursement to survive. Under any contract there are nonreimbursable expenses, and every significant organization has expenses that are not specific to one project. The margin allowed on the cost-plus project is what an organization draws from to pay these expenses.

The cost/cost-plus method still dominates health care provider payment. Some people like cost-plus contracts because they provide high levels of transparency and seem to limit profits. However, there are drawbacks. These bills are often so detailed that the payer can understand only the bottom line.[6] In practice, what is reimbursable, as well as ceilings and

thresholds on the amounts, must be set. Accounting for utilization of shares of resources can be complicated, and approaches must be agreed on. In addition, cost-plus contracting does not reward the organization, in this case the health care provider, for either better quality or finding new ways to provide services more cheaply. In a true cost-plus system, the contract penalizes the providing organization for cutting costs.

Time and Materials. The hourly payment method, common in service industries, is often referred to as **time and materials.** In this case, a provider would be charged a fixed hourly rate covering all the costs except agreed-on materials, which would be billed as incurred. For example, a residential electrician might pass along all costs for fixtures and breakers and charge $85 per hour for his time, which then must cover his vehicle, all his tools, any assistants he might employ, and so forth. Time and materials tends to be the system of choice in cases where the scope of work is not clear to either party. **Per diem** (by the day) reimbursement remains a very common payment method for hospitals (Kaiser Family Foundation, 2002). And although such a system encourages the hospital to work hard to minimize overhead expenses, payers will always worry that the hospital is not looking for ways to increase efficiency.

Fee-for Service. The **fee-for-service** method is common when the scope of work is clear to both sides. It is the oldest form of payment for health services and the predominant system of paying physicians, dentists, and private providers in the Other Professional Services category of the NHE. For example, a dentist will typically have a set price for a cleaning and checkup. If additional services are needed, those will be performed at essentially published prices. In such a system, the risk of inefficiency is born by the provider and the risk of bad advice is born by the customer. Whether a root canal requires 1 hour or 2 hours to perform and whether or not a root canal is the best use of the patient's money, the dentist receives the same payment. The local market and the dentist's perceived reputation in it drives the rates he or she can charge.

According to some observers (Jonas, 1978; Roemer, 1962), in the past this piecework system was a major cause of many of the observed problems in the health care delivery system. Although the patient's risk that he or she overpays for a service is

---

[6]In health care, a cottage industry has formed around the interpretation of medical bills. For fees ranging between $50 and $250 per hour, *claims assistance professionals* or *health-care advocates* will decipher bills, challenge errors, and negotiate discounts (Francis, 2006; Whitehouse, 2006).

reduced, such systems do not reward the providers for better quality service. Nor do they reward the provider for steering the patient toward more efficient services. A frequent complaint is that preventive medicine is completely ignored (Lown, 1998; Medical Reform Group of Ontario, 1980).

Fixed-Price. A service is called **productized** when it can be marketed or sold as a commodity, which implies that a **fixed price** will buy a known quantity of that service. Critically, the known quantity is a customer-centric outcome (or in the case of health care, treatment of a disease or condition on a per-episode basis). This can be compared with the provider-centric fee-for-service system, which focuses on what the provider does, whereas a fixed-price, productized approach is nominally focused on the condition presented by the patient.

The **prospective payment system** (PPS) was adopted for Medicare by the federal government in 1983 for Medicare Part A benefits (i.e., payments to hospitals) as a way to control costs. It can be seen as forcing productization on the hospitals—at least with respect to the patients covered by Medicare. With PPS, the hospital is paid a predetermined rate for each Medicare patient based on the patient's presenting condition. Each patient is classified into a Diagnosis-Related Group (DRG), a preset list created by the Centers for Medicare and Medicaid Services (CMS). Except for certain extremely high-cost patients, the hospital receives a flat rate for the DRG, regardless of the volume of actual services provided to a patient.

In such a system the provider is rewarded for how efficiently the patient is treated. Quality is emphasized to the extent that it affects the efficiency of the treatments for the initial diagnosis. The negative side of this type of system is that it intrinsically rewards providers who exaggerate the reported severity of the diagnosis, because disease classification determines the amount of payment that will be received. Since patients are classified by the same organizations that treat them, there can be what is called **"up-coding."** Also, providers are rewarded for attracting or seeking healthier patients (who otherwise tend to heal faster than sicker ones) and preventive medicine tends to remain a low priority.

Capitation.   **Capitation** is a fixed prepayment per person to the health care provider for an agreed-on array of services. The payment is the same no matter how many services or what type of services each patient actually gets. In theory, such a system encourages the selection of the least expensive treatments as well as promotes services likely to result in the lowest overall cost during the contract period. However, such a system has no reinforcement for promoting the long-term health of the patient. With capitation, providers are likely to be rewarded for enrolling patients least likely to consume many health services, that is, the healthy.

One can also see **global budgeting** (a payment method common to government-run facilities) as a simplified form of capitation—one with only one payer. The provider receives a global budget, which must cover all costs of treatment needed by the eligible population. This is the common way of paying for Veterans Administration hospitals, state mental hospitals, and local health department clinics. In practice, a global budget model tends to resemble the cost model, as the budgets are often negotiated starting with the previous year's cost, and those in operational control are not usually rewarded for coming in under budget (in bureaucracies, coming in under budget is taken as a sign that the budget was set too high).

Value.   Not frequently seen in health care services, **value-based compensation** is the payment model in which the performing organization is rewarded for the value delivered. Value-based systems are most often used when the value is easy to measure and indisputable. For example, personal injury lawyers often offer their services purely for a contingency fee because the value of the lawsuit proceeds is easy to measure.

One of the assumptions of market theory is that the buyer, in this case, the patient, has a sense of the value of what he or she is buying. As Arrow pointed out in 1963, the uncertainties surrounding medicine make it difficult for providers to know the real value of what they are providing and even more difficult for the patient, who is almost certainly at an information disadvantage relative to the provider. On the other hand, if patients started paying for care according to how much it was worth to them economically, the system would tend toward valuing the lives of wealthier people more highly, which most people would find unethical. Finally, in an emergency situation, a patient may not be able to value care until after the care is provided.

Risk Transfer and Good Intentions

The different payment models can be arranged along a continuum representing the financial risk borne by the buyer and the risk borne by the provider. If the payment model with which the patient pays is different from the payment model under which the provider operates (as is possible in a system with third-party payers such as the current U.S. health system), then the possible combinations can be represented as a matrix.

With each combination, any risk not borne by the provider or patient is borne by the third-party payer. One could expect a third-party payer to react to this risk by excluding people or conditions, rejecting charges, capping fees, or otherwise capping coverage and raising premiums.

On the other hand, even when the payment methods match (e.g., the patient and the provider operate under a fee-for-service contract), either side may wish to use an intermediary. The introduction of **Health Savings Accounts** (HSAs) has essentially created an opening for a different type of institution in health care that starts to resemble something like American Express as opposed to United Health. And so one sees banks—experts in low-risk, high-volume transactions such as managing payments for product purchases—entering the health care market.

It should be noted that how we pay for health care has both short-term and long-term implications. The system of payment affects how the principals act in the system today, but also who and where the principals are tomorrow. There is no shortage of physicians in training who vie for residencies in dermatology or cosmetic surgery, but pediatrics is always in need. A simple capitation system will encourage physicians (and other providers) toward healthier patients. Similarly, a system rewarding outcomes may encourage physicians away from riskier cases. The challenge of rewarding for process consistency is that nearly all best practices are contraindicated in some populations.

Third-Party Payers

Insurance (Risk Management). Who should pay for health care? As important as how we pay for health care is who controls the payments. Although ultimately all costs of health care are borne by the people, how the money gets from the people to the providers of goods (antibiotics, vitamins, wheelchairs, etc.) and services (physicians, hospitals, chiropractors) shapes the system. A system where people purchase directly from the providers, just as they purchase cars and hire mechanics, will be very different from one in which the people give their money to the government, which then maintains a health care system much as all governments maintain a military.

Although most people do not need very much health care in a given year, any significant health care incident is likely to be very expensive. Severe illness can easily cost tens of thousands of dollars, and heroic measures (e.g., trauma and organ transplants) can easily cost in the hundreds of thousands of dollars. Some rare conditions can even cost into the millions of dollars to treat (Thomas, 2006; Zhang, 2006). A health care condition requiring $500,000 in treatment would exceed the lifetime income of most people and would be financially devastating for all but a small percent of the population.

As noted earlier, whereas a significant number of people retain their health expenditure rank from year to year, a sizeable number do not. Therefore, most people desire some sort of insurance to protect themselves against wild swings in health care costs. As Glied (2001) pointed out, people do not buy health insurance to insure their health, but rather to insure their ability to pay for (and obtain) health care in the event that their health status changes. Historically, health insurance was intended to cover major medical events (Dranove & Millenson, 2006).

Matching Different Provider and Patient Payment Approaches. The real motivation for having third-party payers is to bridge the gap between how people want to pay for health care and how third-party payers want to be paid. Although there is little need for a third-party payer in a case where a person wants to pay a fixed monthly amount for health care to a provider who is paid on a capitation basis and offers the entire range of medical services, in reality people do not usually have this option.

More often, people obtain their health care from a variety of providers who may be operating under anyone of those aforementioned models, and quite often an individual provider will offer services under multiple and differing charging models. A third-party payer adds value by converting a stream of monthly payments into a stream of service-driven or ailment-driven payments to providers.

Maintaining a Network of Providers.   To maintain this conversion, the third-party payer maintains a **network of providers** with which it has negotiated contracts. These contracts detail which payment models will be used and what rates will be used, as well as other details common to commercial contracts.

Price and Provider Expertise.   With the most extensive databases of patient visits, especially over time, third-party payers have the benefit of expertise. The databases of third-party payers are a wellspring of information for longitudinal studies and better understanding of treatment options. Third-party payers deal with an array of providers daily. They know the going rate for a wide variety of procedures and consultations across geographic regions and quality tiers. They can conduct quantitative quality studies more easily than any other organization. Therefore, it is third-party payers who have the best chance of predicting which providers will offer a good outcome.

SUMMARY

The United States spends more on health care than any other country in the world, both on a gross basis and on a per capita basis. Further, the United States has a uniquely complex financing and payment system (as demonstrated by the information in this chapter). As some have assessed, we creakily crank dollars through the system, which requires enormous amounts of eligibility determination, benefit checking, coinsurance/deductible, calculation/billing/collection, preutilization authorization, utilization review, and so on (Himmelstein & Woolhandler, 2001). Mountains of paperwork are created, astronomical voice and fax/telephone costs are incurred, and untold amounts of computer time and space are used. Huge numbers of staff are required to carry out these activities.

In addition to the high cost related of administration, the U.S. health care system leaves many people without health insurance and, therefore, with much reduced access to health care. As a matter of fact, in 1999, more than 42 million Americans had no health care payment coverage of any kind (Schroeder, 2001). This lack of health insurance has many negative consequences, ranging from personal anxiety, to increased use of emergency rooms (often meaning that care was deferred past the point where it might have been routine—and cheap—to where it

was complex and expensive, with the delay leading to avoidable complications), to growing personal bankruptcy rates (Hoffman et al., 2001).

REFERENCES

Agency for Healthcare Research and Quality (AHRQ). (2006). *Medical Expenditure Panel survey background.* Retrieved December 26, 2006, from: http://www.meps.ahrq.gov/mepsweb/aboutmeps/surveyback.jsp

American Heritage dictionary of the English language. (2000). Boston: Houghton Mifflin.

Arrow, K. J. (1963). Uncertainty and the welfare economics of medical care. *American Economic Review, 53*(5), 941–973.

Baker, D. W., Sudano, J. J., Albert, J. M., Borawski, E. A., & Dor, A. (2001). Lack of health insurance and decline in overall health in late middle age. *New England Journal of Medicine, 345*(24), 1106–1112.

Blue Cross Blue Shield Association (BCBS). (2007). *History of Blue Cross Blue Shield.* Retrieved January 15, 2007, from: http://www.bcbs.com/about/history/

Bureau of Economic Analysis. (2006). *Table 2.5.5. Personal consumption expenditures by type of expenditure.* Washington, DC: Author.

Bureau of Labor Statistics. (2006). Health care (NAICS 62, except 624). In *Career guide to industries, 2006–07 edition* (pp. 231–237). Washington, DC: Bureau of Labor Statistics, U.S. Department of Labor.

Burns, B., Glaun, K., & Lipschutz, D. (2005). *Consumers face inadequate protections concerning Medicare Part D enrollment and/or disenrollment problems.* California Health Advocates. Retrieved March 31, 2007, from http://www.cahealthadvocates.org/_pdf/advocacy/2006/Brief_Inadequate_P5.pdf

Center for Financing, Access, and Cost Trends. (2005). Total expenses for conditions by site of service: United States, 2003. In *Medical Expenditure Panel Survey component data.* Rockville, MD: Agency for Healthcare Research and Quality.

Centers for Medicare and Medicaid Services (CMS). (2007a). *National health care expenditure Web tables.* Retrieved January 15, 2007, from: http://www.cms.hhs.gov/NationalHealthExpendData/downloads/tables.pdf

Centers for Medicare and Medicaid Services (CMS). (2007b). *Nation's health dollar, calendar year 2004: Where it came from.* Retrieved January 15, 2007, from: http://www.cms.hhs.gov/NationalHealthExpendData/downloads/PieChartSourcesExpenditures2004.pdf

Cohen, S. B., & Yu, W. (2006). *The persistence in the level of health expenditures over time: Estimates for the U.S. population, 2002–2003* (Statistical Brief No. 124). Rockville, MD: Agency for Healthcare Research and Quality.

Cunningham, R., & Sherlock, D. B. (2002). Bounceback: Blues thrive as markets cool toward HMOs. *Health Affairs, 21*(1), 24–38.

Dean, K. (1981). Self-care responses to illness: A selected review. *Social Science & Medicine [A], 15*(5), 673–687.

Dranove, D., & Millenson, M. L. (2006). Medical bankruptcy: Myth versus fact. *HealthAffairs, 25*(2), w74–83.

Emanuel, E. J., & Emanuel, L. L. (1994). The economics of dying. The illusion of cost savings at the end of life. *New England Journal of Medicine, 330*(8), 540–544.

Francis, T. (2006, March 20). Escape from claims hell. *Wall Street Journal.*

Franks, P., Clancy, C. M., & Nutting, P. A. (1992). Gatekeeping revisited—protecting patients from overtreatment. *New England Journal of Medicine, 327*(6), 424–429.

Glied, S. A. (2001). Health insurance and market failure since Arrow. *Journal of Health Politics, Policy and Law, 26*(5), 957–965.

Himmelstein, D., & Woolhandler, S. (with Hellander, I.). (2001). *Bleeding the patient.* Monroe, ME: Common Courage Press.

Hoffman, C., Schoen C., Rowland, D., & Davis, K. (2001). Gaps in health coverage among working-age Americans and the consequences. *Journal of Health Care for the Poor and Underserved, 12*(3), 272–289.

Hoffman, E. D., Klees, B. S., & Curtis, C. A. (2000). Overview of the Medicare and Medicaid programs. *Health Care Financing Review, Medicare and Medicaid Statistical Supplement.*

Igelhart, J. K. (1999a). The American health care system: Expenditures. *New England Journal of Medicine, 340*(1), 70–76.

Igelhart, J. K. (1999b). The American health care system: Medicaid. *New England Journal of Medicine, 340*(5), 403–408.

Igelhart, J. K. (1999c). The American health care system: Medicare. *New England Journal of Medicine, 340*(4), 327–332.

Institute of Medicine. (2002). *Unequal treatment: Confronting racial and ethic disparities in health care.* Washington, DC: National Academies Press.

Jonas, S. (1978). *Medical mystery: The training of doctors in the United States.* New York: W. W. Norton.

Kaiser Family Foundation. (2006). *The Medicaid program at a glance.* Retrieved January 15, 2007, from: http://www.kff.org/medicaid/upload/7235.pdf

Kaiser Family Foundation. (2002). *Trends and indicators in the changing health care marketplace. Section 6: Trends in health plan and provider relationships.* Retrieved March 1, 2007, from: http://www.kff.org/insurance/7031/ti2004-6-set.cfm

Lown, B. (1998). Physicians need to fight the business model of medicine. *Hippocrates, 12*(5), 25–28.

Medical Reform Group of Ontario. (1980). *The crisis in health care.* Toronto: Author.

Meier, D. E., & Morrison, R. S. (2002). Autonomy reconsidered. *New England Journal of Medicine, 346*(14), 1061–1066.

Moon, M. (2001). Health policy 2001: Medicare. *New England Journal of Medicine, 344*(12), 928–931.

Roemer, M. I. (1962, Spring). On paying the doctor and the implications of different methods. *Journal of Health and Human Behavior, 3*(1), 4–14.

Rosenbaum, S. (2002). Health policy report: Medicaid. *New England Journal of Medicine, 346*(8), 635–640.

Schroeder, S. A. (2001). Prospects for expanding health insurance coverage. *New England Journal of Medicine, 344*(11), 847–852.

Selden, T. M., Levit, K. R., Cohen, J. W., Zuvekas, S. H., Moeller, J. F., McKusick D., et al. (2001). Reconciling medical expenditure estimates from the MEPS and the NHA, 1996. *Health Care Financing Review, 23*(1), 161–178.

Smith, C., Cowan, C., Heffler, S., Catlin, A., and the National Health Accounts Team. (2006). National health spending in 2004: Recent slowdown led by prescription drug spending. *Health Affairs, 25*(1), 186–196.

Stanton, M. W., & Rutherford, M. K. (2006). The high concentration of U.S. health care expenditures. In *Research in Action* (Issue 19). Rockville, MD: Agency for Healthcare Research and Quality.

Thomas, R. (2006, November 23). Million dollar man: Life slowly returning to normal after struggle with tick bite. *Decatur Daily, IL.*

U.S. Census Bureau. (2005). *Statistical abstract of the United States: 2006.* Washington, DC: U.S. Department of Commerce.

Whitehouse, K. (2006, January 1). How to fight overcharges. *Wall Street Journal.*

Zarabozo, C., Taylor, C., & Hicks, J. (1996). Medicaid managed care: Numbers and trends. *Health Care Financing Review, 17*(3), 243–246.

Zhang, J. (2006, December 5). Amid fight for life, a victim of lupus fights for insurance. *Wall Street Journal.*

CHAPTER 14

Electronic Health Record

What Is an Electronic Medical Record?

Learning Objectives

- Define the medical record
- Discuss the purpose of using electronic medical records versus traditional paper records
- Describe the common health care computer systems
- Define database and its role in the electronic medical record

Key Terms

Biologic markers	Electronic medical record (EMR)	Pen-based input
Clinical data repositories		Picture Archiving and
Coding systems	Indexes	Communication Systems
Computer-based patient record (CPR)	International Classification of Diseases (ICD)	(PACS)
		Presentation level
Data-level integration	Intranet	Server
Database	Legacy systems	Voice recognition technology
Database management systems	Networking	

Reports of the use of computers to support clinical data management activities date back to the late 1950s. Over the years computer systems have been designed that support most major activities related to health care business practices and clinical processes. The most common types of systems are listed in Table 14.1.

Until recently, hospitals led the way in the development of clinical information systems. This was owing, in part, to several factors: 1) the cost of these systems (including personnel) made information technology too expensive for smaller entities, and 2) hospitals had greater needs of meeting regulatory and financial requirements. Hospital Information Systems (HIS) usually have, as their central component, an Admission, Discharge, and Transfer (ADT) system that manages census and patient demographic information. Billing and accounting packages are also frequently included as core components. In many community hospitals, financial and ADT systems along with Laboratory Information Systems (LIS) comprised the complete HIS package until recently. In the last ten years most hospitals, regardless of size, have created fairly complete Information Systems (IS) solutions via integration of departmental systems with the core HIS.

Departmental systems, especially those for Pharmacy, Radiology, and Laboratory, have evolved from a focus on administrative tasks (scheduling, order-entry, billing) to more clinically oriented functions. For example, modern pharmacy systems commonly provide drug interactions, allergy alerts, and drug

Jerome H. Carter, Ch 1, "What is an Electronic Medical Record?", *Electronic Medical Records: A Guide for Clinicians and Administrators.* The American College of Physicians 2001. Used with permission from The American college of Physicians.

Table 14.1 Common Health Care Computer Systems

System Type	Function
Master Patient Index	Registration and assignment of unique identifier
Pharmacy Information System	Medication dispensing, inventory, billing, drug information and interactions
Radiology Information System	Scheduling, billing, results reporting
Picture Archiving System	Storage and presentation of radiologic images
Nursing Information System	Storage and collection of nursing documentation, care planning, administrative information
Hospital Information System	Core system manages hospital census (admission, discharge, transfer) and billing; most often linked to departmental systems (pharmacy, laboratory, etc.)
Chart Management/Medical Records Systems	Assist in the management of paper records and required statistical reporting; used by Medical Records Personnel
Practice Management System	Outpatient system for managing business-related information; may contain some clinical information (CPT, ICD)
Laboratory Information System	Ordering of laboratory tests, results reporting; covers blood bank, pathology, microbiology, etc.

monographs as part of their standard functions. When looking at the evolution of clinical information systems, it is instructive to consider how the end-user has changed over the years. Departmental systems were designed primarily for use by workers within those departments, not health care providers. This drug-interaction information was available only to pharmacists and their staffs, not directly to doctors and nurses. Clinical information systems were labeled as such because they were utilized in areas that supported clinical activities, not because they were intended for use primarily by clinicians.

Of all the systems that fall under the rubric of clinical information systems, only a few are designed primarily for use by health care providers: Intensive Care Unit (ICU) systems, Picture Archiving (PAC) systems, and Electronic Medical Record (EMR) systems. ICU systems monitor a number of physiologic variables and thereby aid in decision making. PAC systems provide access to radiologic images at locations throughout the enterprise. Both have well-defined domains and may work quite well without close integration with other departmental systems. EMRs are quite another story. The EMR is intended to integrate information from all departmental systems and deliver that information to health care providers at or close to the point-of-care. This is no small task.

THE ELECTRONIC MEDICAL RECORD CONCEPT

Aside from having health care providers as primary users, EMRs have a another trait that sets them apart from other clinical information systems; they are de-

signed to capture and represent data that accurately capture the clinical state of the patient. Symptoms, physical examination findings, and treatment plans find their home in EMRs. The EMR, as a concept, is a tool that helps the clinician manage all aspects of patient care. The data-capture functions help to ensure that all pertinent patient data are accurately entered, appropriate for the stated diagnoses, and legible. However, it is the presentation functions that drive the EMR concept. Here reside the means to look at data in new ways, whether they be trends in serum glucose values, medication history, or a list of patients who have not received recommended preventive health interventions. Unlike the paper chart, the EMR is capable of presenting previously stored data in novel ways. Trends may be reviewed for one patient or an entire group. The potential impact on decision making is almost unlimited.

ORIGINS

Early efforts at building what are now referred to as EMRs began in the 1960s with the COSTAR system, developed by Barnett at the Laboratory of Computer Science at Massachusetts General Hospital (1). Subsequent efforts at Duke University (2) and the Regenstrief Institute at Indiana University Medical Center (3) have given rise to robust EMR systems that contain data for thousands of patients. Commercial versions of EMRs are available from over 200 companies. However, despite these successes, EMR technology is not widespread. It has been estimated that only 3% to 5% of doctors have access to or use EMRs on a regular basis (4). Given the nearly forty years of development activity, it is difficult to understand why EMRs are not a more commonly used clinical tool. The answer may lie in the complexity of the issues that surround the design and implementation of these systems.

EMR and CPR Defined

In 1991 the Institute of Medicine (IOM) published a landmark report, "The Computer-Based Patient Record: An Essential Technology for Health Care" (5). This document served to focus attention on the issues surrounding EMR design and implementation. Perhaps one of its more valuable contributions is in the area of terminology.

When perusing publications concerned with EMRs and associated technologies, one is quickly struck by the number of terms used to describe what are often represented as the same entity. *Electronic medical record, electronic patient record, electronic health record, computer-stored patient record, ambulatory medical record,* and *computer-based medical record* are at varying times applied to the same type of system. Are they the same thing? The IOM report suggests very useful definitions, and these will be used for these terms throughout this book. It defines the **CPR (Computer-based Patient Record)** as an

> electronic patient record that resides in a system designed to support users through availability of complete and accurate data, practitioner reminders and alerts, clinical decision support systems, links to bodies of medical knowledge and other aids.

The report goes on to define a CPR system as

> the set of components that form the mechanism by which patient records are created, used, stored, and retrieved ... It includes people, data, rules, procedures, processing and storage devices, and communications and support procedures.

Further amplification was later provided by one of the report's editors, Richard Dick, who states (6):

> The CPR is a representation of all of a patient's data that one would find in ... the paper-based record, but in a coded and structured, machine-readable form. It incorporates a messaging standard for common

representation of all pertinent patient data. Clinical documentation is completed via computer and is coded within the patient's CPR. Stored data are indexed with sufficient detail to support retrieval for patient care delivery, management and analysis.

He then proceeds to discuss the features of EMRs and EPRs:

> The EMR and EPR, which are, in fact reasonably synonymous, are electronic, machine-readable versions of much of the data found in paper-based records, comprising both structured and unstructured patient data from disparate, computerized ancillary systems and document imaging systems. Clinical documentation may originate in either paper records or computerized data; however, the data are not comprehensively coded. One might consider the EMR or EPR as transitional between the paper-based record and the CPR.

The perspective offered by Dick relates the CPR, EMR, and EPR along a continuum based upon, among other factors, the level of granularity of stored data. A true CPR requires that every data item be uniquely coded and individually searchable; an EMR/EPR does not. EMR systems only require that the data be in electronic form. An example may make this point clearer. This chapter is being written using a word processor. Therefore it is in electronic form. However, there is no index to this document that would permit one to answer questions such as how many lines contain the word *almost*. A clinical example might be: "Retrieve all records for patients who have an S3 recorded for their most recent physical exam." In both examples, an indexed database of terms is required to perform an efficient query. Of course, to ensure that all retrieved records actually relate to the same phenomenon and that all records of patients with an S3 are in fact found, some means has to be in place to find records that do not explicitly contain the term S3. Records that have a "third heart sound" or a "summation gallop" recorded as findings would be overlooked. A controlled vocabulary, as well as a mechanism for creating searchable terms, is required. A CPR requires both of these features along with many others. Commercially available systems are EMRs. In fact, the author is unaware of any true CPR system, commercial or otherwise. The EMR, while not the ultimate patient record system, is still a very complex technology.

AN INTRODUCTION TO ELECTRONIC MEDICAL RECORD SYSTEMS

The availability of a standard definition for EMR helps when discussing products and concepts but does little to aid in the evaluation of systems. One reason for this is that an EMR may be a stand-alone product or a virtual system created via integration of existing systems. Two levels of integration are possible: presentation and data level.

At the **presentation level,** users will be able to view data from all connected systems through a common interface. The user may access a single terminal to review patient information. Laboratory work may be reviewed, medications ordered, and so on. Systems like this are quite useful but very limited when users wish to do more than simple data retrieval. These systems only *seem* to be one coherent system because a single interface is utilized to interact with all of its components. Much of the enthusiasm for the Intranets and Web browsers are due to their ability to support, with relative ease, presentation-level system integration.

Data-level integration is much more desirable and considerably more difficult. Data-level integration requires that all system components use a consistent scheme for labeling (coding) data elements and that a mechanism be present for movement of data between systems (from components to the central system). In the case of a hospital system, the central system may be a database on the mainframe or a server with connections to all component systems. Data integration in a mainframe-dominant environment is rarely seen unless all departmental systems are provided by the same IS vendor. **Clinical data repositories** (databases which accept data from a number of departmental systems and combine them into a centrally, searchable form) provide another mechanism for data-level integration.

In the setting of a single hospital or integrated delivery system, system integration is difficult and seldom completely accomplished. Most successful systems achieve only presentation-level integration. The downside to presentation-level integration is the lack of query capability across all systems. For example, it would not be possible to issue a command such as "Find all patients with a diagnosis of conges-tive heart failure who are not taking an ACE inhibitor" because the patient problem list and medication record reside on two different computer systems. The billing system may hold the problem list and the pharmacy system the medication profile. For a system to qualify as an EMR some degree of data-level integration should exist. All references to EMRs in this text will assume the existence of data-level integration (a feature found in all commercially available packages).

Information systems in hospitals or Integrated Delivery Systems (IDS) represent a special problem for EMR implementation due to the presence of **"legacy" systems** (older systems currently in place). These older systems often cannot be easily replaced and so must become part of newer systems. In many instances presentation-level integration is all that is possible. Another issue for hospitals and IDS is that few stand-alone EMR packages bring their own integration headaches and may create as many problems as they solve.

The EMR is one instance in which ambulatory practice sites are in a much better position to implement new technologies than their often wealthier inpatient cousins. First, ambulatory care sites tend to be simpler. ICU and nursing systems are not an issue. Laboratory information systems requirements often are not present (however, obtaining data in electronic form from outside labs can be problematic). Pharmacy function requirements are usually limited to those required by health care providers (prescription writing, drug interactions, etc.). Second, stand-alone systems that support most major EMR functions are available from many vendors.

EMR Building Blocks

Databases. From the preceding discussion it should be clear that databases are the foundation of any EMR system. A **database** is a software program that permits the storage and retrieval of information. Databases can store data in large blocks (documents or images) or as discrete items (numbers or single words). Modern database systems may hold billions of data items. Finding anything quickly would be very difficult if not for the presence of indexes. **Indexes** are ordered files (alphabetical, numeric, or a combination) that indicate exactly where each stored data item may be found.

A database may reside on a single computer (the server) or multiple computers. Data repositories are special types of database programs. All EMRs contain a database of some type. In a stand-alone EMR, the database contains all chart notes, laboratory values, medication lists, problem lists, etc. This is the situation with most commercial systems aimed at outpatient practices. **Database management systems** are software programs that provide all the functions required to manipulate the information stored in databases. In addition, they provide development tools for creating specialized applications such as EMRs. A few such programs dominate the market: Oracle, SQL Server, and Sybase provide the underlying database system for most currently available EMRs.

Data Input Technologies. Data entry is a major EMR implementation issue. The traditional means of interacting with computers, the keyboard, is not feasible for many EMR users. Other data entry methods are being investigated as adjuncts or substitutes for keyboards. The two that have received the most attention are pen and voice-based input.

Pen-based input relies on a pointing device that may operate much like a mouse or it may be used to write actual characters. In the latter case, the computer must learn to decipher what has been written (handwriting recognition) prior to storing it in the database. Success with handwriting recognition has been limited when large amounts of data are entered. As the technology improves, however, this may become a more viable data entry option. Pen-based input (mouse type) is available with many EMR systems and may for some providers be a workable answer to data entry needs (7).

Voice recognition technology has progressed significantly over the last few years. Second-generation voice recognition systems are available that can handle continuous speech (no unnatural pauses between words) with relatively few errors. They are also much more affordable. Voice recognition has yet to be widely adopted as an EMR data-entry mechanism. However, the technology is sufficiently mature to warrant an evaluation (8).

Networking. Even in the setting of a solo practice networking is required to reap the full benefits of an EMR. Until the appearance of the Internet, **networking** referred to the practice of wiring computers directly together in order to permit communication and sharing of resources. Local Area Networking (LAN) is the name given to this practice. LAN technology makes computing more affordable because it permits a build-it-as-you-need-it approach to purchasing and installing hardware and software. The main computer in LAN is referred to as the **server.** Depending upon the amount of computing power required, a server may be a fast personal computer with extra memory or a special computer designed just for this purpose. In either case a server for a small office can be purchased for less than $3000. LANs are constructed by physically connecting computers and other devices using some type of wiring. Wiring an office requires time and a good deal of planning; every time the computers are moved the wiring has to be adjusted accordingly. All things considered, however, LANs are very cost-effective solutions for implementing EMRs.

Internet technologies also provide a means for networking that is very cost-effective and in many cases superior to other ways of sharing information and resources. One important benefit of using the Internet as the networking technology is that it is relatively platform independent. The essential piece of software required for accessing the Internet is referred to as a *browser* (e.g., NetScape Navigator and Miscrosoft Internet Explorer). Any software written to obey the communications and display protocols that govern the Internet will be able to send and receive information from any browser. A server connected to the Internet may be used by any other computer that can establish a connection to the server. Since Internet protocols can be used over standard telephone lines, a virtual network can be established simply by attaching a server to the Internet and making that address known to those with whom you wish to share information. If you wish to limit access to a group of computers or people, it can be accomplished quite easily with an **Intranet** (a system that uses Internet rules but has access restricted to a specific site or group). A growing number of vendors are offering Internet and Intranet EMR applications, and these may prove to be very attractive to smaller practice sites.

Wireless computer capability is also changing the networking equation. Wireless networks rely on radio frequency transmissions to communicate. One great feature of using wireless technology is that users are not tied to one location. No more worrying about wiring schemes and which rooms should have terminals. The cost of wireless technology is decreasing in cost while becoming more powerful. It is worthy of consideration when planning your networking strategy.

Biometrics.   Maintaining the security of the information stored in an EMR is of the utmost importance. The standard mechanism in most EMRs for restricting access to sensitive information is passwords. Passwords can be quite effective if guarded properly. However, they can be easily forgotten or stolen. A newer approach to identifying users is via the use of **biologic markers** (9). Fingerprint and iris scanning technologies are already enjoying fairly widespread use in a number of fields. In fact, iris scanning is reputed to have an error rate of only 1 per 1.2 million scans. Voice and face recognition systems are also available. Biometric identification is superior to passwords in two ways: they cannot be forgotten or stolen. The role of biometric identification for EMR security has yet to be fully determined. Practice sites with many employees may find that biometrics offers a more manageable solution to data security than do traditional passwords.

Storing Clinical Information

EMRs exist to store clinical information. The exact means used to accomplish this task, however, is anything but straightforward. Two fundamental data-related issues must be addressed when implementing an EMR; movement of information between systems and the format to be used for ultimately storing the data. A number of solutions are possible for each task, some sufficiently widespread that it is possible to grant them the status of a "real world" standard. (A number of officially defined standards exist; however, they are not widely used).

Messaging.   Perhaps the most widely accepted standard for messaging between systems in the United States is Health Level 7 (10). HL-7 was initiated in 1986 as a cooperative effort between health care providers and technology vendors. HL-7 is the messaging standard for moving clinical and other types of data (orders, referrals, test results, administrative information, etc.) between computer systems. It supports a range of data types and even includes provisions for handling structured text notes. HL-7 is supported by most commercial EMR and clinical information systems vendors. It is a "must have" for any system under consideration.

Like HL-7, DICOM (Digital Imaging and Communications in Medicine) is another widely used standard (11). It addresses issues related to the processing of imaging data. DICOM is a joint product of the American College of Radiology and the National Electrical Manufacturers Association. All major types of radiologic images are covered in the standard. Due to the massive nature of imaging files and their storage requirements, specialized computer systems, **Picture Archiving and Communications Systems (PACS),** are used. PACS, which are usually found in larger health care facilities, are an important component of any EMR implementation.

The American Society for Testing and Materials (ASTM) also has a major role in defining standards for health care data exchange (12). This organization collaborates with the developers of both HL-7 and DICOM. ASTM Committee E-31 is responsible for health care related standards and has sponsored many publications.

Codes and Classifications.   Once received from another system or via data entry, data must be stored in a manner that permits their use for clinical and research purposes. There are a number of competing "standards" in this area; here they will be considered by area of application.

The EMR is an application aimed primarily at caregivers. Aside from the problem of getting data into the system, the matter of ensuring that when retrieved the data are properly interpreted is a very important issue. The problem list is an essential component of any medical record. A notation of "ESRD" in a patient's progress note would be taken by most internists to mean "end-stage renal disease" but could have another meaning or not be recognized at all by someone from a different medical specialty. **Coding systems** help to reduce ambiguity by offering a common notation for clinical concepts. The codes are chosen by the provider and have standard definitions and representations. The **ICD (International Classification of Diseases)** offers a standard set of codes for capturing diagnostic information and concepts (13). The ICD code set is published by the World Health Organization and is the accepted standard for diagnostic coding in the United States. Of course, this only partially addresses the problem of ambiguity. After all, codes are selected by the clinician. If an incorrect code is entered, the data in the system will be incorrect and may cause harm to the patient. Incorrect codes may result from oversight or errors in clinical judgement. For example, a patient who presents with 2+ pitting edema may be given a code for congestive heart failure when the real problem is peripheral vascular disease. Thus a coding standard does not necessarily mean accurate patient information.

Current Procedural Terminology (14) is a coding system for diagnostic and therapeutic procedures used primarily for billing purposes. The CPT code set is published by the American Medical Association. Most EMR systems utilize CPT and ICD codes as the only means of storing patient data (aside from free-text).

A third coding system commonly found in EMR systems is SNOMED (Systemized Nomenclature of Medicine), a product of the College of American Pathologists (15). SNOMED is a somewhat more complex coding system than either CPT or ICD. Whereas ICD terms are meant to be used as single entities, SNOMED terms may be combined to form more complex concepts. The downside to this expressive freedom is that there are multiple ways to encode the same clinical concept, which may lead to ambiguity.

Aside from the possibility of erroneous entries, the aforementioned coding systems offer only the barest indication of the actual clinical state of the patient. That information is usually found in an uncoded portion of the record—the progress note. The development of a coding scheme for data contained in the progress note is a major area of inquiry. (Most EMR systems make no provision for this.) However, two viable systems do exist.

The Read Clinical Classification codes (16) were developed in the early 1980s by a British physician. They were later adopted by the British National Health Service. The Read codes have the very ambitious goal of providing a term for all concepts that clinicians might enter into a patient's chart. The second system, developed by a private vendor in the United States, is MEDCIN (17), which directly addresses the problem of encoding the progress note. MEDCIN consists of 75,000+ findings that represent clinically valid terms. Neither of these systems is commonly found in commercial systems within the United States, although MEDCIN is licensed by a few major American-based EMR vendors.

The remaining classification systems are usually buried within the EMR out of sight of clinicians, but they are valuable tools for managing clinical data. Laboratory test and clinical observation coding is the aim of LOINC (Logical Observations Identifiers Names and Codes) (18). It has been adopted by a number of major laboratory systems vendors and major medical centers. NDC (the National Drug Code), a system for classifying pharmaceuticals (19), is widely used within the pharmaceutical industry and may play a key role in future EMR implementations.

The significance of these systems to those planning to implement an EMR system is, for the present, dependent upon the anticipated practice environment. Large sites (hospitals, IPAs, etc.) will likely have a number of clinical systems that must be integrated. In such cases, the use of standard coding systems may lower the cost of system implementation and maintenance. HL-7 capability is a must in larger environments and may be quite helpful to those in much smaller practices where transmission of laboratory data is desired. ICD and CPT codes are a feature of all systems due to their role in billing and administrative activities. The role of clinical nomenclatures such as MEDCIN has yet to be defined. However, as it becomes more important to capture granular patient information for use by clinicians and other EMR components (i.e., decision support subsystems), the interest in the use of such systems is sure to increase.

SUMMARY

Over the last 40 to 50 years clinical systems have undergone significant evolution. The Computer-Based Patient Record is the ultimate goal of those who see the value of information systems in the care of patients. The Electronic Medical Record, in its current incarnation, is a valuable tool and a significant step toward the CPR. However, much remains to be done in the areas of data coding, data entry, user interfaces, database design, and security before CPR becomes a reality.

REFERENCES

1. Grossman, J. H., Barnett, G. O., Koespell, T. D. An automated medical record system. JAMA. 1973; 263:1114–20.
2. Stead, W. W., Hammond, W. E. Computer-based medical records: the centerpiece of TMR. MD Computing. 1988; 5:48–62.
3. McDonald, C. J., Blevins, L., Tierney W. M., Martin, D. K. The Regenstrief medical records. MD Computing. 1988; 5:34–47.
4. McCormack J. Wooing physicians to embrace electronic records. Health Data Management. 1999; 7:56–68.
5. Dick, R. S., Steen, E. B., Detmer, D. E. The computer-based patient records an essential technology for health care. The Institute of Medicine, 1991.

6. Andrew, W, Dick, R. Venturing off the beaten path: It's time to blaze new CPR trails. Healthcare Informatics. 1997; 14:35–42.

7. Lussler, Y. A., Maksud, M., Desrulsseaux, B., et al. PureMD: a Computerized Patient Record software for direct data entry by physicians using a keyboard-free pen-based portable computer. In: Proceedings of the Annual Symposium on Computer Applications in Medical Care. Institute of Electrical and Electronics Engineers. Piscataway, NJ; 1992:261–4.

8. Gillespie, G. For physicians talk is cheap. Health Data Management. 1999;7:92–6.

9. http://www.zdnet.com/pcweek/reviews/1027/27bioapp.html

10. www.HL7.org

11. www.nema.org

12. www.astm.org

13. www.vaccines.ch/whosis/icd10/index.html

14. www.ama-assn.org/med-sci/cpt/cpt.htm

15. www.snomed.org/

16. www.schin.ncl.ac.uk/mig/terms.htm

17. www.medicomp.com

18. www.regenstrief.org/loinc/loinc_information.html

19. www.fda.gov/cder/ndc/

Electronic Medical Records

Learning Objectives

- Distinguish between the use of electronic medical records and paper medical records
- Describe the differences between paper charting and electronic charting
- Understand HIPAA compliance with regard to the use of electronic medical records
- Describe the use of personal digital assistants with electronic medical records
- Know the benefits of using electronic medical records

Key Terms

Drop-down menus

Electronic health record (EHR)

Electronic medical record (EMR)

Electronic signature

Health Insurance Portability and Accountability Act (HIPAA)

Indecipherable

Personal digital Assistant

ELECTRONIC MEDICAL RECORDS: CASE STUDY

Walter Reardon is an 80-year-old patient in Dr. Rand's office. Dr. Rand has recently converted his patient files from paper medical records to electronic medical records. David is Dr. Rand's medical assistant. David escorts Mr. Reardon to the examination room and then begins to perform his initial assessment using the electronic medical record he accesses from the computer in the examination room. When he notices this, Mr. Reardon becomes upset, saying he doesn't trust computers and doesn't want his private medical information "out there for everyone to see."

Electronic medical records, sometimes called electronic health records, are part of health care's future. Although electronic medical records have been around since the Mayo Clinic began using them in the 1960s, the technology has been slow to move into ambulatory care. As today's health care providers strive to make health care safer and allow for efficient team communication, electronic records are playing a more prominent role.

In his 2004 State of the Union address, President George W. Bush stated, "By computerizing health records, we can avoid dangerous medical mistakes, reduce costs, and improve care." Shortly after this speech, President Bush outlined a plan to ensure that most Americans have electronic health records by 2014.

Malone, Christine, *Administrative Medical Assisting: Foundations and Practices*, 1st Edition, © 2010. Reprinted by permission of Pearson Education, Inc., Upper Saddle River, NJ.

Box 14.1 Medical Assisting Standards

CAAHEP Entry-Level Standards
- Organize technical information and summaries (cognitive)
- Document patient care (cognitive)
- Document patient education (cognitive)
- Identify systems for organizing medical records (cognitive)
- Describe various types of content maintained in a patient's medical record (cognitive)
- Discuss principles of using Electronic Medical Record (EMR) (cognitive)
- Identify types of records common to the healthcare setting (cognitive)
- Discuss the importance of routine maintenance of office equipment (cognitive)
- Execute data management using electronic healthcare records such as the EMR (psychomotor)
- Use office hardware and software to maintain office systems (psychomotor)
- Use internet to access information related to the medical office (psychomotor)
- Document accurately in the patient record (psychomotor)
- Apply HIPAA rules in regard to privacy/release of information (psychomotor)

ABHES Entry-Level Competencies
- Maintain confidentiality at all times
- Use appropriate guidelines when releasing records or information
- Be cognizant of ethical boundaries
- Evidence a responsible attitude
- Application of electronic technology
- Apply computer concepts for office procedures
- Prepare and maintain medical records

ELECTRONIC MEDICAL RECORDS ARE EASILY ACCESSIBLE

Electronic medical records are simply the portions of patients medical records that are kept on a computer's hard drive or a medical office's computer network rather than on paper. While physicians must retrieve paper files from separate and often large rooms, electronic records are easily accessible on a computer. In large offices where patients may see several different providers, electronic medical records allow physicians easily to locate patients' laboratory results, consultations, X-rays, and examination findings from other providers.

Using **electronic health records (EHRs),** medical offices are able to access any one patient's file from more than one networked computer in the office. For example, the billing office might have the patient's medical record open on a computer screen while they are accessing information needed for coding a specific procedure. At the same time, the physician might have the same patient's file open on a separate computer screen while she inputs treatment notes.

Charting patient information, such as telephone calls, is easily done within the electronic medical record. Typically the software will contain a section for adding information, such as telephone calls or personal conversations that are related to the patient's medical care.

Many medical offices have computer terminals in each examination room, allowing the medical personnel to add information to the patient's electronic medical record, download test results, or research past medication records while the patient is in the room. In some offices, the physician or medical assistant uses a portable electronic tablet to enter patient data into the computer system.

HOW DOES PAPER CHARTING DIFFER FROM ELECTRONIC CHARTING?

With paper charting, the patient's chart is only available to one staff member at a time. The following example illustrates the steps an office using paper charting might take:

1. The patient telephones the medical office and schedules an appointment to see the physician. The receptionist writes down the information the patient gives her, such as the patient's name, address, telephone numbers, insurance information, and the patient's current complaint.
2. Sometime before the patient's appointment, the receptionist or the billing office may call the patient's insurance carrier to verify the patient's benefits.
3. The day before the patient's appointment, the receptionist may call the patient to remind him of his appointment for the next day.
4. The day before the patient's appointment, the receptionist will prepare the new patient's chart. This is typically done by gathering a paper file folder, color-coded labels to identify the patient's last name, and any other paper forms the patient and the medical staff will fill out on that first visit.
5. When the patient arrives for his visit, the receptionist will give the patient the necessary papers to fill out.
6. When the patient is taken back to the examination room, the clinical medical assistant will begin taking vital signs, such as blood pressure, pulse, and temperature, and begin noting this information by writing in the patient's paper medical chart.
7. When the physician sees the patient, she will review the information the patient has filled out along with the information the medical assistant has filled out and begin making notes of her own into the patient's paper chart. If the physician writes a prescription, she will make a note of this in the patient's chart, along with writing the actual prescription on a paper for the patient to take to the pharmacy. In some offices, the physician does not make written notes in the patient's chart and instead dictates her findings into a tape recorder. Those notes will be transcribed by an assistant or a transcription service, then added to the patient's paper chart.

8. If the physician orders X-rays or laboratory tests, the patient's paper chart will be pulled once those reports are returned to the office in order for the physician to review the results along with the patient's chart.

In contrast, here are the steps an office using electronic charting might take:

1. A patient calls the office to schedule a new appointment. The receptionist begins an electronic chart while she has the patient on the telephone, adding information about telephone numbers, insurance information, and symptoms into the software program.
2. Sometime before the patient's appointment, the software may be programmed to confirm electronically the patient's health insurance coverage.
3. The day before the patient's appointment, the software may be programmed to call and remind the patient of his appointment the next day. If not, it may send a reminder for office personnel to make this phone call.
4. When the patient arrives in the office, he may be escorted to an examination room, where a medical assistant will fill out the patient information form on the computer while the patient is present to answer any questions.
5. The medical assistant will then take the patient's vital signs, entering all fathered information into the electronic medical record as she goes.
6. When the physician comes into the room, he will review the patient's information in the electronic medical record and make his own notes there while interviewing and examining the patient. If a prescription is written, the physician will fill this information out in the electronic medical record, including faxing the prescription to the pharmacy the patient chooses. If any laboratory work or X-rays are ordered, the physician or medical assistant will fill this out within the electronic medical record. If the physician wishes to give the patient any educational materials, such as information on reducing cholesterol, this information may be quickly printed from within the computer system, including making a notation within the patient's electronic medical record that the information was given.
7. If laboratory work or X-rays were ordered, the physician will need only to review the patient's electronic medical record on the computer,

which may be done from any computer terminal within the clinic.

MAKING THE CONVERSION FROM PAPER TO ELECTRONIC MEDICAL RECORDS

Though many health care providers and clinical support staff find that the process of changing from paper to electronic medical records format is time consuming, most would agree that once the EMR have been implemented, using the computer rather than writing in the patient's chart by hand saves a great deal of time.

The conversion from paper to electronic medical record format is typically done over a period of time. Some clinics are able to use a scanner to scan documents from the patient's paper medical record to the electronic record. Other clinics may need to enter information from the paper chart to the electronic medical record software being used and the preferences of the medical staff.

Once the information from the paper medical record has been transferred to the electronic medical record, the clinic staff may choose to destroy the paper record. This must be done by shredding the documents contained in the medical record. In some offices, the staff chooses to simply store the paper record in a secure location rather than destroy the file. When documents such as written reports or consultations from other facilities come into the office, these documents are typically added to the electronic medical record using a scanner. If the original document is no longer needed, it can be shredded in order to protect patient privacy.

Training

Any software company that sells electronic medical records software should supply the medical office with a certain amount of training for the staff to learn to use the equipment. This training should be attended by anyone within the office who will be using the software, including the physicians. In addition, a training manual should be supplied for use in training future staff members. Software companies that sell electronic medical record software should also supply the office with contact information to reach a technical support person in the event a question or concern with the new software should arise within the medical clinic.

ELECTRONIC HEALTH RECORDS AND HIPAA COMPLIANCE

Just as with paper medical records, electronic medical records must be kept private. In order to assure patient privacy and compliance with **HIPAA** legislation, all computer users must have their own password to access the patient medical records. With each person having login information, the software can track each entry or deletion and who made it. With paper records, it is not always obvious who last had a record and who made the latest changes if the user is not identified.

Each station must be logged off when the user is away from their desk and computer screens must not be viewable by other patients while private patient information is displayed on the screen. Given the regulations in HIPAA legislation, computerized medical records are just as safe, if not more so, than paper medical records with regard to possible improper disclosure of information.

Backing Up Computers and Electronic Medical Records

In order to remain in compliance with HIPAA regulations, medical offices must use data backup systems to safeguard the information contained on the office computer systems, including patient medical records. This is typically done on a daily basis and in most offices the computer backup system is set to work automatically. By having daily backup files, the medical office will not likely lose computer data, even if the entire computer system goes down.

USING PERSONAL DIGITAL ASSISTANTS WITH ELECTRONIC MEDICAL RECORDS

Depending on the program, electronic records are available via keyboard connected to a computer system or stylus tapped on a notebook computer or on a **personal digital assistant (PDA).** These devices have many of the same functions as a full-size computer and have the added benefit of being small enough for physicians to carry with them from patient to patient. Most electronic medical records systems can be configured to work according to an office's specific needs. One of the many benefits of such systems is the ability to access medical record information from many locations in the health care facility and to quickly search for and retrieve information in the patient's medical record.

OTHER BENEFITS OF ELECTRONIC MEDICAL RECORDS

There are additional benefits to using electronic medical records, which are discussed in the following sections.

Electronic Signatures

An office that uses **electronic medical records** may use an **electronic signature.** In offices where medical notes are dictated and printed for patient files, an electronic signature or rubber-stamp signature may replace handwritten signatures. In these offices, there must be a permanent record of the signer, as well as an original version of the signature on file.

Avoiding Medical Mistakes

Electronic medical records can be used to alert health care providers to possible medication reactions. This is especially helpful when treating patients who are cotreating with several specialists. The EMR software will typically have a safeguard mechanism built in that alerts the prescribing physician to any contraindicated medications a particular patient may have.

One of the most convincing arguments for converting paper medical records to an electronic format is based on patient safety. In 1999, the Institute of Medicine published a report called "To Err Is Human: Building a Safer Health System." This report stated, "At least 44,000 people, and perhaps as many as 98,000 people, die in hospitals every year as a result of medical errors that could have been prevented." One of the Institute's recommendations was to move to electronic medical records. Their conclusions suggested that some medical errors are caused by **indecipherable** handwriting, a

problem that would be eliminated if providers made their entries electronically rather than in handwritten form.

Some states have enacted legislation to address the issue of illegible handwriting and medical errors. In March 2006, Washington State passed a law that requires all prescriptions written by physicians to be submitted electronically to pharmacists or to be printed rather than written in cursive.

Saving Time

The time saved by electronic medical records may be better invested in patient care. Many health care providers believe they spend a great deal of time charting, far more time than they spend on actual patients care. With the cost of health care rising, it makes sense to free up the health care provider's time while decreasing avoidable patient injuries.

Most electronic medical records programs have **"drop-down menus"** that allow the user to choose information or symptoms from a preprogrammed list. For example, when the user inserts a diagnosis of "diabetes," the software may display a list of possible symptoms the patient may be having, such as excessive thirst or frequent urination. Many EMR programs also include lists of possible diagnoses for the physician to choose from based on the symptoms the patient lists. For example if the patient complains of excessive thirst and frequent urination, the program may offer "diabetes" as a possible diagnosis for the physician to choose from.

Electronic medical records allow medical staff easily to transmit patient information to patients' health insurance companies when requested, rather than having to photocopy the paper records and send them via the postal service. It is just as important to follow HIPAA guidelines for releasing medical records electronically as it is for releasing photocopies of the patient's paper medical record.

Health Maintenance

Many medical offices send reminder cards or letters to patients regarding the need for upcoming services. These are typically used to remind patients of the need for a dental exam, a mammogram, a yearly physical, immunizations, or well child check-ups. Using electronic medical records, the administrative

Box 14.2   Correct an Electronic Medical Record

Theory and Rationale

As with a paper medical record, mistakes may be made within an electronic medical record. The medical assistant must be aware of how to make appropriate corrections to the electronic medical record in an accurate manner. Corrections must be made in an accurate manner to avoid lawsuits or other legal issues.

Materials

- Computer with electronic patient medical record

Competency

(Conditions) With the necessary materials, you will be able to **(Task)** correct an electronic medical record **(Standards)** correctly within the time limit set by the instructor.

1. Identify the correct patient electronic medical record where the error was made.
2. Locate the error within the record.
3. Using the rules associated with the software you are using, make the appropriate correction within the medical record.
4. Sign off on the changes as necessary, according to the steps required within the software program.
5. Verify that the change is correct before closing the patient's electronic medical record.

medical assistant can ask the software program to print these reminders.

Using Electronic Medical Records with Diagnostic Equipment

With electronic medical records software, the medical office is able to perform many tests in the office and have the results show immediately within the electronic medical record. This can also be done with digital X-rays, Holter monitors, spirometers, and a number of laboratory tests on blood and urine samples.

Marketing Purposes

Many medical clinics send informational flyers to patients on a regular basis. An example would be a flyer that is sent during flu season and describes the signs and symptoms of the flu along with prevention tips. Part of the prevention tips would be to encourage readers to come into the physician's office for a flu vaccine.

With electronic medical records, the administrative staff is also able to create a list of patients according to specific parameters. For example, if the office has recently welcomed a physician who specializes in allergies to the office, the administrative staff can create a list of patients who have been treated for allergies and use that list to send a letter to patients to let them know of the availability of the new physician.

Communicating between Staff Members

There are times in the medical office when one member of the staff needs to communicate with another staff member about a particular patient. An example would be a patient who has an outstanding balance owing in the medical office. The billing staff member may need to see the patient when he comes into the office for his visit with the physician. Using the electronic medical record, the billing staff member can post an alert that will be seen by the receptionist when she checks the patient in. The alert allows the billing staff member to have the receptionist direct the patient to the billing office prior to his visit with the physician.

Putting Medical Records Online

Some clinics, like Group Health in Washington State, allow patients to look up portions of their electronic medical records via the Internet. Using this password-protected system, patients can access a company's network or intranet for their lab results, dates of immunizations, or medication levels, which can help when patients travel or need to seek emergency care with someone other than their primary care provider. Several Internet-based businesses now offer individuals online storage of medical information, such as immunizations, medications, and surgeries.

MAKING CORRECTIONS IN THE ELECTRONIC MEDICAL RECORD

Just as with paper medical records, medical staff, entering data into the electronic medical record may make mistakes in their entries. When this happens, the mistake must be corrected as soon as possible. With electronic health records, the steps to take to make the correction will depend upon the software. Most often, the user will make the correction by crossing out the error and entering the correct information. The original entry will still be viewable, though it may show on a separate screen or it may show as having a line drawn through the entry.

SUMMARY

- Electronic medical records are the portions of a patient's medical record that are kept on a computer's hard drive or a medical office's computer network rather than on paper.
- Electronic medical records are gaining popularity over conventional paper files because they offer enhanced ease, efficiency, and accessibility.
- With paper charting, the patient's chart is only available to one staff member at a time. Electronic medical records make the patient's chart available to many healthcare team members at the same time.
- The conversion from paper to electronic medical record format is typically done over time. Once paper medical records are converted to electronic versions, those paper records must be appropriately destroyed.
- Medical offices should correct errors in a patient chart according to accepted protocol.
- By using electronic medical records, a medical office is able to perform tasks such as sending reminder post cards more easily than performing these same tasks with paper medical records.
- Other benefits of electronic medical records include using electronic signatures, avoiding medical mistakes, saving time, and communicating between staff members.

CHAPTER **15**

Introduction to Technology in Healthcare

Perspectives on Biological and Medical Technologies

Learning Objectives

- Describe the shift from patient based accounts of symptoms to technology based testing.
- Describe the development of technology and the acceptance of the technology by both healthcare professionals and patients.
- Discuss the role of technology in American medicine.
- Discuss the impact of interposing an instrument between patient and doctor and how it changed the doctor patient relationship.
- Discuss the relationship between the amount of technology and the frequency of use of that technology.

Key Terms

Cloning technology
Iatrogenic illness

Infirmities
Intractable illness

Objective thinker
Subjective evidence

INTRODUCTION

It is in the field of medical technologies, perhaps more than any other area of technological change, where we can readily agree that the tools and processes developed have been predominantly beneficial to humankind. Medicines such as antibiotics, pain relievers, and drug therapies; diagnostic tools such as MRIs, ultra-sound, and even the lowly stethoscope; and life-extending machines such as oxygen tanks, life-support equipment, and kidney dialysis—all of these technologies and scientific breakthroughs have allowed humans to live longer and to survive accidents or illnesses that at one time would have meant certain death. Furthermore, emerging fields such as genetic therapy and advanced neuroscience mean that even **intractable illnesses** or **infirmities** may become a thing of the past.

Why, then, would anyone raise concerns about advances in medical technology? Because, as with every other category of technological development, we can identify both positive and negative outcomes. In other words, the effects of medical technologies, although substantially positive, have also created dilemmas related to costs, access, and the ways that medicine is practiced.

The debate about access to health care that has been waged in the U.S. for many years centers around one essential issue: a growing number of Americans cannot afford private health insurance and do not qualify for public assistance for medical care. As healthcare costs continue to rise,[1] this means that millions of Americans simply cannot afford health care, preventative or otherwise.[2] Developments in new medical technologies have contributed greatly to the rising cost of health care, yet their availability has not necessarily translated into better overall care. Because health care spending represents one of the single biggest categories of spending in the U.S., we must come to terms with the need for a cost-benefit analysis of those expenditures.

In addition to access issues, some new medical technologies have fundamentally challenged our concept of what is meant by "health care." Should some things be ethically off limits? For example, should **cloning technology** be pursued to provide replacement organs, knowing that cloning can also potentially provide replacement people? Should a couple know the genetic particulars of their unborn child, perhaps causing them to face the difficult decision to abort? Even more controversial, should embryos harvested for in vitro fertilization be "graded" and the parents be allowed to choose the "best" one? These questions, by definition, cannot be resolved through technology, but rather must be answered by members of a society who are both technologically literate and ethically engaged.

Most medical procedures carry some risks. Generally speaking, the more intrusive the procedure, the greater the likelihood of complications, which in some cases turn out to be more damaging than the original condition. The statistics on **iatrogenic** (treatment-induced) **illness** and death are sobering. Estimates are that they account for up to 12 percent of office or hospital visits; for somewhere between 44,000 and 98,000 deaths annually in the U.S.; and that the total cost of medical errors of all types is between $37 billion and $50 billion annually.[3] Children and the elderly are at particular risk. This prob-

lem is not confined to the U.S. alone, and is certainly not always a result of high-tech medical care. Nevertheless, medical consumers are cautioned to actively oversee their health care, and to question the necessity of prescribed medicines and procedures.[4]

Another key point regarding the cultural effects of medical technologies is the way this approach to health care has influenced our relationships with our own health. There is less incentive to follow good judgment with regard to exposure to illness, nutrition, exercise, and adequate rest when we believe that there will be treatments for whatever ill health may result. For example, six in ten Americans are estimated to be overweight or obese, and as a nation we spend tens of billions of dollars annually on weight loss products and services. Much of this money is spent on a "never-ending quest for easy solutions" to the problem of being overweight.[5] A technological approach to medical care also may make us less likely to seek out and/or accept traditional or alternative treatments, some of which may be superior to riskier or more costly modern approaches.[6]

THE IDEOLOGY OF MACHINES: MEDICAL TECHNOLOGY

A few years ago, an enterprising company made available a machine called HAGOTH, of which it might be said, this was Technopoly's most ambitious

---

The Ideology of Machines: Medical Technology

Neil Postman provides a historical background to help explain the dominant philosophy of medical practice in the United States, which he characterizes as "aggressive" and much more interventionist than the health care typically provided in other developed nations.

These are two central impacts of medical technology on health care that are highlighted in this excerpt. First is that the focus of medical attention has shifted to the condition and away from the patient. Second, physicians have come to rely more on the information they receive from the medical technologies than they do on the patients themselves. These may seem like subtle points, but an examination of their effects can reveal fundamental changes in how we approach health care and, in fact, how we think about *health* in general. The important question that emerges, then, is whether we are better off from a quality of life standpoint. Does a highly technologized form of health care delivery lead to better overall health? Is this form of care more cost effective than other strategies? Finally, how can the system of health care delivery be improved to achieve greater levels of overall health, at sustainable levels of spending, for all citizens?

Neil Postman, who died in 2003, was a professor of media, culture, and communication, and was the author of numerous essays and books, including *Technopoly: The Surrender of Culture to Technology* (1993), *The Disappearance of Childhood* (1994), *Teaching as a Subversive Activity* (1971), and *Building a Bridge to the 18th Century: How the Past Can Improve Our Future* (2000).

---

hour. The machine cost $1,500, the bargain of the century, for it was able to reveal to its owner whether someone talking on the telephone was telling the truth. It did this by measuring the "stress content" of a human voice as indicated by its oscillations. You connected HAGOTH to your telephone and, in the course of conversation, asked your caller some key question, such as "Where did you go last Saturday night?" HAGOTH had sixteen lights—eight green and eight red—and when the caller replied, HAGOTH went to work. Red lights went on when there was much stress in the voice, green lights when there was little. As an advertisement for HAGOTH said, "Green indicates no stress, hence truthfulness." In other words, according to HAGOTH, it is not possible to speak the truth in a quivering voice or to lie in a steady one—an idea that would doubtless amuse Richard Nixon. At the very least, we must say that HAGOTH'S definition of truthfulness was peculiar, but so precise and exquisitely technical as to command any bureaucrat's admiration. The same may be said of the definition of intelligence as expressed in a standard-brand intelligence test. In fact, an intelligence test works exactly like HAGOTH. You connect a pencil to the fingers of a young person and address some key questions to him or her; from the replies a computer can calculate exactly how much intelligence exists in the young person's brain.[1]

HAGOTH has mercifully disappeared from the market, for what reason I do not know. Perhaps it was sexist or culturally biased or, worse, could not measure oscillations accurately enough. When it comes to machinery, what Technopoly insists upon most is accuracy. The idea embedded in the machine is largely ignored, no matter how peculiar.

Though HAGOTH has disappeared, its idea survives—for example, in the machines called "lie detectors." In America, these are taken very seriously by police officers, lawyers, and corporate executives who ever more frequently insist that their employees be subjected to lie-detector tests. As for intelligence tests, they not only survive but flourish, and have been supplemented by vocational aptitude tests, creativity tests, mental-health tests, sexual-attraction tests, and even marital-compatibility tests. One would think that two people who have lived together for a number of years would have noticed for themselves whether they get along or not. But in Technopoly, these subjective forms of knowledge have no official status, and must be confirmed by tests administered by experts. Individual judgments, after all, are notoriously unreliable, filled

with ambiguity and plagued by doubt, as Frederick W. Taylor warned. Tests and machines are not. Philosophers may agonize over the questions "What is truth?" "What is intelligence?" "What is the good life?" But in Technopoly there is no need for such intellectual struggle. Machines eliminate complexity, doubt, and ambiguity. They work swiftly, they are standardized, and they provide us with numbers that you can see and calculate with. They tell us that when eight green lights go on someone is speaking the truth. That is all there is to it. They tell us that a score of 136 means more brains than a score of 104. This is Technopoly's version of magic.

What is significant about magic is that it directs our attention to the wrong place. And by doing so, evokes in us a sense of wonder rather than understanding. In Technopoly, we are surrounded by the wondrous effects of machines and are encouraged to ignore the ideas embedded in them. Which means we become blind to the ideological meaning of our technologies. In this chapter I will provide examples of how technology directs us to construe the world.

In considering here the ideological biases of medical technology, let us begin with a few relevant facts. Although the U.S. and England have equivalent life-expectancy rates, American doctors perform six times as many cardiac bypass operations per capita as English doctors do. American doctors perform more diagnostic tests than doctors do in France, Germany, or England. An American woman has two to three times the chance of having a hysterectomy as her counterpart in Europe; 60 percent of the hysterectomies performed in America are done on women under the age of forty-four. American doctors do more prostate surgery per capita than do doctors anywhere in Europe, and the United States leads the industrialized world in the rate of cesarean-section operations—50 to 200 percent higher than in most other countries. When American doctors decide to forgo surgery in favor of treatment by drugs, they give higher dosages than doctors elsewhere. They prescribe about twice as many antibiotics as do doctors in the United Kingdom and commonly prescribe antibiotics when bacteria are likely to be present, whereas European doctors tend to prescribe antibiotics only if they know that the infection is caused by bacteria *and* is also serious.[2] American doctors use far more X-rays per patient than do doctors in other countries. In one review of the extent of X-ray use, a radiologist discovered cases in which fifty to one hundred X-rays had been taken of a single patient when five would have been sufficient.

Other surveys have shown that, for almost one-third of the patients, the X-ray could have been omitted or deferred on the basis of available clinical data.[3]

The rest of this chapter could easily be filled with similar statistics and findings. Perhaps American medical practice is best summarized by the following warning, given by Dr. David E. Rogers in a presidential address to the Association of American Physicians:

> As our interventions have become more searching, they have also become more costly and more hazardous. Thus, today it is not unusual to find a fragile elder who walked into the hospital, [and became] slightly confused, dehydrated, and somewhat the worse for wear an the third hospital day because his first 48 hours in the hospital were spent undergoing a staggering series of exhausting diagnostic studies in various laboratories or in the radiology suite.[4]

None of this is surprising to anyone familiar with American medicine, which is notorious for its characteristic "aggressiveness." The question is, why? There are three interrelated reasons, all relevant to the imposition of machinery. The first has to do with the American character, which I have previously discussed as being so congenial to the sovereignty of technology. In *Medicine and Culture*, Lynn Payer describes it in the following way:

> The once seemingly limitless lands gave rise to a spirit that anything was possible if only the natural environment . . . could be conquered. Disease could also be conquered, but only by aggressively ferreting it out diagnostically and just as aggressively treating it, preferably by taking something out rather than adding something to increase the resistance.[5]

To add substance to this claim, Ms. Payer quotes Oliver Wendell Holmes as saying, with his customary sarcasm:

> How could a people which has a revolution once in four years, which has contrived the Bowie Knife and the revolver . . . which insists in sending out yachts and horses and boys to outsail, outrun, outfight and checkmate all the rest of creation; how could such a people be content with any but "heroic" practice? What wonder that the stars and stripes wave over doses of ninety grams of sulphate of quinine and that the American eagle screams with delight

> to see three drachms [180 grains] of calomel given at a single mouthful?[6]

The spirit of attack mocked here by Holmes was given impetus even before the American Revolution by Dr. Benjamin Rush, perhaps the most influential medical man of his age. Rush believed that medicine had been hindered by doctors placing "undue reliance upon the powers of nature in curing disease," and specifically blamed Hippocrates and his tradition for this lapse. Rush had considerable success in curing patients of yellow fever by prescribing large quantities of mercury and performing purges and bloodletting. (His success was probably due to the fact that the patients either had mild cases of yellow fever or didn't have it at all.) In any event, Rush was particularly enthusiastic about bleeding patients, perhaps because he believed that the body contained about twenty-five pints of blood, which is more than twice the average actual amount. He advised other doctors to continue bleeding a patient until four-fifths of the body's blood was removed. Although Rush was not in attendance during George Washington's final days, Washington was bled seven times on the night he died, which, no doubt, had something to do with why he died. All of this occurred, mind you, 153 years after Harvey discovered that blood circulates throughout the body.

Putting aside the question of the available medical knowledge of the day, Rush was a powerful advocate of action—indeed, gave additional evidence of his aggressive nature by being one of the signers of the Declaration of Independence. He persuaded both doctors and patients that American diseases were tougher than European diseases and required tougher treatment. "Desperate diseases require desperate remedies" was a phrase repeated many times in American medical journals in the nineteenth century. The Americans, who considered European methods to be mild and passive—one might even say effeminate—met the challenge by eagerly succumbing to the influence of Rush: they accepted the imperatives to intervene, to mistrust nature, to use the most aggressive therapies available. The idea, as Ms. Payer suggests, was to conquer both a continent and the diseases its weather and poisonous flora and fauna inflicted.

So, from the outset, American medicine was attracted to new technologies. Far from being "neutral," technology was to be the weapon with which disease and illness would be vanquished. The weapons were not long in coming. The most significant of the early medical technologies was the stethoscope, invented (one might almost say discovered) by the French physician René-Théophile-Hyacinthe Laënnec in 1816. The circumstances surrounding the invention are worth mentioning.

Working at the Necker Hospital in Paris, Laënnec was examining a young woman with a puzzling heart disorder. He tried to use percussion and palpation (pressing the hand upon the body in hope of detecting internal abnormalities), but the patient's obesity made this ineffective. He next considered auscultation (placing his ear on the patient's chest to hear the heart beat), but the patient's youth and sex discouraged him. Laënnec then remembered that sound traveling through solid bodies is amplified. He rolled some sheets of paper into a cylinder, placed one end on the patient's chest and the other to his ear. *Voilà!* The sounds he heard were clear and distinct. "From this moment," he later wrote, "I imagined that the circumstance might furnish means for enabling us to ascertain the character, not only of the action of the heart, but of every species of sound produced by the motion of all the thoracic viscera." Laënnec worked to improve the instrument, eventually using a rounded piece of wood, and called it a "stethoscope," from the Greek words for "chest" and "I view."[7]

For all its simplicity, Laënnec's invention proved extraordinarily useful, particularly in the accuracy with which it helped to diagnose lung diseases like tuberculosis. Chest diseases of many kinds were no longer concealed: the physician with a stethoscope could, as it were, conduct an autopsy on the patient while the patient was still alive.

But it should not be supposed that all doctors or patients were enthusiastic about the instrument. Patients were often frightened at the sight of a stethoscope, assuming that its presence implied imminent surgery, since, at the time, only surgeons used instruments, not physicians. Doctors had several objections, ranging from the trivial to the significant. Among the trivial was the inconvenience of carrying the stethoscope, a problem some doctors solved by carrying it, crosswise, inside their top hats. This was not without its occasional embarrassments—an Edinburgh medical student was accused of possessing a dangerous weapon when his stethoscope fell out of his hat during a snowball fight. A somewhat less trivial objection raised by doctors was that if they used an instrument they would be mistaken for surgeons, who were then considered mere craftsmen. The distinction between physicians and surgeons

was unmistakable then, and entirely favorable to physicians, whose intellect, knowledge, and insight were profoundly admired. It is perhaps to be expected that Oliver Wendell Holmes, professor of anatomy at Harvard and always a skeptic about aggressiveness in medicine, raised objections about the overzealous use of the stethoscope; he did so, in characteristic fashion, by writing a comic ballad, "The Stethoscope Song," in which a physician makes several false diagnoses because insects have nested in his stethoscope.

But a serious objection raised by physicians, and one which has resonated throughout the centuries of technological development in medicine, is that interposing an instrument between patient and doctor would transform the practice of medicine; the traditional methods of questioning patients, taking their reports seriously, and making careful observations of exterior symptoms would become increasingly irrelevant. Doctors would lose their ability to conduct skillful examinations and rely more on machinery than on their own experience and insight. In his detailed book *Medicine and the Reign of Technology*, Stanley Joel Reiser compares the effects of the stethoscope to the effects of the printing press on Western culture. The printed book, he argues, helped to create the detached and **objective thinker.** Similarly, the stethoscope

> helped to create the objective physician, who could move away from involvement with the patient's experiences and sensations, to a more detached relation, less with the patient but more with the sounds from within the body. Undistracted by the motives and beliefs of the patient, the auscultator [another term for the stethoscope] could make a diagnosis from sounds that he alone heard emanating from body organs, sounds that he believed to be objective, bias-free representations of the disease process.[8]

Here we have expressed two of the key *ideas* promoted by the stethoscope: Medicine is about disease, not the patient. And, what the patient knows is untrustworthy; what the machine knows is reliable.

The stethoscope could not by itself have made such ideas stick, especially because of the resistance to them, even in America, by doctors whose training and relationship to their patients led them to oppose mechanical interpositions. But the ideas were amplified with each new instrument added to the doctor's arsenal: the ophthalmoscope (invented by Hermann von Helmholtz in 1850), which allowed doctors to see into the eye; the laryngoscope (designed by Johann Czermak, a Polish professor of physiology, in 1857), which allowed doctors to inspect the larynx and other parts of the throat, as well as the nose; and, of course, the X-ray (developed by Wilhelm Roentgen in 1895), which could penetrate most substances but not bones. "If the hand be held before the fluorescent screen," Roentgen wrote, "the shadow shows the bones darkly with only faint outlines of the surrounding tissues." Roentgen was able to reproduce this effect on photographic plates and make the first X-ray of a human being, his wife's hand.

By the turn of the century, medicine was well on its way to almost total reliance on technology, especially after the development of diagnostic laboratories and the discovery and use of antibiotics in the 1940s. Medical practice had entered a new stage. The first had been characterized by direct communication with the patient's experiences based on the patient's reports, and the doctor's questions and observations. The second was characterized by direct communication with patients' bodies through physical examination, including the use of carefully selected technologies. The stage we are now in is characterized by indirect communication with the patient's experience and body through technical machinery. In this stage, we see the emergence of specialists—for example, pathologists and radiologists—who interpret the meaning of technical information and have no connection whatsoever with the patient, only with tissue and photographs. It is to be expected that, as medical practice moved from one stage to another, doctors tended to lose the skills and insights that predominated in the previous stage. Reiser sums up what this means:

> So, without realizing what has happened, the physician in the last two centuries has gradually relinquished his unsatisfactory attachment to **subjective evidence**—what the patient says—only to substitute a devotion to technological evidence—what the machine says. He has thus exchanged one partial view of disease for another. As the physician makes greater use of the technology of diagnosis, he perceives his patient more and more indirectly through a screen of machines and specialists; he also relinquishes control over more and more of the diagnostic process. These circumstances tend to estrange him from his patient and from his own judgment.[9]

There is still another reason why the modern physician is estranged from his own judgment. To put it in the words of a doctor who remains skilled in examining his patients and in evaluating their histories: "Everyone who has a headache wants and expects a CAT scan." He went on to say that roughly six out of every ten CAT scans he orders are unnecessary, with no basis in the clinical evidence and the patient's reported experience and sensations. Why are they done? As a protection against malpractice suits. Which is to say, as medical practice has moved into the stage of total reliance on machine-generated information, so have the patients. Put simply, if a patient does not obtain relief from a doctor who has failed to use all the available technological resources, including drugs, the doctor is deemed vulnerable to the charge of incompetence. The situation is compounded by the fact that the personal relationship between doctor and patient now, in contrast to a century ago, has become so arid that the patient is not restrained by intimacy or empathy from appealing to the courts. Moreover, doctors are reimbursed by medical-insurance agencies on the basis of what they *do*, not on the amount of time they spend with patients. Nontechnological medicine is time-consuming. It is more profitable to do a CAT scan on a patient with a headache than to spend time getting information about his or her experiences and sensations.

What all this means is that even restrained and selective technological medicine becomes very difficult to do, economically undesirable, and possibly professionally catastrophic. The culture itself—its courts, its bureaucracies, its insurance system, the training of doctors, patients' expectations—is organized to support technological treatments. There are no longer methods of treating illness; there is only one method-the technological one. Medical competence is now defined by the quantity and variety of machinery brought to bear on disease.

As I remarked, three interrelated reasons converged to create this situation. The American character was biased toward an aggressive approach and was well prepared to accommodate medical technology; the nineteenth-century technocracies, obsessed with invention and imbued with the idea of progress, initiated a series of remarkable and wondrous inventions; and the culture reoriented itself to ensure that technological aggressiveness became the basis of medical practice. The ideas promoted by this domination of technology can be summed up as follows: Nature is an implacable enemy that can be subdued only by technical means; the problems created by technological solutions (doctors call these "side effects") can be solved only by the further application of technology (we all know the joke about an amazing new drug that cures nothing but has interesting side effects); medical practice must focus on disease, not on the patient (which is why it is possible to say that the operation or therapy was successful but the patient died); and information coming from the patient cannot be taken as seriously as information coming from a machine, from which it follows that a doctor's judgment, based on insight and experience, is less worthwhile than the calculations of his machinery.

Do these ideas lead to better medicine? In some respects, yes; in some respects, no. The answer tends to be "yes" when one considers how doctors now use lasers to remove cataracts quickly, painlessly, and safely; or how they can remove a gall-bladder by using a small television camera (a laparoscope) inserted through an equally small puncture in the abdomen to guide the surgeon's instruments to the diseased organ through still another small puncture, thus making it unnecessary to cut open the abdomen. Of course, those who are inclined to answer "no" to the question will ask how many laparoscopic cholecystectomies are performed *because* of the existence of the technology. This is a crucial point.

Consider the case of cesarean sections. Close to one out of every four Americans is now born by C-section. Through modern technology, American doctors can deliver babies who would have died otherwise. As Dr. Laurence Horowitz notes in *Taking Charge of Your Medical Fate*, ". . . the proper goal of C-sections is to improve the chances of babies at risk, and that goal has been achieved."[10] But C-sections are a surgical procedure, and when they are done routinely as an elective option, there is considerable and unnecessary danger; the chances of a woman's dying during a C-section delivery are two to four times greater than during a normal vaginal delivery. In other words, C-sections can and do save the lives of babies at risk, but when they are done for other reasons—for example, for the convenience of doctor or mother—they pose an unnecessary threat to health, and even life.

To take another example: a surgical procedure known as carotid endarterectomy is used to clean out clogged arteries, thus reducing the likelihood of stroke. In 1987, more than one hundred thousand Americans had this operation. It is now established that the risks involved in such surgery outweigh the risks of suffering a stroke. Horowitz again: "In other words, for certain categories of patients, the operation may actually kill more people than it saves."[11] To take still another example: about seventy-eight thousand people every year get cancer from medical

and dental X-rays. In a single generation, it is estimated, radiation will induce 2.34 million cancers.[12]

Examples of this kind can be given with appalling ease. But in the interests of fairness the question about the value of technology in medicine is better phrased in the following way: Would American medicine be better were it not so totally reliant on the technological imperative? Here the answer is clearly, yes. We know, for example, from a Harvard Medical School study which focused on the year 1984 (no Orwellian reference intended), that in New York State alone there were thirty-six thousand cases of medical negligence, including seven thousand deaths related in some way to negligence. Although the study does not give figures on what kinds of negligence were found, the example is provided of doctors prescribing penicillin without asking the patients whether they were hypersensitive to the drug. We can assume that many of the deaths resulted not only from careless prescriptions and the doctors' ignorance of their patients' histories but also from unnecessary surgery. In other words, iatrogenics (treatment-induced illness) is now a major concern for the profession, and an even greater concern for the patient. Doctors themselves feel restricted and dominated by the requirement to use all available technology. And patients may be justifiably worried by reports that quite possibly close to 40 percent of the operations performed in America are not necessary. In *Health Shock*, Martin Weitz cites the calculations of Professor John McKinlay that more deaths are caused by surgery each year in the United States than the annual number of deaths during the wars in Korea and Vietnam. As early as 1974, a Senate investigation into unnecessary surgery reported that American doctors had performed 2.4 million unnecessary operations, causing 11,900 deaths and costing about $3.9 billion.[13] We also know that, in spite of advanced technology (quite possibly because of it), the infant-survival rate in the United States ranks only fourteenth in the world, and it is no exaggeration to say that American hospitals are commonly regarded as among the most dangerous places in the nation. It is also well documented that, wherever doctor strikes have occurred, the mortality rate declines.

There are, one may be sure, very few doctors who are satisfied with technology's stranglehold on medical practice. And there are far too many patients who have been its serious victims. What conclusions may we draw? First, technology is not a neutral element in the practice of medicine: doctors do not merely use technologies but are used by them. Second, technology creates its own imperatives and, at the same time, creates a wide-ranging social system to reinforce its imperatives. And third, technology changes the practice of medicine by redefining what doctors are, redirecting where they focus their attention, and reconceptualizing how they view their patients and illness.

Like some well-known diseases, the problems that have arisen as a result of the reign of technology came slowly and were barely perceptible at the start. As technology grew, so did the influence of drug companies and the manufacturers of medical instruments. As the training of doctors changed, so did the expectations of patients. As the increase in surgical procedures multiplied, so did the diagnoses which made them seem necessary. Through it all, the question of what was being *undone* had a low priority if it was asked at all. The Zeitgeist of the age placed such a question in a range somewhere between peevishness and irrelevance. In a growing Technopoly, there is no time or inclination to speak of technological debits.

AUTHOR CITATIONS

1. I am not sure whether the company still exists, but by way of proving that it at least once did, here is the address of the HAGOTH Corporation as I once knew it: 85 NW Alder Place, Department C, Issaquah, Washington 98027.
2. All these facts and more may be found in: Payer, L. *Medicine and Culture: Varieties of Treatment in the United States, England, West Germany, and France.* New York: Penguin Books, 1988; or in: Inlander, C. B.; Levin, L. S.; and Weiner, E. *Medicine on Trial: The Appalling Story of Medical Ineptitude and the Arrogance that Overlooks It.* New York: Pantheon Books, 1988.
3. Reiser, S. J. *Medicine and the Reign of Technology.* Cambridge University Press, 1978, (p. 160).
4. Ibid., p. 161.
5. Payer, p. 127.
6. Quoted in ibid.
7. For a fascinating account of Laënnec's invention, see Reiser.
8. Ibid., p. 38.
9. Ibid., p. 230.
10. Horowitz, L. C., M. D. *Taking Charge of Your Medical Fate.* New York: Random House, 1988, (p. 31).
11. Ibid., p. 80.
12. Cited in Inlander et al., p. 106.
13. Cited in ibid., p. 113.

ENDNOTES

1. According to the National Coalition on Health Care, "in 2008, total national health expenditures were expected to rise 6.9 percent—two times the rate of inflation. Total spending was $2.4 trillion in 2007, or $7900 per person. Total health care spending represented 17 percent of the gross domestic product (GOP). . . . U.S. health care spending is expected to increase at similar levels for the next decade, reaching $4.3 trillion in 2017, or 20 percent of GOP." (From *Health Insurance Costs:* http://www.nchc.org/facts/cost.shtml.)
2. According to the Centers for Disease Control (CDC), over 43 million Americans were without any form of health insurance in 2006, and for more than half of these individuals cost was the primary factor (see: http://www.cdc.gov/Features/Uninsured/).
3. Cook, Dawn M. 2001. Iatrogenic illness: A primer for nurses. *MedSurge Nursing.* 10(3): 139–146.
4. Moser, Marvin. The Patient as a Consumer. In Barry L. Zaret, Marvin Moser, and Lawrence S. Cohen (Eds.), *Yale University School of Medicine Heart Book.* New York: William Morrow and Company, Inc. pp. 359–362.
5. Federal Trade Commission. 2002. *Weight loss advertising: An analysis of current trends.* Available: http://www.ftc.gov/bcp/reports/weightloss.pdf.
6. See, for example, the World Health Organization's overview of traditional medicine at: http://www.who.int/topics/traditional_medicine/en/.

CHAPTER **16**

Telehealth

Telehealth: I Can See the Highway, but Where Is the Ramp?

INTRODUCTION

In a remote village in Central America, an otherwise unmanaged child's infection could take a turn for worse without the long-distance diagnostic capacity made possible by the installation of a telemedicine system between Zacapa, Guatemala, and Houston, Texas, where subspecialists in the field of pediatric dermatology can view the wound and prescribe critically needed treatment for the child thousands of miles away. Recent developments in the telecommunications and information technology fields hold the promise of improved access to, and the better utilization of, healthcare-related resources. In addition to these developments, the deployment of interactive distance training programs offers an opportunity to decrease the knowledge gap between the leading academic medical centers, and remote healthcare practitioners, who find themselves pressed to deliver quality care that meets the needs of their communities· in an environment of limited resources and competing priorities.

Worldwide electronic networking, in which telemedicine is a unique tool, has created new opportunities for imagining the possibility of a more efficient, accessible, and integrated healthcare delivery system. Telemedicine is the tool by which more and more communities in need are able to overcome barriers to the delivery of quality healthcare services to their locality. Recent developments in modern telecommunications, medical equipment, and information technology tools present a radical opportunity to change the healthcare delivery infrastructure from the ground up. The implementation of telehealth programs in areas of need is supported by enthusiastic approaches, if not always with enough site-specific planning or sustain ability tools.[1]

There is a need to understand how to optimally select, implement, and sustain the advantages offered through intelligent communications that limitlessly extends the boundary of our senses, records, activities, collaboration, and outreach. This understanding includes the engineering plans for system design and support.

THE TELEHEALTH EVOLUTION

Telehealth is not a new entity, as most may think. Rather, it is the product of over 70 years of historical evolution. The April 1924 issue of the *Radio News Magazine* showed a drawing of a physician viewing a patient over a shortwave radio set that included a television like display. More realistically, the early programs in the 1950s and 1960s were highlighted with some success by the Nebraska Psychiatric In-state, Massachusetts General Hospital, and Boston's Logan International Airport link.[2] However, these programs lacked the ability to deliver sustained satisfaction to the healthcare providers or to the patients involved. Following the invention of the color television and the launching of communications satellites in 1965, Dr. Michael DeBakey, the cardiovascular surgeon at the Baylor College of Medicine, started to incorporate video tools into the medical training program. That same year, Dr. DeBakey made the first live broadcast of cardiac surgery from Methodist Hospital at the Texas Medical Center to Europe, utilizing satellite transmission. Colleagues in Amsterdam viewed and listened as Dr. DeBakey mentored the procedure, an altogether new technique for teaching cardiac surgical intervention. The investment of the United States Army and of the federal government in the late 1980s and early 1990s in the integration of better telemedicine tools placed a focus on rural communities and the need to extend care to internationally deployed forces. These efforts provided the initial impetus for today's telemedicine programs.

The new modality, namely the Internet, provided another example of how the barrier of distance can be overcome by having access to tools that enjoy, by now, a much more ubiquitous communications platform to transmit information between any two distant locations at any time. In 1983, the first use of the Internet to disseminate medical information between participants took place at the Texas Medical Center and demonstrated the potential for scientific interactions that were untried before then. Not only can we now use satellites and telephone lines in order to deliver medical information, but we have also added the Internet and the provision for communication between two single points, as well as the ability to share information among multiple sites simultaneously, at an affordable cost.

The early applications of video engineering were essentially an attempt to overcome intra-hospital information-flow *bottlenecks*. The connection with remote rural communities was not attempted until sufficient experience had accumulated with intra-hospital transmission of video, with the available telecommunications services including the "last mile," the point between the shared infrastructure and user connectivity. Thus, in 1993 we began to take advantage of these opportunities and reach out with our educational and clinical programs beyond the confines of the Texas Medical Center, reaching out 400 miles southwest of Houston to McAllen, Texas, near the Mexican border. The program then, as today, focused on the extension of pediatric subspecialty expertise to communities in need.[3] The growing acceptance of telemedical-based services is changing the way healthcare is delivered and provides opportunities not available before.

In a recent survey conducted by *Telemedicine Journal* of telemedicine service providers, almost 70 percent of the responders cited the need to increase access to specialty care as the major motivation for initiating remote interactive clinical service; while 33 percent of the responders cited cost savings as the primary methodology for measuring the success of such a service.[4] While the service can be administered in a variety of platforms, the need to accommodate clinical requirements and appreciate technological limitations is universal. However, these requirements and limitations change from one program to another and from one location to another. Successful development and implementation of telemedicine service depends on the ability to focus on and address specific clinical needs, the integration of infrastructure with existing platforms, and the availability of a reliable and sufficient end-to-end broadband telecommunications service. In addition, sensitivity to cultural preferences and compliance with legal issues has an impact on performance as well.

THE HIGHWAY

Interactive devices and advanced telecommunications technologies are transforming every aspect of our life, and medicine is no exception. From virtual classrooms to simulation centers, and from pharmaceutical supply dispensers to artificial organ replacements and remote surgical procedures, advances are generating breakthrough applications that improve quality of life for an ever-growing number of people. Healthcare providers and educators, as constituents of this transformation era, enjoy new opportunities created for their active and critical participation in this transformation. When we review the positive impact that the integration of ostensibly independent patient-care services have on the efficient management of the total quality and safety of care, of education, and of collaborative research, it is not surprising that telehealth systems deployment is on the rise. The forces that drive this phenomenon include the following:

- The positive impact of vast knowledge sharing
- The need to instill prevention behavior as well as to manage the entire disease encounter
- The desire to increase standards for quality of care over a wider geographically disbursed community
- The escalation of customer expectations
- Globalization of healthcare and its support services
- An increase in patient and provider convenience
- User acceptance of the technological highway competency

Telehealth can be envisioned as the delivery of healthcare services through the use of advanced communication technologies, informatics and computers, video instrumentations, and medical devices, to exchange information and/or to facilitate collaboration that overcomes barriers like distance, time, and social and cultural dissimilarity.[5] Telemedicine and eHealth are considered additional nomenclatures of the same strategy as telehealth, but with variation in the intensity level of the collaboration and the knowledge level of the communicating parties. Specific systems and applications include the following.

SYSTEMS

Systems vary according to the type and latency of the telecommunication infrastructure deployed. The format ranges from radio communication and telephone to the Internet and satellites that connect collaborating parties in real-time, messaging style, or with e-mail. Furthermore, the telehealth system can be designed for use in a large conference room, in a studio, office, or at home, or it can be mobile. It can accommodate one-way, two-way, or multiple simultaneous sessions with the communicating parties having unrestricted access to health information. The system also provides authentication identifying specific care providers or consumers. The quality of the presentation itself, the image and sound, must meet minimum criteria for the designated service in order to be valid and professionally acceptable.

Radiology, dermatology, and cardiology services require better image resolution than other services. It is important to establish an ongoing technology management program that will ensure that the image quality will not deteriorate with changes in the display monitor, the camera, or the communication network. In addition, the placement of systems at home or in a remote village must include appropriate user training and man-machine interfaces (human engineering) that are adequate for the skill level of the user. Simple troubleshooting guidelines are always useful and should be available at implementation.

APPLICATIONS

The applications vary according to the format and scope of services included within the telehealth program. They facilitate functions such as the following:

- Interactions for the delivery of healthcare services
- Consultation or validation
- Prevention
- Diagnosis
- Treatment
- Emergency and disaster impacted area
- Transferring healthcare data
- Information
- Prescription
- Registration
- Networking and messaging
- Education
- Professional
- Consumers
- Support services
- Collaborative research
- Utilization of interactive audio, video, laboratory instrumentation, and telecommunications systems to accelerate or enhance outcomes.

The following applications are used in the delivery of those functions:

- Initial screening and evaluation of patients
- Triage decisions and pre-transfer assessments

- Remote medical and surgical follow-up
- Prescription translation, authorization and medications review
- Consultation for primary care encounters
- Extension of subspecialty care consultation, referral, and planning
- Local management of chronic diseases and conditions
- Expansion of diagnostic expertise, knowledge and work-ups
- Remote coverage of in-hospital care (intensive care area)
- Expert review of diagnostic images
- Remote surgical procedures under unique conditions (combat, space)
- Wider access to preventive medicine behavior and consumer education
- Recruitment and retention of participants pool of candidates for various research protocols

When building or expanding the telehealth highway, it is clear that the benefits from facilitating the quality and safety of these functions mandate expert planning and support. The combination of information technology and telecommunications, together with clinical instrumentation and video systems, creates an opportunity for clinical engineers (CE) and biomedical equipment technicians (BMET) to expand their own expertise, and therefore affect the quality and safety of the overall system.

HIGHWAY DESIGN

Telehealth practice is the use of information, audiovisual, and communication technologies to provide and support health services when distance and time separate the participants.[5] In its simplest form, a telemedicine program consists of a site where a consulting physician is located (the hub) and a remote location or locations (the spoke) where the referring physician and the patient are present. The interaction or consultation between the two peers can take the form of a session, where medical information and treatment history are exchanged, for a primary diagnosis or as validation of a treatment plan, or as a second opinion session. The central hub can serve one or many spokes located at remote sites. The peer-to-peer review can be practiced in two different modalities; in **real-time (synchronous)** or in **delayed time (asynchronous),** known as the **store-and-forward mode.** In addition to different system components, the main difference between the modalities is the time span associated with concluding the consultation protocol and the requirements for wider communication bandwidth.[6]

Telehealth practices can be categorized into a variety of modalities according to type of services provided, as already described. Telemedical encounters can focus on clinical, educational, or administrative programs. A program that provides clinical encounters must comply with a variety of regulatory and professional guidelines and must adhere to policies and procedures quite different than those required for the provision of educational programs, nonpatient care, and services. Another categorization can be by the types or the size of network deployed, such as a point-to-point system, or a hub and multiple spokes system. However, the most popular categorization is done by time span within which the telemedical encounter begins, is reviewed, and completed.

Most of the telehealth programs operate in synchronous mode, or in what is known as an interactive, real-time full-motion encounter. The other modality, **store-and-forward,** is an **asynchronous mode** where the referring physician and the patient do not have to be present at the time of the consultation together with the specialist. Rather, the referring physician gathers the patient information over a period of time utilizing a battery of diagnostic instruments, ranging from electronic stethoscope and X-ray images to images of pathological slides or cine fluoroscopy.

Other patient information, such as echocardiograms, can be incorporated, as well as dictation of patient symptoms, family history, vital signs, and demographics. This information is then packaged and moved as a completed file—an electronic portfolio of the patient—to the consulting physician address at the hub. The transmission is encrypted to protect privacy and provide confidentiality of information. The consulting physician, after being alerted to the arrival of a new electronic file, will open the portfolio, review it, and then render a diagnosis and an opinion as to the management of this condition. The consultant will then send it back to the referring physician for action.

There are some advantages to the store-and-forward modality. The patient is not constrained by the schedules of the referring and the consulting physicians, and the cost of telecommunications is minimal. However, a real-time interactive mode allows for high presentation quality and the opportunity to have multiple subspecialists participate simultaneously in management of the condition; all of which permits an earlier and quicker decision-making process. Another important feature of real-time interactive dialogue is the increased possibilities for building trust and cultural bridges, which another modality may not facilitate as quickly.

With the increase of clinical applications, the minimum feature level and fidelity provided by the various types of telehealth equipment and communication systems must be accurately assessed, in order to effectively match capability with service needs, especially when on-demand response is involved. There is a critical opportunity for engineers and clinicians to participate in this process by defining the appropriate fidelity level that will best accommodate the clinical requirement.

There are additional important barriers still to overcome.[7] These are the critical financial, legal, and technical barriers in telehealth that require understanding and solution:

- Reimbursement for investment in space and technology, for professional components, and administrative components
- Liability
- Licensure
- Scheduling issues
- Equality/universality of care and medication
- Patient/doctor and institution relationships
- Appropriateness of remote application
- Patient and provider resistance
- Abuse/over utilization
- Confidentiality/privacy
- Fraud

THE RAMP

Once the objectives and the scope of the program are clearly defined, and we move beyond the clinical goals, other challenges must be addressed. These challenges include financial, return-on-investment projection, legal issues, social and cultural issues, and engineering issues. For a successful telehealth strategy, all of these challenges must be carefully considered because, together, they impact the whole expected outcome. *If telehealth is going to become a staple of healthcare practice on our planet, a massive reengineering of the national and international telecommunications infrastructure, licensure and reimbursement legislation, as well as collaborative clinical practices will be required.* There are

several hundred telemedicine programs in operation today. It is estimated that the majority are less than 10 years old, representing a relatively new modality in the healthcare delivery system. The vast majority of healthcare providers are still debating the appropriate entry course and the consequent regulatory and sustainability issues.

It is an opportune time for clinical engineers and BMETs to learn why and how telehealth programs operate, as well as what kind of engineering support is required for the technological components. Such programs have unique features; their sustain ability depends on expertise in systems engineering, telecommunication, satellite connectivity, video and audio processing, privacy and confidentiality, interface standards and biomedical equipment operation. Early adaptors will be positioned to move into an interesting and promising career that may be looking down a great highway. It is important to gain understanding of the telecommunications and video presentation that are integral parts of the telehealth functions.

THE TELECOMMUNICATIONS COMPONENT

One of the fastest-changing fields, telecommunications enables existing and new platforms for the exchange of information and to support interaction through unique applications, including the medical peripherals. Thus, the management of telemedicine programs must incorporate the understanding of telecommunications technologies and the optimization of this component. The convergence of digital and analog transmission methods and the advantages of the various networking technologies require the ability to evaluate and match network needs with the capabilities of the available infrastructure. Clinical requirements must be matched with technical capacity and be supported by financial sustainability to influence design and implementation decisions for selecting the platform to be employed.

There are many modes of communications to support speed and bandwidth, which range from the narrowband used for the plain old telephone system to the wideband application supported by integrated services digital network and satellite communications. Various selectable bandwidths, availability, and level of service should all be considered. In selecting a telecommunications technology, one needs to clearly know how the network will be designed, what protocols are expected to be used, how much and how often data will be transmitted, and what the budget is for this program. The communication highway consists of a variety of transmission mediums, essentially made up of telephone lines and Internet protocol (IP), or a combination of these platforms.[8] Video compression, a coding technique used to reduce the bandwidth required for the transmission of video images, is a developing science. Recent developments are awaiting validation of their clinical acceptance and are still largely unsubstantiated by a conclusive body of research. There is a multitude of opinion on the topic, but very little hard data. The science of visual perception is unique in that it is a subjective function of the brain as well as the eye. No two individuals perceive the exact same image in exactly the same way. The threshold of persistence of vision and the measurable speed at which a motion picture or video screen ceases to flicker and begins to "move" may vary significantly among different observers under different lighting conditions. The eye and brain are thought to generally retain a visual impression for approximately 1/30th of a second. When viewed as a continuum, this collective retention is "seen" by the viewer as uninterrupted motion. It is significantly important, therefore, that the effect of the compression technique chosen for a telemedicine system will not further modify the assessment of the medical conditions being viewed.

TRANSMISSION CONDITIONS EVALUATION

The evaluation of high-end telehealth systems requires the commitment of many resources. There is a continual need to evaluate new, evolving platforms, systems, and technologies for an optimal match between patient and physician needs on the one hand, and technological capability on the other. This will permit optimal display fidelity and refined, sustained performance under varied conditions.

As an example, the impact of changing technical transmission specifications such as those presented in global telecommunications was evaluated in our biomedical engineering laboratory, several years ago. We conducted an evaluation to determine the magnitude of variation in video processing between systems. Our test was subjective in that our panel of experts scored competitors based on their own impressions and perceptions of "quality." Our testing protocol provided for a single video source to simul-

taneously broadcast its signal to two video-conferencing systems. The video-conferencing systems were designed to communicate with the video source at different bandwidths. The communication with the video source was in real-time, over a protocol H.320 full T1 carrier service (1.544 Mbps) down to a one-quarter T1 (386 Kbps). The video source was changed from an ultrasound examination of a patient's cardiac condition to a simulated patient with advanced Parkinson's disease. Other rapid and sudden movements against a large white background, such as a downhill ski race, were used as well. A panel of senior medical subspecialists observed the presentations and related their ability to render a medical opinion based on the quality of the displayed video and fidelity of the audio.

For slow-moving events, such as an examination of skin conditions, a small fraction of a T1 line was acceptable for rendering an opinion. However, for ultrasound examination and downhill skiing, the panel opinion was that only presentation quality of one-half T1 or better was sufficient to determine minute changes in the conditions presented. Proper lighting and the positioning of the camera during patient examination were also noted as critical for successful assessment of clinical conditions. Finally, the resolution and overall size of the video screen were determined to have impact on the clinical acceptance of the telemedical encounter as well. The closer the display area was to a real-life size, the more the panel felt it was acceptable. Consequently, we conducted telemedical encounters with content including significant motion only through one-half T1 or better and employed television sets with the diagonal measure of 31 inches.

All video sources were calibrated as to level and connected via 1 x 8 video switcher (selector). This enabled the selection of the various sources utilized in the evaluation at the request of the panel members. The output of the selector was passed to a distribution amplifier (D/A) to compensate for losses resulting from the division of the video signals into two paths. The video signals were then passed to the two transmission CODECs, "A" and "B" (compressor/decompressor); equal lengths of transmission lines connected the CODECs at the "near end," used for analog to digital conversion, and subsequent compression and transmission of the signals to the CODECs at the "far end" used for reception, decompression and digital to analog conversion.

The output analog information from the two *far-end* CODECs were connected to individual multisync monitors (A and B). The monitors, both of the same manufacturer and model, had been, prior to the evaluation, calibrated using an NTSC laboratory grade color bar generator and photometric color temperature and luminance meters. This calibration ensured that both monitors were objectively as similar as possible in terms of picture quality. In addition, to provide a better side-by-side comparison of the two systems under evaluation, a split-screen monitor was employed. Video information from both CODEC sources was split and sent through a switcher, enabling the side-by-side viewing of video information on a single monitor. Immediately prior to the tests and evaluation, the clinical engineer in charge ensured integrity of the *double-blind* nature of the evaluation by making the final connections from the outputs of CODECs A and B to the monitor chain.

This information was kept confidential until the evaluations were completed. Resolution of these issues will extend our ability to exchange information and to increase interoperability with legacy systems. This will extend our capacity to engage in this evolution and to determine when it presents sufficient fidelity to deploy this service in the clinical setting. Finally, one must review the legal aspects and regulatory guidelines that can influence equipment selection for the test described above in both the domestic and global aspects

SAME PROBLEMS, DIFFERENT SOLUTION

As is the case in many of the recently integrated systems that are becoming part of the biomedical field, telehealth presents to some extent the same problems—however, with a different solution. The Center for TeleHealth (CTH), one of the first telemedicine programs to focus solely on the extension of pediatrics subspecialty services, is the result of a collaborative program between the Texas Children's Hospital and the Baylor College of Medicine.

Although the Center was created specifically to link the institution's expertise to remote communities in Texas, as well as to global communities in need, it would not have gained executive and medical faculty support without the success of its initial applications, which were the result of applying video and communications engineering concepts to solving intra-hospital problems. It required the installation of a video network for the transmission of real-

time information of echocardiography images to the locations where the experts were available, the cardiology reading area. Soon, other problems were solved with a similar measure of success. The subspecialty coverage of a remote clinical area, the newborn nursery, successfully tested the provision of remote video monitoring of babies by neonatalogists.[2]

New knowledge is being discovered and acquired at an accelerated pace, specifically in the field of diagnostic and therapeutic medicine, within the cluster of major academic medical centers. However, care providers who practice in rural or remote areas, or in overburdened urban clinics, have yet to realize how best to absorb and deploy this new information. Soon, the increased availability of electronic patient medical records will ease and facilitate the integration of Telehealth-based medical services.

Telehealth is providing a unique opportunity to restructure the methodology for the dissemination of knowledge used in today's healthcare delivery system in a way that will distribute specific competencies to the most needed environment—leading to the optimal practice at the point of care. This focus will allow our society to move from a reactive mode of delivering care toward life-long health management where individual accountability, preventive medicine, and customized wellness programs are integral components of a new health management methodology.

SUMMARY

Telehealth is an emerging industry with the arsenal to revolutionize the delivery of health-related information and care for the benefit of healthcare systems, providers, and consumers. The application of electronically connected parties for the provision of healthcare and training already shows some very exciting possibilities. Future expansion of telehealth systems will help to deliver services to benefit providers' networks, economy, and patients. Recent developments and improvements in standards in the telecommunications and information technology fields hold the promise of improved access to, and better utilization of, healthcare-related resources. There is now a critical opportunity for clinical engineers and BMETs to participate in supporting telehealth programs. This can be accomplished by demonstrating skill sets which assert and establish a quantifiable level of service in order to ensure an appropriate match between the fidelity of acquiring and delivering sound and video levels and the clinical requirements of a specific medical encounter.

Telemedical services can be deployed in a variety of platforms. Those platforms continue to improve the capture, transmission, and presentation of medical information. The deployment of anyone platform, or combination of platforms, is dependent upon such conditions as clinical needs, level of staff training, legal and cultural constraints, limitations of telecommunications infrastructure, regional economics, and the stage of technological development. Therefore, some applications are better suited than others to support the needs of distant healthcare providers. Telehealth systems must be tailored to the needs of the participating healthcare system. Usually, a tiered approach consisting of various levels of professionally trained staff, a mixture of real-time and store-and-forward technologies, availability of wide bandwidth, and reasonable frame rate are the optimal solution.

With proper planning and the anticipated advances in computing power, direct medical digital imaging and telecommunications will continue to increase the cost-effectiveness and expand the scope of telehealth services. In addition to the information available on the Internet, the two telehealth modalities of practice now emerging are the real-time intereactive mode and the store-and-forward mode. The combination of these modalities with the capabilities to exchange health information as supported by the new telecommunications infrastructures places telehealth at a central position for improving access to quality healthcare by all.

We must continue to endeavor to remove penalties—financial, legislative, and regulatory[6]—in order to permit everyone in need to reach their goal by finding the ramp and getting on the telehealth highway. We need, however, to identify and to quantify the contribution of this transformation to the betterment of health for all. This challenge is going to be the next biggest obstacle for the field of telehealth. Dr. Michael DeBakey put it best: "These technologies will allow us to improve the standards of healthcare around the world . . . providing an important opportunity for distant learning and for the dissemination of medical knowledge and support of this goal."[8]

ENDNOTES

1. D. Perednia, "Summary of the 1999 ATSP Report of Telemedicine in the U.S." Proceedings of the TeleHealth 2000 Conference, HIMSS, October 31 to November 3, 2000, Los Angeles, CA.
2. J. Reid, *A Telemedicine Primer: Understanding the Issues,* Iowa Innovative Medical Communications, 1996.
3. L. Adcock, Y. David, et al., "Telemedicine Examination of Newborn Infants: How Accurate the Technology" Society for Pediatric Research, Proceedings of the Annual Meeting, May 1999, San Francisco, California.
4. D. R. Dakins, "Telemedicine in Review," TeleHealth—Steps to Successful Implementation, Conference Proceedings, HIMSS, September 25–27, 1997, Dallas, Texas.
5. American Telemedicine Association, http://www.atmeda.org/.
6. M. J. Field (ed.), *A Guide to Assessing Telecommunications for Healthcare* Institute of Medicine, National Academy of Medicine, 1996.
7. The Center for Telehealth & E-Health Law (CTeL), Washington, D.C., www.ctl.org.
8. Meeting notes from the Center for TeleHealth at Texas Children's Hospital, Houston, Texas, http://www.texaschildrenshospital.org/Professionals/Telehealth/Default.aspx.

Accidental communication—also known as unintentional communication; happens when you do not know or realize that you are communicating. (Communication 1)

Acculturation—is almost always a host culture influencing a newcomer who has moved into its environment. (Culture)

Accuracy—knowing the difference between reasoning and rationalizing, what is true and what seems true, and opinion and fact. (Critical thinking)

Activities of daily living (ADLs)—the ability to perform common tasks such a feeding, bathing, dressing, toileting, and transferring. (Health)

Activity tracks—component of multiple sequence model that entails task, relational, and topical tracks. (Team)

Acupuncture—Chinese medicine treatment in which tiny needles are inserted into specific points in the body to alleviate pain and relieve various physical, mental, and emotional conditions. (History)

Acute distress—stress that is intense but doesn't last long. (Stress)

Adaptor—element of nonverbal communication that is considered to be body language such as crossing your arms. (Communication 2)

Adult foster home—also called adult foster care; a setting such as a family-style home that provides 24-hour personal care, meals, and supervision for a small number of residents. (History)

Affect display—element of nonverbal communication that involves facial expressions. (Communication 2)

Alphabetic filing—arranging of names or titles according to the sequence of letters in the alphabet. (Medical records)

Alternative medicine—health care systems, practices, and products that have not traditionally been performed by practitioners of Western medicine; practices used instead of conventional medicine. (History)

Ambulatory services—health care services that do not require hospitalization; also known as outpatient services. (History)

Amoral—lacking or indifferent to moral standards. (Ethics)

Analysis level—fourth level on Bloom's Taxonomy of Thinking and Learning characterized by being able to break the information down into parts and then look at the relationships among the parts. (Critical thinking)

Appeal to authority—support views by citing experts; if person is truly expert in the field for which they are being cited, then testimony is probably valid; views cited though are sometimes not that of experts in their field. (Critical thinking)

Appeal to fear—premise based on a treat, or "swinging the big stick." (Critical thinking)

Appeal to ignorance—relies on claims that if no proof is offered that something is true, then it must be false, or conversely, that if no proof is offered that something is false, then it must be true. (Critical thinking)

Appeal to the masses—fallacy that occurs when support for the premise is offered in the form, "It must be right because everybody else does it." (Critical thinking)

Appeal to the person—occurs when a person offers a rebuttal to an argument by criticizing or denigrating its presenter rather than constructing a rebuttal based on the argument presented. (Critical thinking)

Appeal to tradition—used as an unsound premise to argue that something is true based on an established tradition. (Critical thinking)

Application level—third level on Bloom's Taxonomy of Thinking and Learning characterized by being able to construct knowledge by taking previously learned information and applying it in a new and different way to solve problems. (Critical thinking)

Applied ethics—the practical application of moral standards that concern benefiting the patient. Therefore the medical practitioner must adhere to certain ethical standards and codes of conduct. (Ethics)

Arbitration—process by which the parties in a dispute submit their differences to the judgment of an impartial party. (Legal)

Arguments—a form of thinking in which reasons (statements and facts) are given in support of a conclusion. (Critical thinking)

Assessment—process of determining the health needs of a community. (Public health)

Assisted living residence—facility that provides housing, meals, and personal care to individuals who need help with daily living activities but do not need daily nursing care; may also be referred to as supportive housing, residential long-term care facilities, adult residential care facilities, board-and-care, and rest homes. (History)

Assurance—process of making sure that correct actions are taken to protect community health. (Public health)

Asynchronous time—delayed time; example: use of email to send and receive images used in telemedicine. (Telehealth)

Authoritarian style—style of leadership that involves the leader being very directive in terms of the group goals and procedures, the division of work, and deciding the outcome of conflict. (Team)

Baby boomers—name given to those people born in the immediate post World War II era; refers to people born between 1944 and 1964. (Economics)

Begging the question—also referred to as arguing in a circle; a conclusion is used as one of the premises. (Critical thinking)

Beneficence—action of helping others and performing actions that would result in benefit to another person. (Ethics)

Beneficiary—the person receiving the benefits from the health care insurance. (Economics)

Bioethicists—specialists in the field of bioethics who give thought to ethical concerns that often examine the more abstract dimensions of ethical issues and dilemmas. (Ethics)

Bioethics—a field resulting from modern medical advances and research. (Ethic)

Biologic markers—a new approach to identifying users; includes fingerprint and iris scanning technologies, and voice and face recognition systems. (EMR 1)

Block grants—money granted by the national government to a state government with few restrictions on its spending. (Public health)

Boards of health—the policymaking bodies for a state's Department of Health. (Public health)

Breakpoints—components of the multiple sequence model that are interruptions in an activity track. (Team)

Capitation—fixed prepayment per person to the health care provider for an agreed-on array of services; the payment remains the same no matter how many services or what type of services each patient actually receives. (Economics)

Case—term used in health statistics to refer to each person who has a disease. (Public health)

Categorical grant—money granted by the national government which has strict or specific provisions on the way it is to be spent. (Public health)

Center for Disease Control (CDC)—works with state health departments and other community organizations to monitor disease, help prevent outbreaks, maintain national health statistics, and operate disease prevention and health promotion programs. (Public health)

Centers for Medicare and Medicaid Services (CMS)—provides health care insurance through third-party carriers for about one in every four Americans. (Public health)

Character—develops through interactions of temperament with the environment. (Personality)

Charity care—term providers use when they have borne the burden for the cost of providing care. (Economics)

Chiropractic—health care practice based on the belief that pressure on the nerves leaving the spinal column causes pain and dysfunction of the body part served by that nerve. (History)

Chronic stress—stress that is not as intense as acute stress but it lingers for prolonged periods of time. (Stress)

Clinical data repositories—databases which accept data from a number of departmental systems and combine them into a centrally, searchable form. (EMR 1)

Cloning technology—producing a cell or organism that is genetically identical to the original from which the material to make the duplicate was derived. (Technology intro)

Coding systems—standardized definitions and representations. (EMR 1)

Cohesiveness—feeling of "oneness" in a group, being "close-knit," bound to one another, and united as members of a team. (Team)

Coinsurance—a provision in a member's coverage that limits the amount of coverage by the health plan to a certain percentage, commonly 80%. Any additional costs are paid out-of-pocket. (Economics)

Communicable disease—disease that spreads from person to person; another term for infectious disease. (Public health)

Communication—process of a source stimulating meaning in the mind of a receiver by means of verbal and nonverbal messages. (Communication 1)

Comparable worth—also known as pay equality, a theory that extends equal pay requirements to all persons who are doing equal work. (Ethics)

Compassion—the ability to have a gentle, caring attitude toward patients and fellow employees. (Ethics)

Complementary and alternative medicine (CAM)—health care practices, products, and approaches to health care that have not traditionally been performed in conventional medical offices; practices used together with conventional medicine. (History) and (Economics)

Comprehension level—second level on Bloom's Taxonomy of Thinking and Learning characterized by being able to classify, describe, discuss, explain and recognize information; you are in the process of interpreting information. (Critical thinking)

Computer-based patient record (CPR)—electronic patient record that resides in a system designed to support user through availability of complete and accurate data, practitioner reminders and alerts, clinical decision support systems, links to bodies of knowledge and other aids. (EMR 1)

Conclusions—sixth step in critical thinking where you finalize your decision; you should not reach a conclusion unless you have sufficient evidence to support that decision. (Critical thinking)

Confidentiality—also known as privacy, the ability to safeguard another person's confidences or information. (Ethics)

Conflict—antagonistic state or action as of divergent ideas, interests, or persons. (Team)

Conformity—type of group influence; a change in the individual brought about by pressure (real or imagined) for the person to behave in a manner advocated by the group. (Team)

Consciousness-raising groups—groups designed to increase persons' awareness of characteristics and concerns in order to stimulate action. (Team)

Construction—as used in critical thinking means our unique view or perception of the world which is based on our thoughts and beliefs; first step in critical thinking. (Critical Thinking)

Content communicator—this means that you say what you mean and mean what you say. (Communication 2)

Content level of message—what we have said. (Communication 1)

Continuing care community—provides a variety of living arrangements that support lifestyles as they change from independent living to the need for regular medical and nursing care. (History)

Cooperators—get what they want and where they want to go by getting along with others; are law abiding and accommodating with those around them. (Personality)

Cost-plus basis—when an organization is reimbursed for actual costs plus an additional percentage of those costs. (Economics)

Counteractive influence—behavior in functional group decision making where a member corrects a fallacious conclusion by another group member. (Team)

Critical thinking—thinking that moves you beyond simple observations and passive reporting of those observations; is an active, conscious, cognitive process in which there is always intent to learn; is a process by which we analyze and evaluate information to make good sense out of all the information we are continually bombarded with. (Critical thinking)

Cross-cultural—between cultures. (Culture)

Cultural competency—understanding, valuing, and incorporating the cultural differences of America's diverse population and examining one's own health related values and beliefs so as to respond appropriately to and directly serve the unique needs of the populations whose cultures may be different from the prevailing culture. (Culture)

Culture—an interlinked web of symbols; a learned set of shared perceptions about beliefs, values, and norms that affect the behaviors of a relatively large group of people. (Culture)

Culture empathy/sensitivity—maintaining your preference for your own culture (remain ethnocentric) but learning to understand how other cultures see things from their vantage points rather than through the evaluative filter of your belief system. (Culture)

Culture shock—the trauma you experience when you move into a culture different from your home culture. (Culture)

Curative medical care—medical care that helps to cure an already ill or infected person. (Public health)

Customers—people interacting with you and other health care professionals during course of the day; can be patients, vendors, other employees or staff. (Professionalism)

Data-level integration—requires that all system components use a consistent scheme for labeling (coding) data elements and that a mechanism be present for movement of data between systems. (EMR 1)

Database management systems—software programs that provide all the functions required to manipulate the information stored in databases. (EMR 1)

Database—a software program that permits the storage and retrieval of information; data can be stored in large blocks (documents or images) or as discrete items (numbers or single words). (EMR 1)

Decision-making group—type of task-oriented group that problem solves plus decides what solution will be implemented, when and how the solution will be implemented, how progress will be monitored, and how changes in the solution will be handled. (Team)

Declarative knowledge—knowing facts and concepts. (Critical thinking)

Decoding—the interpreting and evaluating of the source's message by the receiver. (Communication 1)

Decorum—showing appropriate professional standards in conduct and appearance; the good appearance and professional behavior you show on the job. (Professionalism)

Deductible—the amount a patient must pay out-of-pocket, usually annually on a calendar-year basis, before insurance will begin to cover costs. (Economics)

Defendants—the parties against whom a legal complaint is being filed. (Legal)

Delays—type of breakpoint in the small group decision-making process that occurs when the group cycles back to rework an issue. (Team)

Democratic style—style of leadership that involves viewing all issues (including goals, procedures, and work assignments) as matters to be discussed and decided upon by the group. (Team)

Deontological ethical theory—asserts that at least some actions are right or wrong and, thus, we have a duty or obligation to perform them or refrain from performing them, without consideration of the consequences. (Ethics)

Depositions—questions that are asked to obtain additional information, and designated experts are asked to provide their opinions and the justifications for those opinions; depositions are taken prior to a case going to trial. (Legal)

Diagnosis-Related Group (DRG)—groups of inpatient discharges with final diagnoses that are similar clinically and in resource consumption; used as a basis of payment by the Medicare program, and as a result, widely accepted by other payers. (Economics)

Dialogue—style of conflict resolution in which a person exchanges opinions, attitudes, facts, and ideas in an attempt to see both sides and approach solution with an open mind. (Communication 2)

Disruptions—type of breakpoint in the small group decision-making process that occurs when there is a major disagreement or when the decision-making process agreed upon by the group fails. (Team)

Distress—bad stress or unhealthy stress and pertains to the definition of the rate of wear and tear on the body. (Stress)

Donut hole—pertains to Medicare Part D prescription drug plan, the donut hole is when Medicare temporarily stops paying for a person's prescriptions and that person will have to pay the entire cost of their medications. (Economics)

Drop-down menus—in an electronic medical records program, allows the user to choose information or symptoms from a preprogrammed list. (EMR 2)

Drug resistant—describes when a disease or bacteria is not affected or stopped by the use of common antibiotics and other drugs. (Public health)

Dual eligibles—population subset that is eligible for both Medicaid and Medicare. (Economics)

Dualism—simplest stage in levels of thinking characterized by students viewing knowledge as a factual quality dispensed by authorities. (Critical thinking)

Due process—the entitlement for employees of the government and public companies to have certain procedures followed when they believe their rights are in jeopardy. (Ethics)

Duty-based ethics—focuses on performing one's duty to various people and institutions such as parents, employers, employees, and customers (patients). (Ethics)

Electronic health records (EHR)—information about patients that is recorded and stored on computer. (Medical records)

Electronic health records—electronic medical records that allow medical offices to access any one patient's file from more than one networked computer in the office. (EMR 2)

Electronic medical records—the portions of patients medical records that are kept on a computer's hard drive or a medical office's computer network. (EMR 2)

Electronic signature—electronic version of a person's signature to be used in electronic medical records. (EMR 2)

Emotional health—sometimes called mental health, refers to our ability to feel and express the full range of emotions in an appropriate and controlled manner. (Stress)

Empathy—the ability to understand the feelings of others without actually experiencing their pain or distress. (Ethics)

Encoding—process of conceiving an idea, determining your intent, and selecting the meaning you wish to express. (Communication 1)

Enculturation—learning our native culture; allows us to learn from others and know what choices are suitable for specific circumstances; passing on one's culture to the children through a learning process. (Culture)

Environmental health—refers to external factors or factors that occur outside the person that may affect what is going on inside; it is one dimension over which we probably have the least amount of control. (Stress)

Epidemiology—the study of the nature, cause, control, and determinants of the frequency of disease, disability, and death in human populations; also the study of the history of a disease and its distribution throughout a society. (Public health)

Epidemic—term used to describe a disease that is widespread in a population. (Public health)

Episode-of-care basis—care of a patient by a health care facility or provider for a specific medical problem or condition; can be a single continuous encounter or a series of encounters for a specific problem with brief separations from care. (Economics)

Equivocation—occurs when the conclusion does not follow from the premises due to using the same word to mean two different things. (Critical thinking)

Ethics—set of personal principles that guide a person in making decisions. These principles are based on religious teaching, community morals, and upbringing. (Professionalism) and (Ethics)

Ethics committees—group of professionals within an organization or agencies who examine ethical issues relating to patient care; can serve in an advisory capacity to patients, families, and staff for case review of difficult ethical issues, especially when there is a lack of agreement as to what is in the patient's best interest. (Ethics)

Ethnocentrism—the view that the customs and practices of one's own culture are superior to those of other cultures; is a source of cultural identity. (Culture)

Ethnorelativism—relations that are mediated by empathy, the ability to temporarily shift one's frame of reference to see the world 'as if' through the eyes of another person. (Culture)

Eustress— [yōō´stres] considered to be a good stress or healthy stress. (Stress)

Evaluation level—sixth and final level on Bloom's Taxonomy of Thinking and Learning characterized by being able to judge the validity of the information. (Critical thinking)

Expanding consciousness—a theory developed by Margaret Newman to assist patients in making their lives as meaningful as possible focusing on their possibilities rather than their limitations. (History)

Expert witness—a witness who has knowledge not normally possessed by the average person concerning the topic that he is to testify about. (Legal)

Expressive communication—characterized by messages that express how the sender feels at a given time. (Communication 1)

Extrovert—a person who gets their energy from outside themselves—friends and family. (Personality)

Face-to-face communication—preferred form of human communication; source and receiver are interchangeable; communication occurs "in person". (Communication 1)

Fairness—treating everyone the same. (Ethics)

Fallacy—an instance of incorrect reasoning. (Critical thinking)

False cause—fallacies that occur when a causal relationship is assumed despite a lack of evidence to support that relationship. (Critical thinking)

False dilemma—known as the either/or fallacy, it presumes that there are only two alternative from which to choose when in actuality there are more than two. (Critical thinking)

Faulty analogy—type of fallacy committed when there is a claim that things that have similar qualities in some respects will have similarities in other respects. (Critical thinking)

Fee-for-service—a billing system in which a health care provider charges a patient a set amount for each service used. (Economics)

Feeling—a value function; to make a value judgment about objects such as how we like or feel about them; learning style is interactive and collaborative. (Personality)

Fidelity—loyalty and faithfulness to others; implies that we will perform our duty. (Ethics)

Food and Drug Administration (FDA)—assures the safety and efficacy of food, cosmetics, and medications. (History) and (Public health)

Forgiven debt—term providers used when they have borne the burden for the cost of providing care. (Economics)

Foundation—type of non-profit organization that raises money and then distributes it to other organizations in support of their programs. (Public health)

Functional approach to leadership—focuses on the leadership behaviors needed by a group to accomplish its goals, not on specific individuals. (Team)

Gene therapy—the insertion of normal DNA into cells to correct a genetic defect or to treat certain diseases. (History)

Gentleness—mild, tender-hearted approach to other people. (Ethics)

Global budgeting—payment method common to government-run facilities; simplified form of capitation; one with only one provider. (Economics)

Goodness of fit—concept describing an interaction that results when properties of the environment and its expectations and demands are in accord with the organism's own capabilities, motivations, and styles of behavior. (Personality)

Gross Domestic Product (GPD)—the market value of everything produced by all the people and all the companies in a country; includes the total consumer, investment and government spending, along with the value of exports, the value of imports is then deducted from total. (Economics)

Groupthink—communication process that sometimes develops when members of a group begin thinking similarly, greatly reducing the probability that the group will reach an effect decision. (Team)

Hasty generalizations—premise often seen when people stereotype others. (Critical thinking)

Health—state of complete physical, mental, and social well-being and not merely the absence of disease or infirmity. (Health) and (Public health)

Health Insurance Portability and Accountability Act (HIPAA)—legislation that addresses patient privacy. (EMR 2)

Health Resources and Services Administration (HRSA)—provides access to health care services for low-income and uninsured people or for people who live in areas where health care is not easily available. (Public health)

Health Savings Accounts (HSA)—creating an account for individuals who have high-deductible health plans (HDHP) to help them save for medical expenses not covered under that plan; contributions can be made by both the individual or the employer; there is a maximum yearly limit. (Economics)

Hippocratic Oath—2500-year-old statement of ethics that requires equality for humankind. (Culture)

Holistic health—your overall state of wellness on all levels of your being: physical, emotional, mental, and spiritual. It covers the health of your entire being and extends to your resources, environment, and relationships. (History) and (Stress)

Homeopathy—a health care practice that is based on the idea that "like cures like." Disorders are treated with very small amounts of the natural substances that cause symptoms of the same disorder in health people. (History)

Homeostasis—maintaining an internal equilibrium. (Stress)

Honesty—the quality of truthfulness, no matter the situation. (Ethics)

Hospice—a facility or service that offers palliative (relieves but does not cure) care and support to dying patients and their families. (History)

Hostile aggression—style of conflict resolution in which a person uses intimidation to get his or her point across. (Communication 2)

Hourly payment method—also referred to as time and materials; provider charges a fixed hourly rate covering all the costs except agreed-on materials which are billed as incurred. (Economics)

Humility—acquiring an unpretentious and humble manner; being entirely honest with ourselves; recognizing one's own limits. (Ethics)

Iatrogenic—treatment-induced illness. (Technology intro)

Idea-generating group—type of task-oriented group that seeks to discover a variety of solutions, approaches, perspectives, consequences, etc., for a topic. (Team)

Identify—in critical thinking this refers to identifying core issues and information; this is the third stage of the critical thinking process and you try to make sense of all the pieces, not just the ones that happen to fit your own preconceived pattern. (Critical thinking)

Illness—any state that is diagnosed as such by a competent professional. (Health)

Indecipherable—unreadable. (EMR 2)

Indemnity plan—type of insurance traditionally provided by both Blue Cross-Blue Shield and the commercial insurance companies before the advent of managed care; commonly used in both fee-for-service private medical practice and item-of-service hospital reimbursement. (Economics)

Indexes—ordered files (alphabetical, numeric, or a combination) that indicate exactly where each stored data item may be found. (EMR 1)

Infectious disease—a disease that can spread from person to person (versus a genetic disease or a disease that is not contagious). (Public health)

Infirmity—a weakness or ailment usually brought on by old age. (Technology intro)

Informed consent—part of the principle of autonomy; means patients must be informed and understand what they are told before they can provide consent for treatment. (Ethics)

Inpatient—admitted to and treated within a hospital. (History)

Insight—fifth step in critical thinking when you sit back and detach yourself from all the information you have processed to allow new meanings to emerge that will provide a new awareness. (Critical thinking)

Insufficient premises—premises that do not eliminate reasonable grounds for doubt; includes hasty generalizations, faulty analogy, and false cause. (Critical thinking)

Integrative medicine—combines treatments from conventional medicine with complementary and/or alternative medicine for which there is high quality scientific evidence of safety and effectiveness; also call integrated medicine. (History)

Integrity—the unwavering adherence to one's principles. (Ethics)

Intellectual health—refers to our ability to have an open mind and learn new things. (Stress)

Interactive real-time full-motion encounter—synchronous mode used in most of the telehealth programs. (Telehealth)

Intercultural—between cultures. (Culture)

Interethnic—between ethnic groups. (Culture)

Intermediate nursing care facility (INCF)—a type of nursing home that provides personal care, social services, and regular nursing care for individuals who do not require 24-hour nursing but are unable to care for themselves. (History)

Internal equilibrium—our physiological state when our body is functioning normally and all is well physically. (Stress)

International Classification of Diseases (ICD)—offers a standard set of codes for capturing diagnostic information and concepts. (EMR 1)

International—in relation to cultural communication refers to information passed on from government representatives of different cultures. (Culture)

Interpersonal communication—communication that occurs between two people; most important element is that it is "two-way" with the source (sender) becoming the receiver and vice versa. (Communication 1)

Interracial—between racial groups. (Culture)

Intractable illness—illness that is difficult to cure or alleviate the symptoms. (Technology intro)

Intracultural—within the same culture. (Culture)

Intranet—a system that uses Internet rules but has access restricted to a specific site or group. (EMR 1)

Introvert—a person who gets their energy from within themselves. (Personality)

Intuitive—a possibility function; see the possibilities inherent in objects; learning style is creating and experimenting. (Personality)

Irrelevant premises—premises that are not logically related to the conclusion; can also be fallacious; includes equivocation; appeal to the person, appeal to authority; appeal to the masses; appeal to tradition; appeal to ignorance; and appeal to fear. (Critical thinking)

Judger—people who prefer to orient their lives as structured, organized, scheduled, planned, and controlled with the ability to make decisions quickly. (Personality)

Justice—fairness in all our actions with other people; carefully analyzing how to balance our behavior and be fair to all. (Ethics)

Knowledge level—lowest level on Bloom's Taxonomy of Thinking and Learning characterized by the memorization of a lot of information in a short amount of time; you might do okay, but will most likely forget most of the information soon after taking the test. (Critical thinking)

Laissez-faire style—style of leadership that involves a minimum of involvement by the leader in the group activity. (Team)

Laws—rules or actions prescribed by an authority such as the federal government and the court system that have a binding legal force. (Ethics)

Learning groups—groups whose major purpose is to acquire more information and understanding of a topic. (Team)

Legacy systems—older systems current in use in a facility that often cannot be easily replaced but must become part of new systems. (EMR 1)

Lens—last step of critical thinking where you can view issues from multiple perspectives; offers a more encompassing view of the world around you. (Critical thinking)

Litigious—excessively inclined to sue. (Ethics)

Local health department—serves an individual county, city, or region; is responsible for the delivery of services mandated by the state or by local statute; can be independent or part of a state department of health. (Public health)

Loyalty—a sense of faithfulness or commitment to a person or persons. (Ethics)

Luxury MCO plan—provides unrestricted choice of physician without prior authorization and without additional payment beyond deductible; when available is at an extra cost and usually only available to higher paid employees. (Economics)

Managed care—a system of health care delivery that influences or controls utilization of services and costs of services by providing both the financing of care and the health services for covered individuals; uses financial incentives and management controls to spur providers to give appropriate, cost-effective care; emphasizes prevention, early intervention, and outpatient care to contain costs and improve health status among covered individuals. (Economics)

Managed care organization (MCO)—grouping of physicians, hospitals and affiliated other providers which provide health care services under managed care. (Economics)

Massage therapy—manipulation of soft tissues by rubbing or kneading to achieve health benefits. (History)

Mediation—form of alternative dispute resolution (ADR), aims to assist two (or more) disputants in reaching an agreement. (Legal)

Medicaid—a joint federal/state/local program of health care for individuals whose income and resources are insufficient to pay for their care; governed by Title XIX of the federal Social Security Act and administered by the states; major source of payment for nursing home care of the elderly. (History) and (Economics)

Medical communication—communication between health provider and patient or colleague. (Communication 1)

Medical etiquette—standards of professional behavior that physicians practice in the relationship or conduct with other physicians. (Ethics)

Medical ethics—concerns questions specifically related to the practice of medicine. (Ethics)

Medical law—addresses the legal rights and obligations that affect patients and protect individual rights, including those of healthcare employees. (Ethics)

Medical model of health—model of health in which health is understood first as a biological state and that illness is any state that has been diagnosed as such by a competent professional. (Health)

Medical practice acts—established in all 50 states by statutes, apply specifically to the way medicine is practiced in a particular state; define the meaning of the "practice of medicine" as well as requirements and methods for licensure. (Ethics)

Medically indigent—persons in an income range deemed not to be low enough to qualify them for income, but low enough to make paying for health services a heavy burden. (Economics)

Medicare—a federal entitlement program of medical and health care coverage for the elderly and disabled, and persons with end-stage renal disease, governed by Title XVIII of the federal Social Security Act. (Economics)

Medicare Part A—hospital insurance which also covers skilled nursing facility care on a very limited basis. (Economics)

Medicare Part B—supplementary medical insurance which covers physician and certain other health professional services, hospital outpatient care, and certain other services. (Economics)

Medicare Part C—Medicare+Choice which permits Medicare beneficiaries to enroll in MCOs (managed care organization). (Economics)

Medicare Part D—Medicare Prescription Drug Coverage which was designed to lower the costs of prescription medication for Medicare beneficiaries. (Economics)

Metacognition—knowing what knowledge to use to control one's situation (e.g., how to make plans, ask questions, analyze the effectiveness of learning strategies, initiate change). (Critical thinking)

Mirror technique—paraphrasing what your partner is saying in a conflict (or any) situation. (Communication 2)

Monitoring—the regular review of disease data to determine changes in disease levels. (Public health)

Moral hazard—the change in an individual's behavior that results from having insurance coverage, which modifies costs of misfortune. (Economics)

Multidimensional concept of health—looking at health across the three dimensions of absence of disease, social functioning, and psychological health. (Health)

Multiple sequence model—model of group decision making that suggests groups can have different patterns of sequences because they can take various paths to a decision. (Team)

Multiplicity—second stage in levels of thinking characterized by students recognizing the complexity of knowledge (can understand there is more than one perspective on a topic) and believes knowledge to be subjective. (Critical thinking)

National health expenditures (NHE)—calculated by the Centers for Medicare and Medicaid Services (CMS), Office of Actuary, National Health Statistics Group, this number is comprised of two major categories: Health Services and Supplies; and Investments; most expenditures fall within Health Services and Supplies and most of these are for personal health care. (Economics)

National Institutes of Health (NIH)—twenty-seven institutes and centers that conduct and support all types of medical research. (History) and (Economics)

Networking—the practice of wiring computers directly together in order to permit communication and sharing resources. (EMR 1)

Network of providers—approved providers under negotiated contracts for the people covered by a particular insurance. (Economics)

Noise—any physical or psychological stimulus that distracts the receiver from focusing on the communication process. (Communication 1)

Nonverbal communication—includes touch, adaptors (body language), regulators (body movements), affect displays (facial expressions), paralanguage (pitch, tone, volume of voice). (Communication 2)

Nursing home—facility for the care of individuals who do not require hospitalization but who do need general nursing care and assistance performing daily living activities. (History)

Occupational health—has to do with all the dimensions of health (physical, social, emotional, intellectual, spiritual, environmental) but as they relate to your place of employment. (Health) and (Stress)

Objective thinker—person who bases conclusions on facts and observations and not emotions and feelings. (Technology intro)

Osteopathy—health care practices based on the belief that the body can protect itself against disease if the musculoskeletal system, especially the spine, is in good order. (History)

Out-of-pocket—direct payments to providers for noninsured services, extra payments to providers of insurance-covered or managed care-covered services that bill at an amount higher than the insurance/managed care company pays for that service, and deductibles and coinsurance on health insurance/managed care benefits. (Economics)

Outpatient services—health care services that do not require hospitalization; also referred to as ambulatory services. (History)

Pacers—type of breakpoint in the small group decision-making process that determines how a discussion moves along. (Team)

Palliative—reducing pain or severity of a disease or condition rather than curing it. (History)

Pandemic—a rapidly spreading disease that attacks many people at the same time; often refers to disease striking on a global level. (History) and (Public health)

Paralanguage—the pitch, tone, and volume of your voice and the rate at which you speak; perhaps the most influential of nonverbal communication. (Communication 2)

Pen-based input—relies on a pointing device that my operate much like a mouse or it may be used to write actual characters (EMR 1)

Perceiver—people who prefer to allow their environment to be spontaneous, adaptive and responsive to a variety of situations, and who change decisions easily so others have difficulty knowing their positions on issues. (Personality)

Perception—how we view and interpret an event or situation. (Stress)

Percipient witness—a witness who testifies about things she or he actually perceived. For example, an eyewitness. (Legal)

Per diem payment—reimbursement rates that are paid to providers for each day of services provided to a patient, based on the patient's illness or condition. (Economics)

Perseverance—persisting with a task or idea even against obstacles; steady determination to get the job done. (Ethics)

Persona—preferred personality preference. (Personality)

Personal digital assistant (PDA)—small handheld computers that have many of the same functions as a full-sized computer. (EMR2)

Personality—the distinct composite of personal qualities; they are the attributes or distinctive characteristics of a person. (Personality)

Personality type—developed by using one's personality preferences; develop from individual experiences in the near environment, primarily the family system. (Personality)

Persuasion—style of conflict resolution in which people do whatever is needed to get a point across and to persuade the other person to agree with them. (Communication 2)

Philosophical stressor—comes from not living in congruence with your philosophy or your values and beliefs. (Stress)

Physical health—your ability to adequately perform normal activities of daily living. (Health) and (Stress)

Physiological stressor—pertains to one's level of physical comfort, or lack thereof, and usually stems from illness, injury, or environmental factors such as weather or noise. (Stress)

Picture Archiving and Communications Systems (PACS)—specialized computer system for the storing and retrieval of images in a radiologic department. (EMR 1)

Plagiarism—using someone else's words or ideas, may be both unethical and illegal depending on the circumstances. (Ethics)

Policy development—process of making a collective decision about what needs to be done to protect the community's health. (Public health)

Precedent—the decision of the case acts as a model for any future cases in which the facts are the same. (Ethics)

Prejudice—refers to prejudgment and is based on stereotypes; judgments made in advance of the time when they are used; to prejudge a person or the person's behavior based on very limited information about the culture or subculture. (Culture)

Premises—the reasons of an argument. (Critical thinking)

Presentation level—the ability to view data from all connected systems through a common interface. (EMR 1)

Preventative medicine—the ordering of unnecessary tests and procedures by physicians in order to protect themselves from a lawsuit; they can then say "I did everything that I could to treat the patient." (Ethics)

Prevention efforts—health programs and behaviors that prevent illness from occurring. (Public health)

Principle of autonomy—people have the right to make decisions about their own life. (Ethics)

Principle of beneficence—also known as the principle of doing good; we must not harm patients while we are trying to help them. (Ethics)

Principle of nonmaleficence—"First, do no harm." A warning to all members of the healthcare profession to not only do good for the patient, but also to do no harm in the process. (Ethics)

Privacy—also known as confidentiality, the ability to safeguard another person's confidences or information. (Ethics)

Private acceptance—a second type of conformity where the person behaves as suggested by the group because the group produces a change in the person's beliefs and attitudes. (Team)

Private sector—not state controlled and is run for profit; can include private health insurance companies. (Economics)

Problem solving—having the ability and skills to apply knowledge to pragmatic problems encountered in all areas of your life. (Critical thinking)

Problem-solving group—type of task-oriented group that attempts to develop a solution to a problem by analyzing it thoroughly. (Team)

Procedural knowledge—also known as strategic knowledge; knowing how to use declarative knowledge to do something. (Critical thinking)

Productized—when a service can be marketed or sold as a commodity, which implies that a fixed price will buy a known quantity of that service. (Economics)

Professional conduct—exhibiting a business manner and attitude in the workplace setting. (Professionalism)

Professionalism—displaying competence expect in area of training. (Professionalism)

Prospective payment system (PPS)—seen as forcing productization on hospitals with respect to patients covered by Medicare; hospital is paid a predetermined rate for each Medicare patient based on the patient's presenting condition; see DRG. (Economics)

Psychiatric hospital—a facility that offers treatment to individuals with mental, emotional, and behavioral disorders. (History)

Psychological model of health—relies on the individual himself or herself to provide an assessment of his or her own health. (Health)

Psychological stressor—stems from within yourself and pertains to your subconscious perception of yourself or your feelings of self-worth, or lack thereof; basically have to do with your relationship with yourself and/or your level of self-esteem. (Stress)

Psychosomatic—disorders, including physical illness, caused by mental or emotional factors. (History)

Public compliance—when individual behaves in the way desired by the group only when being observed by group members because the person does not really believe in the behavior. (Team)

Quality assurance (QA)—gathering and evaluating information about the services provided, as well as the results achieved, and comparing this information with an accepted standard. (Ethics)

Public health—involves the well-being of all of us as we live together in neighborhoods, communities, states, and countries. (Public health)

Public sector—funding of health care through federal, state, and local governments. (Economics)

Quality of life—refers to the person's ability to enjoy normal life activities. Some medical treatments can seriously impair quality of life without providing appreciable benefit, while others greatly enhance quality of life. (Health)

Quarantine—forced isolation of a person to prevent a disease from spreading. (Public health)

Real time interactive mode—providing telehealthcare in real time (synchronous time); often using interactive videoconferencing. (Telehealth)

Refocus—in critical thinking this means that you have acknowledged some of your own biases, and have refocused your attention so you can hear alternative viewpoints; second step of critical thinking. (Critical thinking)

Regulator—element of nonverbal communication that involves body movements that are used to regulate or manipulate conversation. (Communication 2)

Reimbursement—how hospitals describe payment received for services they have already provided. (Economics)

Relational activity track—decision-making track in which the group activities emphasize the relationships among the group members that pertain to how the group works. (Team)

Relational level of message—the emotional expression of how we feel about the other person or our relationship with that other person. (Communication 1)

Relativism—last stage in levels of thinking characterized by students reaching an understanding that some views make greater sense than other views. (Critical thinking)

Respect—implies the ability to consider and honor another person's beliefs and opinions. (Ethics)

Responsibility—sense of accountability for one's actions; implies dependability. (Ethics)

Rhetorical communication—communication that has a specific goal in mind; most common type of communication and represents the majority of our interactions. (Communication 1)

Rights-based ethics—also known as natural rights, ethical theory places the primary emphasis on a person's individual rights; rights belong to all people purely by virtue of their being human. (Ethics)

Rule-out definition—when looking for the presences of abnormal signs or symptoms and none are present, it is possible to rule out ill health. (Health)

SARS—Severe Acute Respiratory syndrome associated with coronavirus. (Public Health)

SF-36—the 36 item Short-Form Health Survey developed to compare the health outcomes over time of patients enrolled in alternative health care delivery systems. (Health)

Sanctity of life—sacredness of human life; protection of all human beings; advocating for people who cannot speak out for themselves. (Ethics)

Sensor—the reality function; are influential doers and action oriented; learning style is hands on. (Personality)

Server—the main computer in a local area network. (EMR 1)

Sexual harassment—the unwelcome sexual advances, requests for sexual favors, and other verbal or physical conduct of a sexual nature when the conduct is made either explicitly or implicitly a term or condition of an individual's employment. (Ethics)

Shadow—non-preferred personality preference. (Personality)

Skilled nursing facility (SNF)—a type of nursing home that provides nursing and rehabilitation services on a 24-hour basis; includes regular medical care for patients with long-term illnesses and those recovering from illness, injury, or surgery. (History)

Small-group communication—communication in gatherings that vary in size from about three to fifteen persons. A group is considered small if members are able to switch roles from receiver to source with relative ease. (Team)

Social health—is measured by your ability to have satisfying relationships as well as the overall quality of your interaction with others. (Stress)

Sociocultural model of health—looks at health as reflecting the extent to which an individual is able to maintain a normal level of functioning within his or her social context; health focuses more on what a person is able to do with his or her body than on the physiological state of that person's body. (Health)

Sociological stressor—stressor that stems from relationships or interactions with others and can be very stressful. (Stress)

Spend down—using a person's money and assets for care in order to qualify for Medicaid. (Economics)

Spiritual health—refers to having a strong sense of meaning, purpose, and direction in life. (Stress)

State Children's Health Insurance Program (SCHIP)—provides health coverage for uninsured children who are not eligible for Medicaid. (Economics)

State health department—government agency charged with promoting the public's health and implementing public health law. (Public health)

Statute of limitations—the certain period of time in which a complaint must be filed; will vary between jurisdictions. (Legal)

Stereotyping—a generalization; a way of trying to make sense out of infinite variations in our environment. (Culture)

Store and forward technology—asynchronous mode where physician and patient do not have to be present at the time of the consultation; often involves the transmission of images. (Telehealth)

Strategic knowledge—also known as procedural knowledge; knowing how to use declarative knowledge to do something. (Critical thinking)

Stressors—an event or situation that threatens to bring us out of physical and/or emotional equilibrium. (Stress)

Stress—a chain reaction involving multiple components, affecting us both psychologically and physically. (Stress)

Style approach to leadership—leadership approach that focuses on the different ways or styles people use to lead others. (Team)

Subculture—smaller cultural groups that exist within large cultural groups. (Culture)

Subjective information—information derived from personal feelings and emotions, how a person perceives it. (Technology info)

Subpoena—formal document that orders a named individual to appear before a duly authorized body at a fixed time to give testimony. (Legal)

Subpoena duces tecum—a writ commanding a person to produce in court certain designated documents or evidence. (Legal)

Substance Abuse and Mental Health Services Administration (SAMSHA)—works to improve the availability and quality of substance abuse prevention, addiction treatment, and mental health services. (Public health)

Surrender—conflict resolution style in which a person immediately gives in to avoid conflict. (Communication 2)

Surveillance—the continuous search for and documentation of disease in public health. (Public health)

Sympathy—feeling sorry for or pitying someone else. (Ethics)

Synchronous time—in real-time; the sending and receiving information in real-time at a distance; example interactive videoconferencing. (Telehealth)

Synthesis level—fifth level on Bloom's Taxonomy of Thinking and Learning characterized by being able to bring together all the bits of information that you have analyzed to create a new pattern or whole. (Critical thinking)

Targeted drug therapy—use of drugs to block the growth and spread of cancer cells by preventing them from dividing or by destroying them. (History)

Task activity track—decision-making track in which the group engages to accomplish its task. (Team)

Task-oriented group—groups that have a particular job to do. (Team)

Taxonomy—classification system; Bloom's Taxonomy was developed to explain how we think and learn. (Critical thinking)

Telemedicine—delivering of health utilizing computers and telecommunications networks to people at a distance. (Telehealth)

Teleological theory—asserts that an action is right or wrong depending on whether it produces good or bad consequences. (Ethics)

Temperament—our inborn form of human nature. (Personality)

Therapy groups—groups that have the purpose of helping individuals solve personal problems. Most common are encounter groups, T-groups, and sensitivity groups, all of which hope to promote personal growth. (Team)

Think through—fourth step of critical thinking that requires you to think through all the information gathered and to distinguish between what is fact and what is fiction and what is relevant and what is not relevant. (Critical thinking)

Thinking—the logical function; interpret thoughts through information, analysis and by making sense out of facts or concepts. (Personality)

Third-party payer—when someone other than the patient or provider pays for the healthcare services. (Economics)

Tolerance—respect for those whose opinions, practices, race, religion, and nationality differ from our own; requires a fair and objective attitude. (Ethics)

Topical activity track—decision-making track made up of the content of the issues and arguments of concern to the group at various times in the discussion. (Team)

Touch—element of nonverbal communication that involves physical contact. (Communication 2)

Trait approach to leadership—assumes that leaders have traits that distinguish them from followers. (Team)

Typewatching—one way of observing people's behaviors and their reactions the environment. (Personality)

Unacceptable premises—premises that are as incredible as the claim they are supposed to support; includes false dilemma and begging the question. (Critical thinking)

Unitary sequence model—model of group decision making that identifies stages that groups go through as they move toward a decision. (Team)

Up-coding—exaggerating the reported severity of the diagnosis to increase the amount of payment received. (Economics)

Utilitarianism—ethical theory based on the principle of the greatest good for the greatest number; is concerned with the impact of actions, or final outcomes, on the welfare of society as a whole. (Ethics)

Utilitarians—go after what they want in the most effective way possible; live with the law, but go outside of the group to pursue their ambitions. (Personality)

Value-based compensation—payment model in which the preforming organization is rewarded for the value delivered; most often used when the value is easy to measure and indisputable. (Economics)

Validity—the relationship between the premises and the conclusion. (Critical thinking)

Verbal communication—refers only to the actual words spoken. (Communication 2)

Virtual-based ethics—ethics based on persons and not necessarily on the decisions or principles that are involved. (Ethics)

Vital statistics—the number of occurrences related to a specific event (e.g., births and deaths) for purposes of reporting. (History) and (Public health)

Voice recognition technology—using specialized software to take the spoken word and transcribe it into a document such as an electronic medical record (EMR 1)

Wellness—promotion of health through preventive measures and the practice of good health habits; when the body is in a state of homeostasis. (History) and (Health)

Withdrawal—conflict resolution style in which a person avoids conflict altogether. (Communication 2)

Work—an effort applied toward some end goal. (Ethics)

World Health Organization—responsible for providing leadership on global health matters, shaping the health research agenda, setting norms and standards, articulating evidence-based policy options, providing technical support to countries and monitoring and assessing health trends. Taken from the WHO website. (Health)

Xenophobia—ethnocentric behavior to the extent that there is a fear of strangers. (Culture)

Yerkes-Dodson Principle—also known as the Good Stress-Bad Stress Curve, states that too little stress as well as too much stress is unhealthy. (Stress)